SUCCESS!

for the Nursing Assistant

A Complete Review

SUCCESS!

for the **Nursing Assistant**

A Complete Review

Eileen Heinze

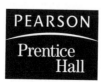

PEARSON

Prentice
Hall

Upper Saddle River, New Jersey 07458

Library of Congress Cataloging-in-Publication Data

Heinze, Eileen.
  Success! for the nursing assistant : a complete review / Eileen Heinze.
    p. ; cm.
  Includes bibliographical references and index.
  ISBN 0-13-114494-4
  1. Nurses aides'--Examinations, questions, etc.   I. Title.
  [DNLM: 1. Long-Term Care--methods--United States--Examination
Questions. 2. Nurses' Aides--United States. 3. Certification--United
States--Examination Questions. 4. Clinical Competence--standards
--United States--Examination Questions.   WY 18.2 H472s 2005]
  RT84.H47 2005
  610.73'06'98--dc22

2005025311

Publisher: Julie Levin Alexander
Executive Assistant: Regina Bruno
Editor in Chief: Maura Connor
Executive Editor: Debbie Yarnell
Managing Development Editor: Marilyn Meserve
Development Editor: Sheba Jalaluddin
Supplements Editor: Michael Giacobbe
Director of Manufacturing and Production: Bruce Johnson
Managing Production Editor: Patrick Walsh
Production Liaison: Mary C. Treacy
Production Editor: Shelley Creager, TechBooks/GTS
Manufacturing Manager: Ilene Sanford
Manufacturing Buyer: Pat Brown
Director of Marketing: Karen Allman
Marketing Manager: Francisco Del Castillo
Marketing Coordinator: Michael Sirinides
Marketing Assistant: Patricia Linard
Media Product Manager: John J. Jordan
Media Production Editor: Amy Peltier
Media Project Manager: Tina Rudowski
Senior Design Coordinator: Maria Guglielmo-Walsh
Cover Design: Anthony Gemmellaro
Composition: TechBooks/GTS York, PA Campus
Printer/Binder: Courier Wesford
Cover Printer: Phoenix Color

Pearson Education LTD.
Pearson Education Singapore, Pte. Ltd
Pearson Education, Canada, Ltd
Pearson Education—Japan
Pearson Education, Upper Saddle River, New Jersey

Pearson Education Australia PTY, Limited
Pearson Education North Asia Ltd
Pearson Educación de Mexico, S.A. de C.V.
Pearson Education Malaysia, Pte. Ltd

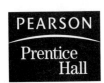

10 9 8 7 6 5 4 3 2 1
ISBN 0-13-114494-4

Anyone who has worked in a long-term care facility, or even just visited, has seen how important the CNAs are to the residents. CNAs are the first people the residents see when they open their eyes in the morning and the last ones they see when they close their eyes at night. Everything CNAs do or say or think or feel directly affects every moment of a resident's existence. CNAs must have a strong personal and emotional commitment to do the job they have chosen. Hour after hour, on weekends and holidays, CNAs cope with illnesses, disabilities, emergencies, and death. They bathe, dress, feed, and lift the people we love: our parents, our grandparents, our friends. Most important, they listen to, comfort, soothe, and console with empathy and compassion. They are the hands, the eyes, and the heart of health care. To CNAs, I offer my respect and admiration.

Contents

Preface

Success! for the Nursing Assistant is designed to help nursing assistants prepare for certification testing.

Students bring diverse life experiences and beliefs into the classroom. *Success! for the Nursing Assistant,* designed to meet the needs of students of various ages, educational backgrounds, and cultures, is succinct, understandable, logical, and useful. Chapter outlines, questions, and rationales are designed to improve critical thinking skills and enhance problem solving. Nursing assistants will be better prepared to make informed choices and respond appropriately to residents' needs and behaviors regardless of their personal beliefs or traditions.

Success! for the Nursing Assistant consists of five sections covering these main topics:

I. Working in Long-Term Care
II. The Resident
III. Body Structure and Function
IV. Activities of Daily Living
V. Residents with Special Needs

Each section is divided into chapters that address specific subjects within the topic. Each chapter is followed by 10 scenario-based, selected response questions to encourage critical thinking, integrating knowledge from current and previous chapters. This format requires the student to prove knowledge of the material plus the logic and reason necessary to respond correctly. The student must know the terminology, understand the concept, determine the principle, and select the correct response. Residents' rights and needs, proper procedure, the nursing assistant's scope of practice, safety, and infection control are incorporated throughout the questions. A separate section of skills checklists allows the student to review the skills required for certification.

Success! for the Nursing Assistant contains a marginal glossary of terms, providing the student with the ability to quickly access the meaning of terms during the study process.

A Student CD-ROM is packaged **free** with the textbook. It provides an interactive study program that allows students to practice answering Certification Review Exam-style Questions with feedback for incorrect answers. It also contains a 100-question comprehensive practice test and an Audio Glossary. In addition, a **free** online study guide, **www.prenhall.com/heinze**, is designed to help students apply the concepts presented in the book. Chapter-specific modules include an Audio Glossary, Certification Review Exam-style Questions, Case Studies, Medialinks as well as a 100-question comprehensive practice test.

The 100-question comprehensive practice test gives students the opportunity to realistically test their knowledge. Test questions are designed to be culture free by eliminating idioms and clichés. The questions integrate knowledge learned from all chapters. When information is associated and related, the student learns by reason rather than by rote.

Appendix A lists important procedures in an easy and concise checklist format for review and successful testing. Appendix B provides references for additional information about each question at the end of the chapters. Students can learn more about the topic and improve your understanding of the material to increase their confidence and success when testing.

Success! for the Nursing Assistant provides students with the opportunity to:

- enhance their knowledge of required material
- improved test-taking skills
- reduce test anxiety through practice and preparation

Success! for the Nursing Assistant is written for and directed toward the learner but can also be used by the instructor as a course outline. The text may be used in lieu of class notes and handouts to simplify studying for the student and minimize preparation time for the instructor.

All nursing staff responsible for supervising certified nursing assistants can benefit by reviewing *Success! for the Nursing Assistant* for a better understanding of the CNA's scope of practice and level of knowledge.

Acknowledgments

My thanks to Barbara Krawiec for providing this opportunity and for her trust and guidance.

Special thanks to Sheba Jalaluddin for her patience, support and encouragement which was offered with persistence and a wonderful sense of humor.

With deepest gratitude, I acknowledge the contributions of Irene Lawson, BA, MA who offered essential research, indispensable coordination, and inspiration.

To Pamela Davis, RN, BS, I offer my appreciation for taking charge, offering advice, and doing what was necessary to make everything work.

My gratitude to Kathryn E. Goodge, RN and Stacey Wiszowaty, RN, BSN for offering input and insight.

For taking the time to read and advise, I thank Thomas Devine, MD, Douglas B. Dick, RPh, and Benjamin August, Dipl.Bichem. ZMBE, Institute of Cell Biology,University Hospital, Muenster Germany

Lynette Murphy, Millie Moncilovich, Joseph Shaffer, BA, AS, Julie Gannon, Lavonne Will, and Valerie Johnson, I thank each of you for being honest, critical, thorough, and supportive.

I want to especially mention Sheryl Morrison, RN who looked forward to this project with anticipation and enthusiasm. Her short life was filled with so many accomplishments as a nurse, a teacher, an artist, and a friend. I will always be inspired by her courage, spirit, wit, and wisdom. Sheryl, we miss you.

REVIEWERS

Judith Bateman, RN, MSN
Clinical Instructor
Black Hawk College
Moline, IL

Beth Anne Batturs, RN, MSN
Director, Nursing Program
Anne Arundel Community College
Arnold, MD

Doris A. Clark, RN, BC, BSN, MSN
PN Faculty
Harrison Center for Career Education
Washington, DC

Winifred Guariglia, RN MSN, CS, GNP
Professor
Bergen College
Paramus, NJ

Donna C. Henry, RN, MS, CHTP
Associate Dean of Nursing/Allied Health
Olney Central College
Olney, IL

Georgette Howard, RN, MN
Nursing Assistant Program Coordinator
Glendale Community College
Glendale, AZ

Linda J. Jaskowiak
Program Administrator
Quality Healthcare Options, Inc.
Wauwatosa, WI

Cherry A Karl, RN, MSN, MA
Associate Professor of Nursing
Anne Arundel Community College
Arnold, MD

Debra Lewis, MSN, RN
Director of Health Sciences
San Joaquin Delta College
Stockton, CA

Alexandra D. McFall, RN, BSN
Instructor
Harrisburg Area Community College
Harrisburg, PA

Valerie Moore, RN, MS
Nurse Assistant Program Director
Illinois Central College
Peoria, IL

Rosemary Smith, RN BS
Coordinator, Patient Care Technician Program
Cedar Valley College
Lancaster, TX

Kathie Zimmerman, RN
Director of Nurse Aide Training
Harrisburg Area Community College
Harrisburg, PA

Information

CERTIFICATION

Since the Omnibus Budget Reconciliation Act (OBRA), nursing assistants who work in long-term care facilities have been required to pass both a state-approved training program and a nurse aide competency evaluation consisting of a written test and a skills evaluation. Each state determines who will administer the tests and where the tests will be given. Presently, written tests approved by most states range from 60 to 150 questions. The percentage of questions that must be answered correctly to pass the test varies from state to state. The nursing assistant must be given three attempts to successfully pass each test.

Skills evaluation must be done in a facility or laboratory setting that reflects the normal resident environment. Skills must be selected from the curriculum for nurse aide training. Each state must follow the federal guidelines but may include additional regulations regarding resident care. Therefore, nursing assistants must be aware of the specific regulations in their state.

If a CNA moves to a different state, the regulatory agency in that state determines what the CNA must do to be included on that registry. States will place CNAs on their registry if they are currently on a registry in another state, have worked at least one 8-hour shift within the past 24 months, and have no complaints against them. Some states also require CNAs to pass a test or even take another training program. Because the required curriculum is federally mandated, *Success! for the Nursing Assistant* is a valuable resource book that can be used as a study guide before applying for testing in other states.

REQUIRED CURRICULUM

All nursing assistant training programs and tests must cover the curriculum as outlined in the Federal Code of Regulations, and include:

- Communication and interpersonal skills; infection control; safety and emergency procedures, including the Heimlich maneuver; promoting residents' independence; respecting residents' rights.

- Basic nursing skills: taking and recording vital signs; measuring and recording height and weight; caring for the residents' environment; recognizing abnormal changes in body functioning and the importance of reporting such changes to a supervisor; caring for residents when death is imminent.
- Personal care skills: bathing; grooming, including mouth care; dressing; toileting; assisting with eating and hydration; proper feeding techniques; skin care; transfers; positioning and turning.
- Mental health and social service needs: modifying the aide's behavior in response to residents' behavior; awareness of developmental tasks associated with the aging process; how to respond to resident behavior; allowing the resident to make personal choices; providing and reinforcing other behavior consistent with the resident's dignity; using the resident's family as a source of emotional support.
- Care of cognitively impaired residents: techniques for addressing the unique needs and behaviors of individuals with dementia; communicating with cognitively impaired residents; understanding the behavior of cognitively impaired residents; appropriate responses to the behavior of cognitively impaired residents; and methods of reducing the effects of cognitive impairments.
- Basic restorative services: training the resident in self-care according to his or her abilities; use of assistive devices in transferring, ambulation, eating, and dressing; maintenance of range of motion; proper turning and positioning in bed and chair; bowel and bladder training; care and use of prosthetic and orthotic devices.
- Residents' rights: provide privacy and maintain confidentiality; promote the residents' right to make personal choices to accommodate their needs; give assistance in resolving grievances and disputes; provide needed assistance in getting to and participating in resident and family groups and other activities; maintain care and security of residents' personal possessions; promote the residents' right to be free from abuse, mistreatment, and neglect, and the need to report any instances of such treatment to appropriate facility staff; avoid the need for restraints in accordance with current professional standards.

I Working in Long Term Care

CHAPTER

1

The Health Care System and Long Term Care

chapter outline

I. THE HEALTH CARE SYSTEM

A. In the United States the health care system includes:

Acute illness—an illness that starts suddenly and may last a short time

1. general hospitals, which provide treatment for **acute illnesses:**
   a. Stay is short.
   b. Patients are very ill.
   c. Medical problems may be unstable.
   d. Complex treatment is required.
2. specialty hospitals, which provide care for one group or one condition:
   a. children's hospitals
   b. women's hospitals
   c. AIDS centers
   d. cancer centers
   e. psychiatric hospitals
3. home health agencies, which provide care and treatment in the home, including:
   a. nursing care
   b. medical treatments

ADLs—routine activities (bathing; mouth, nail, hair care; eating, dressing, moving, toileting)

   c. assistance with **activities of daily living (ADLs)**
   d. meal preparation
   e. housekeeping
   f. therapies

Palliative care—care given to provide comfort without cure

4. hospice programs, which provide **palliative care** for dying residents and support for their families, focusing on:
   a. resident comfort
   b. pain management
   c. quality of life
   d. emotional support for family
   e. grief counseling

Chronic illness—an illness that starts slowly and may last a long time

ICFMR—intermediate care facility for those with mental retardation

Developmental disability—inability to develop normally due to a birth defect, injury, or illness

Mental retardation—low intellect and learning skills

5. long-term care (LTC) facilities, which provide care for people of all ages with chronic medical problems and need for supervision:
   a. Patients are usually called *residents*.
   b. Residents have **chronic illnesses** or permanent disabilities.
   c. Residents may be in the facility for weeks or the rest of their life.
   d. Facilities may be called *nursing homes, skilled nursing facilities, extended care facilities, rehabilitation centers,* or *convalescent centers*.
   e. Specialized long-term care facilities **(ICFMR)** provide care for those with **developmental disabilities,** some of whom have **mental retardation.**

B. Sources for payment of health care costs include:
1. government programs:
   a. Medicare—for persons over age 65 and some persons under age 65 with disabilities
   b. Medicaid—for low-income persons
2. private insurance
3. people who pay for health care services themselves

C. Facilities must provide quality care to all residents regardless of the source of payment.

II. LONG-TERM CARE

A. The purpose of long-term care is to:
1. provide care based on the residents' needs
2. prevent injury, disease, and loss of function
3. provide rehabilitation and **restorative care**

Restorative care—nursing care given to help the resident reach and maintain the highest level of function and independence

B. Long-term care facilities follow federal and state regulations.
1. Regulations protect the residents and ensure quality of care.
2. OBRA (Omnibus Budget Reconciliation Act) is the federal law that:
   a. provides for the safety, happiness, and well-being of elderly residents
   b. outlines residents' rights
   c. requires training for nursing assistants
3. State survey teams inspect facilities to enforce federal rules.
4. Additional inspections are conducted by federal teams and local organizations (fire and local health departments).

C. The organization of long-term care facilities creates lines of authority and responsibility.
1. The medical director oversees the medical care of all residents and reviews medical procedures.
2. The administrator manages all departments and determines **policies.** Departments may include:

Policy—describes what will be done

   a. nursing
   b. medical records
   c. housekeeping
   d. social services
   e. dietary
   f. activities
   g. business office
   h. therapy

Procedure—describes how something is to be done

Job description—describes the duties of each type of worker in the facility

3. The directors of each department develop **procedures** and **job descriptions.**
4. The chain of command is the order of authority and problem solving within a facility.
   a. Employees take problems, questions, and reports to the person directly above them on the chain.
   b. Following the chain keeps communication flowing through all departments.

III. THE HEALTH CARE TEAM

A. The health care team is responsible for:
   1. identifying each resident's needs
   2. communicating information to all team members
   3. developing a plan of care to meet the resident's needs

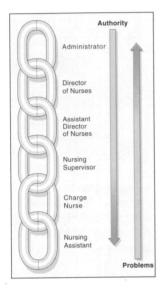

Figure 1–1 An example of a nursing department chart. Always follow the chain of command. (Source: From *The Long-Term Care Nursing Assistant* [2nd ed., p. 4], by P. Grubbs and B. Blasband, 2000, Upper Saddle River, NJ: Prentice Hall. Reprinted by permission.)

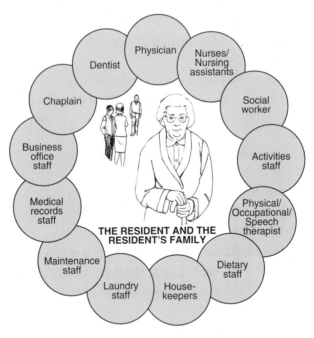

Figure 1–2 All members of the health care team work with the resident and with each other. (Source: From *The Long-Term Care Nursing Assistant* [2nd ed., p. 5], by P. Grubbs and B. Blasband, 2000, Upper Saddle River, NJ: Prentice Hall. Reprinted by permission.)

B. The health care team includes everyone who provides care, services, or support for the resident:
   1. *resident's family*—contributes information about the resident
   2. *physician*—**diagnoses** illness and prescribes treatment
   3. *nursing staff*—monitors health, identifies needs, assists with ADLs, carries out doctor's orders

Diagnosis—the resident's disease or medical condition as determined by the physician

4. *social worker*—counsels and arranges services
5. *activities director*—plans and implements activities
6. *dietician*—monitors nutritional status of the resident and plans menus and special diets
7. *physical therapist*—works with muscle groups to increase the resident's physical abilities
8. *occupational therapist*—works to improve the resident's ability to perform activities of daily living
9. *speech therapist*—works with resident who has difficulty with speech, communication, and swallowing
10. *respiratory therapist*—provides breathing treatments
11. *dentist*—provides routine and emergency dental care
12. *podiatrist*—provides foot care for the resident
13. *optometrist*—provides eye care for the resident
14. *housekeeping staff*—keep resident's environment neat and sanitary
15. *maintenance staff*—keep resident's environment in good repair
16. *spiritual counselor*—provides spiritual guidance and coordinates religious services
17. *guardian, health care representative*—makes decisions if resident is not able

IV. HEALTH CARE PLAN

A. The resident's care plan is a written plan that outlines all of the resident's needs, including:
1. physical
2. psychological
3. social
4. spiritual
5. **cultural**

B. Health care team members complete the Minimum Data Set (MDS). The MDS is used to develop the care plan.

C. The care plan includes:
1. identification of the resident's needs
2. short-term and long-term goals for the resident
3. the action required to reach each goal
4. the people responsible for assessing each goal

D. The care plan is reviewed and evaluated regularly by the health care team.

E. The care plan establishes guidelines for all team members so continuity of care is achieved.

Cultural need—a need based on a person's heritage or belief, including food restrictions or preferences, dress preferences, activities, and so on

MDS—a form used to identify the physical, mental, and social needs of the resident

V. THE CERTIFIED NURSING ASSISTANT

A. The certified nursing assistant (CNA) is a very important member of the health care team.

B. The CNA's supervisor is the nurse.

C. The CNA contributes to the resident's care plan by:
1. **observing**
2. **reporting**
3. **recording**

D. The CNA provides direct care to the resident.

Observing—gathering information about a resident by using your senses

Reporting—verbally informing the nurse about resident care and your observations

Recording—writing down information in the resident's medical record about resident care you have given and observations you have made

DIRECTIONS

A brief description of a resident is given followed by 10 questions related to the resident. Each question has four possible answers. Read each question and all answer choices carefully. Choose the one best answer.

Mrs. Michelle Adams is 61 years old. She was admitted to the long-term care facility three days ago. She is recovering from a fractured hip.

1. Mrs. Adams does not qualify for Medicare payment because she is:
   A. not sick enough
   B. under the age of 65
   C. able to help herself
   D. a new resident

2. Mrs. Adams was transferred to a long-term care facility because she needs:
   A. complex treatments
   B. palliative care
   C. restorative care
   D. emergency care

3. You notice that Mrs. Adams is not speaking with other residents. You would:
   A. ignore it
   B. tell her she is rude
   C. tell the nurse
   D. invite residents to her room

4. When you help Mrs. Adams bathe, move, or comb her hair, you are assisting her with:
   A. pain management
   B. activities of daily living
   C. rehabilitation
   D. adjustment

5. You encourage Mrs. Adams to participate in her own care so she will:
   A. be less work for you
   B. have something to do
   C. reach her highest level of function
   D. have nothing to complain about

6. Mrs. Adams's spiritual advisor comes to visit. The spiritual advisor:
   A. provides information about the resident
   B. treats disease and illness
   C. makes decisions if the resident is not able
   D. is a part of the health care team

7. The physical therapist comes to talk to Mrs. Adams. The physical therapist will help her with:
   A. activities of daily living
   B. speech problems
   C. breathing problems
   D. regaining strength and mobility

8. The health care team is developing a care plan for Mrs. Adams. You read the care plan so you:
   A. can tell her family how to treat her
   B. understand her illness
   C. know how to take care of her
   D. can answer questions about her condition

9. You contribute to Mrs. Adams's care plan by:
   A. observing and reporting
   B. assessing the resident's medical condition
   C. attending care plan meetings and acting as her advocate
   D. reporting all confidential information that she has told you

10. You understand that following federal and state regulations is important because:
    A. if you don't, you will lose your job
    B. regulations protect the residents and ensure quality of care
    C. a survey team may come into the building
    D. you want to be a good example for others

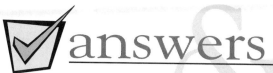

answers & rationales

1.

B. Medicare benefits are available to those age 65 and older. Age is the main qualifying factor for Medicare eligibility.

2.

C. The long-term care facility provides restorative care to help residents regain or achieve their highest level of function. Complex treatments and emergency care are provided at hospitals. Palliative care focuses on comfort rather than cure and is the hospice approach to care.

3.

C. As a nursing assistant it is your responsibility to tell the nurse about any unmet needs the resident may have. The nurse will assess the resident and share information with other members of the health care team.

4.

B. ADLs include bathing, moving, and combing hair. It is important that the resident be encouraged to perform activities of daily living to maintain a satisfying quality of life.

5.

C. Self-care helps the resident reach the highest level of function and independence, possible for that resident. Being able to perform ADLs, also improves self-esteem, confidence, and emotional well-being.

6.

D. Spiritual advisors are a part of the health care team. Spiritual advisors provide guidance and help residents find meaning in their lives.

7.

D. The physical therapist helps residents strengthen muscles and improve mobility to reach their highest level of function and independence. Occupational therapists help residents perform ADLs independently. Speech therapists help residents with speech communication. Respiratory therapists provide breathing treatments.

8.

C. All members of the health care team, including the nursing assistant, read the care plan to learn about the resident's needs and how to meet those needs. Consistent care can then be provided for the resident.

9.

A. By reporting your observations to the nurse you are contributing to care planning. The nursing assistant usually sees the resident more than any other team member.

10.

B. You follow federal and state regulations to protect residents and ensure quality of care. Federal regulations aim to guarantee a basic standard of care for residents. Each state must enforce these regulations.

Role and Responsibilities of the Certified Nursing Assistant

2

chapter outline

I. REQUIREMENTS FOR CERTIFICATION

A. Each state must:
1. outline the duties and responsibilities of nursing assistants
2. maintain a list of all registered nursing assistants (**Nursing Assistant Registry**)
3. have a training and evaluation program that consists of:
   a. at least 75 hours of training
   b. at least 16 hours of supervised practical training in a laboratory or clinical setting
   c. a curriculum that includes basic nursing skills, personal care skills, basic restorative services, residents' rights, infection control, and safety and emergency practices
   d. a competency evaluation that includes a written test and a skills demonstration with at least three attempts to pass

> **Nursing Assistant Registry**—official record of names of all certified nursing assistants in a state

B. The employer must:
1. provide **continuing education** for all nursing assistants
2. conduct performance evaluations

C. The CNA must work at least one 8-hour shift every 24 months. If the CNAs do not meet this federal requirement they:
1. lose certification
2. must take the training program and competency evaluation again

> **Continuing education**—educational training related to job performance provided by the employer

II. JOB DESCRIPTION

A. The nursing assistant is supervised by the nurse.
B. The nursing assistant's job description includes:
1. assisting residents with ADLs
2. making residents physically and **emotionally** comfortable
3. assisting residents with mobility and activities
4. meeting the residents' **psychological** and **social needs**
5. keeping the residents' environment safe and clean
6. measuring **vital signs**
7. providing support services
8. assisting the nurse by observing, reporting, and recording

> **Emotions**—feelings including joy, sorrow, fear, hate, and love
>
> **Psychological**—pertaining to the mind and mental state
>
> **Social needs**—the need for approval, acceptance, and involvement with others
>
> **Vital signs**—the measurement of body temperature, pulse, respirations, and blood pressure

III. SCOPE OF PRACTICE

A. Nursing assistants may perform only those duties that are within their scope of practice.

> **Scope of practice**—the activities that can legally be performed by the nursing assistant

B. The duties of the nursing assistant are outlined in the nursing assistant's job description.

C. CNAs:

1. may NOT give medications
2. may NOT prescribe treatments or medications
3. may NOT take oral or phone orders from a doctor
4. may NOT insert or remove tubes from a resident's body
5. may NOT perform sterile procedures
6. may NOT perform a procedure for which they were not trained
7. may NOT start, adjust, or discontinue an **IV**
8. may NOT suction a resident
9. may NOT discuss a resident's diagnosis, treatment, or behavior with anyone but the nurse
10. may NOT supervise other nursing assistants

IV (intravenous)—into the vein

IV. CODE OF ETHICS

Code of ethics—rules of conduct for a particular group

A. Ethical behavior includes:

1. performing duties to the best of your ability
2. being loyal to your employer and coworkers
3. being honest, truthful, and **accountable**
4. carrying out your supervisor's instructions
5. performing only those duties within your scope of practice
6. respecting all residents without discrimination, regardless of their beliefs, backgrounds, or opinions
7. assisting any resident in need whether or not you are assigned to the resident
8. keeping confidential all personal and medical information about residents
9. providing privacy during procedures
10. providing care that is free from abuse, mistreatment, or neglect
11. safeguarding residents' property from damage, loss, and theft
12. reporting accidents or errors to the supervisor immediately
13. reporting to work as scheduled

Accountability—being legally responsible for what is done or not done

B. Nursing assistants are responsible by law for their actions and behaviors.

1. Legal terms include:
   a. assault—a threat to do bodily harm
   b. battery—touching another person's body without permission
   c. false imprisonment—restraining or restricting a person's movements unnecessarily

Laws—rules of conduct that are decided by the government and enforced by the courts

     d. invasion of privacy—exposing a resident's body

     e. breaching confidentiality—revealing information about a person

     f. negligence—failure to give proper care, which results in physical or emotional harm

     g. slander—a false statement that damages another person's reputation

     h. libel—a *written* false statement that damages another person's reputation

2. The resident's health record is a legal document.

     a. Documentation must be accurate.

     b. The health record is admissible in court.

C. Nursing assistants are ethically and legally responsible for respecting the residents' rights, which include the right to:

Residents' rights—a list of rights and freedoms of residents as mandated by OBRA

1. civil and religious liberties
2. file complaints without fear
3. be informed of his or her rights and the rules of the facility upon admission
4. inspect his or her records
5. be informed of his or her medical condition and treatment and to take part in care planning
6. refuse medical treatment
7. receive information from agencies of inspection
8. be informed of responsibility for charges and services
9. manage his or her own financial affairs
10. receive adequate and appropriate health care
11. be free from unnecessary physical restraints and drugs
12. be free from verbal, mental, sexual, or physical abuse
13. personal privacy and confidentiality of information
14. be treated courteously, fairly, and with dignity
15. send and promptly receive mail that is unopened
16. have private communication with any person of choice
17. receive visitors at any reasonable hour
18. have immediate access to family and friends
19. choose a personal physician
20. have access to private use of a telephone
21. participate in social, religious, and group activities of choice
22. and use personal possessions and clothing as space permits
23. equal policies and practices regardless of source of payment
24. privacy during visits and be able to share a room when a married couple resides in the same facility

D. The nursing assistant may not discriminate against any resident because of

1. age
2. sex
3. religion
4. race
5. ethnic origin
6. handicap

E. The nursing assistant is responsible for keeping health information private and secure according to HIPAA regulations.

HIPAA (Health Insurance Portability and Accountability Act)—law to help keep health information private and secure

1. Discuss resident health information only with the nurse.
2. Secure all documentation regarding resident information.

F. The nursing assistant is responsible for reporting incidents involving residents, visitors, or employees.

Incidents—any unusual events such as accidents, errors, or thefts that occur in a health care facility

1. Report to the nurse immediately.
2. Note the date, time, and location of the incident.
3. State what you observed.
4. Assist the nurse as requested.

V. PERSONAL QUALITIES

A. Nursing assistants should be:

1. sensitive to the feelings of others
2. trustworthy, dependable, and honest
3. cheerful and enthusiastic
4. **courteous** and respectful
5. **empathetic**
6. able to cooperate with others
7. considerate of others
8. patient, kind, and self-controlled
9. willing to learn
10. flexible
11. able to understand their own strengths, weaknesses, and feelings
12. positive in their attitude and have positive **self-esteem**

Courteous—putting the needs of others before your own

Empathy—the ability to realize how you would feel in another's place

Self-esteem—one's opinion of oneself

B. Nursing assistants must maintain their own health.

1. Get adequate rest.
2. Eat a well-balanced diet.
3. Exercise regularly.
4. Use good body mechanics.
5. Avoid drugs, alcohol, and tobacco.
6. Get regular medical, dental, and eye checkups.

7. Identify and manage stress by:
   a. taking time to have fun
   b. thinking a problem through before worrying
   c. being willing to accept change
   d. relaxing when possible

C. Nursing assistants should maintain good personal hygiene.

1. Bathe or shower daily.
2. Use a deodorant.
3. Brush teeth twice a day.
4. Keep hair clean and neat.
5. Keep nails clean and short.
6. Wash hands frequently.

Hygiene—rules for health and cleanliness

D. Nursing assistants should dress professionally.

1. Wear a clean, neat, properly fitting uniform.
2. Change underclothes daily.
3. Wear clean, comfortable shoes with nonskid soles.
4. Limit amount of jewelry worn.
5. Wear a name tag or facility badge.
6. Women should wear little or no makeup.
7. Keep hair neat, pulled back, or pinned up.
8. Do not use perfume.
9. Men should shave daily or keep beard neatly trimmed.
10. Wear a watch with a second hand.
11. Carry a pad of paper and a pen.

Why?
— Nonskid soles prevent falls.
— Jewelry attracts pathogens and can scratch the resident.
— The resident and family have a right to know you by name and title.
— Hair attracts pathogens and spreads infection.
— Residents may be sensitive to strong smells.
— A watch with a second hand is needed to accurately measure vital signs.
— Record care given and observations made on paper so you remember to report all information to the nurse.

E. Nursing assistants should manage time efficiently.

1. Understand your assignment and the needs of each resident.
2. Prioritize your work:
   a. Do the most important things first.
   b. Respond to the resident immediately.
3. Set goals.
4. Work as a team.
5. Help others and ask for help when needed.
6. Report unfinished assignments to the nurse.

Efficient—performing your job well with the least waste of time, effort, or resources

DIRECTIONS A brief description of a resident is given followed by 10 questions related to the resident. Each question has four possible answers. Read each question and all answer choices carefully. Choose the one best answer.

Mr. John Barton is 63 years old. He is recovering from surgery and will go home when therapy is completed.

1. When caring for Mr. Barton, you limit the amount of jewelry you wear because:
   A. wearing jewelry is not professional
   B. Mr. Barton may not like the jewelry
   C. jewelry attracts pathogens and may scratch him
   D. wearing jewelry is against facility policy

2. Mr. Barton's doctor removes a surgical dressing and tells you to put on a new sterile dressing. You should:
   A. do as the doctor orders
   B. tell the doctor that you will get the nurse
   C. ask the doctor to do it herself
   D. get another nursing assistant to help you

3. Mr. Barton's doctor tells him that he cannot go home soon. You realize how you would feel if you were in his place. You are:
   A. courteous
   B. patient
   C. empathetic
   D. flexible

4. Mr. Barton tells you that he wants to see the facility's last inspection report. You should:
   A. ask him what is wrong
   B. get him the inspection report and notify the nurse
   C. explain that he is just angry about the doctor's visit and needs to calm down
   D. inform him that inspection results are for the facility staff only

5. Mr. Barton's family comes to visit while you are working in his room. You should:
   A. tell them to come back later
   B. understand that he has a right to immediate access to family and friends
   C. ask Mr. Barton if he wants them to stay
   D. tell the nurse to ask the visitors to leave

6. Mr. Barton tells you stories about his family and asks you not to tell anyone. You should:
   A. tell the nurse
   B. keep the information confidential
   C. let his family know what he is saying
   D. tell him to stop talking about his family

7. Mr. Barton is visiting with his family. The nurse hands you his medication and tells you to give it to Mr. Barton when his family leaves. You should:
   A. tell the nurse that giving medication is not within your scope of practice
   B. give the medication
   C. tell the doctor what the nurse is doing
   D. ask Mr. Barton's family to give him the medication

8. After completing Mr. Barton's care, you:
   A. offer to help other staff on your team
   B. stand at the nurse's station
   C. take a break
   D. report to the doctor

9. Mr. Barton is sleeping. If you think his position is unsafe, you should:

   A. put the side rails up before leaving the room

   B. ask the nurse if his side rails can be raised

   C. put a restraint on him

   D. stay with him until he wakes up

10. You are not able to finish your assignments by the end of your shift. You should:

   A. tell the nurse that you finished so you won't get in trouble

   B. tell the nursing assistants on the next shift to finish for you

   C. stay until you are finished and then go home

   D. report to the nurse so the tasks can be assigned to the next shift

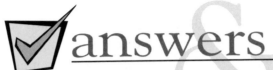

answers & rationales

1.

C. Jewelry attracts pathogens and may scratch the resident. When care is being given, a nursing assistant should be aware of infection control procedures. Wearing jewelry may cause the spread of infection and put the safety of the resident at risk.

2.

B. If a doctor asks you to perform a procedure for which you are not trained or that is not within your scope of practice, report to the nurse. Reporting a team member's need to the nurse is an important part of the nursing assistant's job. Changing a sterile dressing is not within the CNA's scope of practice.

3.

C. Empathy is the ability to realize how you would feel in another's place. Courtesy is putting the needs of others before your own. Patience is the ability to wait or endure without complaint. Flexibility is the ability to be adjustable to change.

4.

B. The resident has the right to see facility inspection reports. The nursing assistant has the responsibility to report the resident's request to the nurse.

5.

B. Resident rights, as outlined in federal regulations, give the resident the right to immediate access to family and friends. Postpone routine care until after visitors leave.

6.

B. A resident should feel confident that personal and medical information will remain private. Personal information should be shared only as needed to provide proper care and treatment.

7.

A. If the nurse asks you to give a resident medication, tell the nurse that you are not able to perform duties outside your scope of practice. A nursing assistant's scope of practice includes the skills you are legally permitted to perform. Certain duties are not performed by the CNA, including giving medications.

8.

A. Teamwork means helping other team members whenever possible. The health care team works best when everyone cooperates.

9.

B. Ask the nurse or check the resident's care plan to see if you can raise the side rails. Use of side rails requires a doctor's order. Using side rails without a doctor's order is considered false imprisonment.

10.

D. Report incomplete assignments to the nurse. The nurse will report what needs to be completed to the next shift.

CHAPTER

3 Communication and Interpersonal Skills

chapter outline

I. EFFECTIVE COMMUNICATION

A. The nursing assistant must effectively communicate with:

Communication—the exchange of thoughts, messages, ideas, and feelings by speech, signals, gestures, or writing between two or more people

1. residents
2. families
3. visitors
4. staff

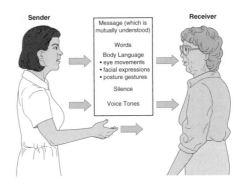

Figure 3–1   The communication process. (Source: From *The Long-Term Care Nursing Assistant* [2nd ed., p. 88], by P. Grubbs and B. Blasband, 2000, Upper Saddle River, NJ: Prentice Hall. Reprinted by permission.)

B. Elements of communication include:

1. the sender who sends clear information
2. the receiver who actively listens
3. a message that is understandable
4. **feedback** that lets the sender know the message was received

Feedback—the verbal or non-verbal responses a listener makes to the sender's message

Verbal communication—communication that uses spoken or written words

Nonverbal communication—communication without words

C. Communication may be verbal or nonverbal.

1. **Verbal communication** includes:
   a. words spoken (conversations or reporting)
   b. written words (charting or documentation)
2. **Nonverbal communication** includes:
   a. facial expression
   b. tone of voice
   c. posture
   d. gestures

D. Messages are received by actively listening.

1. Show interest and concern.
2. Do not interrupt the speaker.
3. Be patient.
4. Give verbal feedback (ask questions, restate what was said).
5. Give nonverbal feedback (nod, smile).

6. Be **nonjudgmental.**
7. Do not use phrases like "don't worry" or "everything will be okay."

E. To communicate effectively:

1. Speak slowly and clearly.
2. Use a gentle tone.
3. Face the other person.
4. Maintain eye contact.
5. Use words that the person understands.
6. Be specific.
7. Give facts rather than opinions.
8. Be brief but complete.
9. Be **logical.**

F. Barriers to effective communication include:

1. language
2. use of **clichés**
3. questions that can be answered with yes or no responses
4. cultural differences including beliefs and practices
5. age
6. life experiences
7. poor communication skills
8. illness
9. sensory impairment, especially hearing, vision, or speech
10. **cognitive impairment**
11. failure to listen to feedback
12. distractions
13. using words with more than one meaning
14. chewing gum

II. GUIDELINES FOR IMPROVING COMMUNICATION

A. To improve communication with the elderly:

1. Address residents by titles or names that they prefer.
2. Be aware of **sensory impairments.**
3. Ask questions.
4. Encourage residents to talk about themselves.
5. Avoid the use of **slang** or medical terms.
6. Know and respect the differences between generations.
7. Understand your own attitude toward the elderly.
8. Speak to elderly residents as adults.
9. Encourage and assist with the use of hearing aids, glasses, and dentures to improve communication.

Nonjudgmental—not judging another person based on your own personal opinions and beliefs

Logic—correct reasoning

Clichés—familiar or overused phrases said with little or no thought (examples: you'll be all right, don't worry, etc.)

Cognitive impairment—diminished mental processes such as memory, judgment, and perception

Sensory impairment—diminished ability to hear, see, feel, smell, or taste

Slang—informal language that is outside standard usage

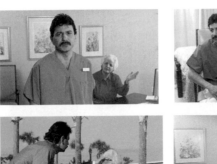
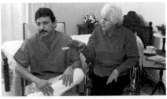
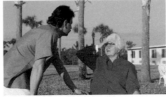
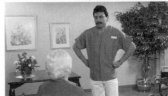

Figure 3–2 Can you identify the barriers to communication in each photograph? (Source: From *The Long-Term Care Nursing Assistant* [2nd ed., p. 93], by P. Grubbs and B. Blasband, 2000, Upper Saddle River, NJ: Prentice Hall. Reprinted by permission.)

B. To improve communication with nonambulatory residents:

1. Sit at eye level with the resident.
2. Speak to the resident.
3. Include the resident in the conversation.
4. Avoid talking about the resident as if he or she is not there.
5. Avoid blocking the resident's view.

Why?
Many nonambulatory residents communicate normally and will be offended if you speak to others as if the resident is not there or cannot understand.

C. To improve communication with culturally diverse residents:

1. Learn about the resident's culture.
2. Be aware of differences in personal space requirements, privacy issues, and levels of formality.
3. Understand and accept family interactions.
4. Know that hand gestures may have different meanings.
5. Do not be judgmental.
6. Respect the customs and beliefs of all residents.

D. To improve communication with vision-impaired residents:

1. Announce yourself when you enter the room.
2. Use touch when appropriate.
3. Allow the resident to touch and handle objects.
4. Identify yourself by name and title when starting a conversation.
5. Provide good lighting.
6. Avoid glare.
7. Face the resident.
8. Explain everything you are going to do.

Why?
— A vision-impaired resident may be unable to identify you by sight.
— Glare will diminish the resident's vision.

9. Be sure the person's glasses are clean.
10. Describe the surroundings.
11. Describe the location of personal items.
12. Describe the location of food at mealtime using the clock method.
13. Describe the new location of items that must be moved.
14. Allow the person to take your arm when walking.

E. To improve communication with hearing-impaired residents:

1. Approach the residents from the front so they can see you.
2. Speak into the better ear.
3. Encourage residents to wear a hearing aid if ordered.
4. Check the hearing aid batteries.
5. Face the resident when speaking.
6. Do not exaggerate your lip movements.
7. Explain everything, one step at a time.
8. Speak slowly and clearly.
9. Do not shout.
10. Use written messages when necessary.

F. To improve communication with speech-impaired residents:

1. Treat the resident as an adult.
2. Speak in a normal voice.
3. Do not speak or fill in words for the **aphasic** resident.
    a. The aphasic resident may:
      • not be able to understand what is said
      • understand but lack the ability to communicate accurately
      • speak with normal rhythm but no meaningful words
    b. Aphasia may:
      • involve the loss of control of muscles needed for speech
      • leave muscle control intact but eliminate the memory of how to form words
4. Allow time for a response.
5. Do not correct or criticize.
6. Be relaxed.
7. Ask questions that can be answered with simple words.
8. Use key words like "eat," "sit."
9. Encourage those who can draw or write to do so.
10. Stand where the resident can see you when you talk.
11. Don't assume that the resident understands you.
12. Speak in simple sentences.
13. Include the resident in the conversation.
14. Be sensitive to the resident's feelings.

Why?
Your body movements are a form of communication to a vision-impaired resident who can feel the speed and movement of your body.

Why?
Hearing-impaired residents may become startled if they do not see you and know that you are there.

Why?
Exaggerated lip movements make it difficult for the resident to read your lips.

Aphasia—the loss of the ability to express oneself, usually caused by brain damage

G. To improve communication with residents with developmental disabilities:

1. Approach each resident as an individual.
2. Treat each resident with respect and dignity.
3. Offer praise and encouragement.
4. Treat residents as adults regardless of their behavior.
5. Use short, simple sentences.
6. Repeat actions and words to ensure understanding.
7. Use words appropriate to each resident's developmental level.

H. To improve communication with a cognitively impaired resident:

1. Give one short, simple direction at a time.
2. Do not try to explain, reason, or argue.
3. Offer simple choices.
4. Give the resident time to respond.
5. Maintain eye contact and use body language.
6. Watch the resident's facial expression and body language for clues to feelings and moods.
7. If the resident becomes agitated, remain calm and speak softly or stop speaking and approach the resident at a later time.
8. Show respect to the resident.
9. Encourage conversation.

Why?
A variety of choices will increase confusion and frustration for the cognitively impaired resident.

I. To improve communication with a dying resident:

1. Speak in a normal tone.
2. Do not whisper.
3. Don't say things you wouldn't want the resident to hear.
4. Continue to talk to and touch the resident even if he or she is unconscious.
5. If speech is difficult, ask questions that can be answered with yes or no.

Why?
Hearing may be the last sense that is lost.

J. To improve communication with visitors:

1. Be positive.
2. Be helpful and friendly.
3. Maintain confidentiality.
4. Never argue with visitors.
5. Remain calm if visitors become angry.
6. Listen to what is being said.
7. Be courteous and empathetic.
8. Treat visitors as guests.
9. Refer questions about the resident's condition to the nurse.
10. Ask if you can help.

III. SPECIAL FORMS OF COMMUNICATION

A. The call signal is an important means of communication for the resident.

1. Answer the call signal quickly.
2. Knock before entering the resident's room.
3. Turn off the call signal.
4. Ask the resident what is needed.
5. Always place the call signal within the resident's reach on the unaffected side.
6. If the call signal is ignored, the resident can feel helpless and isolated.
7. Help residents with impairments to learn to use the call signal.
8. Listen for verbal calls from residents who are unable to use a call signal.

B. When answering the phone:

1. Identify yourself by name, title, and unit.
2. Speak slowly and clearly.
3. Always be courteous.
4. Take a message by noting:
   a. date and time
   b. caller's name, spelled correctly
   c. caller's telephone number
   d. any message
   e. your name
5. Be certain that the message gets to the right person.

C. Use the intercom only when necessary.

1. Remember that an intercom announcement can be a distraction.
2. Never give personal information over the intercom.
3. Keep the announcement brief.
4. Speak slowly and clearly.

IV. INTERPERSONAL SKILLS

A. Interpersonal skills include:

1. *empathy*—the ability to put yourself in another's place
2. *respect*—recognition of the worth of another person
3. *genuineness*—being yourself
4. *warmth*—demonstrating concern and affection
5. *caring*—compassion; understanding the fears, problems, and distress of another
6. *courtesy*—putting the needs of others before your own
7. *emotional control*—remaining calm when others upset you
8. *tact*—the ability to say or do the right thing at the right time

B. Use good interpersonal skills when communicating with residents and visitors.

1. Ask for suggestions.
2. Listen to complaints.
3. Get all the facts.
4. Do not take sides.
5. Answer questions or refer questions to the nurse.

C. Stress can affect interpersonal skills. Signs of stress include:

1. difficulty relaxing or slowing down
2. overreacting to small events or problems
3. having trouble sleeping
4. increase in the use of alcohol or drugs to "relax"
5. weight gain or loss
6. feeling very weak and tired
7. having a short attention span
8. having trouble getting out of bed and going to work
9. headaches and neck aches

DIRECTIONS

A brief description of a resident is given followed by 10 questions related to the resident. Each question has four possible answers. Read each question and all answer choices carefully. Choose the one best answer.

Mrs. Martha Miller is a new resident. She is 88 years old and vision impaired.

1. Mrs. Miller is crying. She tells you that she is afraid her daughter will never visit. She says that she wants to go home. You should:
   A. ask her why she is so upset
   B. tell her that everything will be okay
   C. encourage her to talk about her feelings
   D. explain that she lives here now

2. Other residents ask you why Mrs. Miller is so sad. You should:
   A. tell them that it is none of their business
   B. explain Mrs. Miller's problems to them
   C. tell them that you cannot discuss it
   D. tell them you cannot share any secrets

3. Two weeks later, Mrs. Miller's daughter comes to visit. You should:
   A. tell her what her mother said
   B. ignore her since she is not your problem
   C. encourage her to take Mrs. Miller home
   D. be tactful and make her feel welcome

4. Mrs. Miller's daughter complains about the facility and her mother's care. You should:
   A. listen to her and tell her you will get the nurse to talk to her
   B. tell her that she is the biggest problem
   C. ask her why she hasn't been to see her mother sooner
   D. walk away from her

5. Because she is vision impaired, Mrs. Miller holds your arm when walking. For her, your body movement is a form of:
   A. body language
   B. communication
   C. safety
   D. control

6. As soon as you leave the room, Mrs. Miller puts her call signal on. You should:
   A. respond immediately
   B. ignore it
   C. ask someone else to answer
   D. wait 10 minutes and then answer

7. Light is very important when communicating with Mrs. Miller. The light should be:
   A. behind her and shining on you
   B. as bright as possible
   C. dim so it doesn't hurt her eyes
   D. behind you and shining on her

8. Several residents are in Mrs. Miller's room talking to her. You should:
   A. join the conversation
   B. tell them to leave the room
   C. explain to them how to communicate
   D. leave them alone

9. Mrs. Miller's doctor arrives and asks you how she is doing. You should tell him:
   A. about her problems
   B. that you are a CNA
   C. you will get the nurse
   D. she is doing better

10. Mrs. Miller tells you that everyone calls her Aunt Martha. She asks you to do the same. You:

    A. do as she asks

    B. tell her you must call her Mrs. Miller

    C. ask other nursing assistants what they call her

    D. refer to her as madam from now on

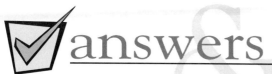
answers & rationales

1.

C. Encouraging a resident to talk about her concerns helps improve the resident's self-esteem.

2.

C. Do not discuss a resident's problems with other residents. Information about a resident must be kept confidential and should only be discussed with the nurse. Keeping information confidential helps residents develop trust in you.

3.

D. When family visits the resident, be pleasant and tactful. Tact is the ability to do and say the right thing at the right time. Family and friends who feel welcome are more likely to visit and support the resident. Never judge the family's behavior.

4.

A. Listen carefully to a visitor's complaints, obtain the facts, and tell the visitor that you will report to the nurse. Listening attentively to complaints lowers tension and is a good first step toward solving problems.

5.

B. We communicate in many ways, including touch and movement. The vision impaired resident can feel your body movements and translate them into messages about speed and direction.

6.

A. A nursing assistant must respond to a call signal immediately. Failure to answer call signals sends a message to residents that they are not important. Residents may use the call signal as a way to determine if staff cares.

7.

A. When communicating with a resident who is vision impaired, the light should be behind the resident and shining on the nursing assistant, eliminating glare, and enabling the resident to see as well as possible.

8.

D. Residents have the right to immediate access to family and friends. If there is no reason for concern, there is no reason for intervention. Leave the residents alone.

9.

C. The nursing assistant works under the supervision of a nurse. The nursing assistant gives information about a resident to the nurse. If other members of the health care team need the information, the nurse will tell them.

10.

A. The resident should decide what she prefers to be called. Persons of different cultures have different standards regarding how people should be addressed. Always address residents by the names and titles they prefer.

Observing, Reporting, and Recording

chapter outline

I. OBSERVING

A. Observation includes:

1. watching
2. listening
3. talking
4. asking questions

Observation—gathering information about the resident by noticing any changes

B. Objective observations are changes noticed by the nursing assistant through the senses of:

1. sight
   a. how a resident performs an activity
   b. body posture and movement
   c. shape and form of body parts
   d. skin
   e. breathing
   f. bowel movement
   g. urine
   h. vomitus
   i. drainage
   j. bleeding
   k. facial expressions
   l. unusual actions
2. hearing
   a. body sounds
   b. verbal complaints
   c. speech problems
   d. confused speech
3. smell
   a. any unusual odors
   b. sweet odors
4. touch
   a. skin
   b. pulse
   c. response to touch

Objective observations—facts observed and not distorted by personal feelings or opinions

C. Subjective observations are statements by the resident.

1. Report observations to the nurse.
2. Carry paper and pen and write down observations so you do not forget them.

Subjective observations—information stated by the resident about how he or she is feeling

Reporting—communicating observations and information to the nurse

II. REPORTING

A. Objective reporting includes:
1. reporting exactly and accurately what you measure or observe
2. what the resident says

B. Subjective reporting includes giving your opinion about what you observed.

C. The nursing assistant reports directly to the nurse:
1. Report resident's name, room number, and bed number.
2. Report as soon as possible.
3. Report the time you made the observation.
4. Report the location of the observation.
5. Report exactly and only what you observe.

D. Report acute changes immediately, including:
1. any sudden change in the resident's condition
2. severe pain
3. seizures
4. loss of consciousness
5. signs of shock
6. signs of hemorrhage
7. difficulty breathing
8. a fall or other accident
9. injuries
10. change in vital signs

Recording—documenting information about the resident

III. RECORDING

A. The resident's chart:
1. is a written account of that resident's condition, treatment, and care
2. is a method of communication among staff
3. includes personal, confidential information about that resident
4. is a legal document that can be used in a court of law
5. may contain the admission sheet, nurses' notes, doctors' notes and orders, history and physical examination, lab and X-ray reports, ADL sheets, care plan

B. When recording information about a resident:
1. Document care only after it is provided.
2. Document throughout the shift when care is provided.
3. Write or print **legibly.**
4. Document entries in **chronological order** and include the date and time.
5. Be sure the page includes the resident's name, room number, and physician's name.

Legible—able to be read

Chronological order—the order in which events occurred

6. Document objective observations.
7. Be specific.
8. Give complete information.
9. Check spelling and grammar.
10. Do not leave areas blank or skip lines.
11. Never use ditto marks.
12. Never document for another team member.
13. Always include your signature and title.
14. Write with nonerasable ink.
15. Never erase, use correction fluid, or scribble out errors.
16. Correct an error by:
    a. drawing a single line through it, writing "error," and signing your name and title
    b. charting the correct entry and signing it
17. Keep resident information confidential.
18. Learn and use approved medical abbreviations.

IV. ABBREVIATIONS

Related to Time

a.c.	before meals	a.m.	morning
p.c.	after meals	p.m.	afternoon or evening
q.d.	every day	h.s.	hour of sleep (bedtime)
b.i.d.	two times a day	n.o.c.	night
t.i.d.	three times a day	stat	immediately
q.i.d.	four times a day	P.R.N.	as necessary
q.o.d.	every other day	D/C	discontinue or stop
q.h.	every hour	c̄	with
min.	minute	s̄	without

Related to Diagnostic Terms and Body Parts

abd.	abdomen	nephro	kidney
ax	axilla	O.D.	right eye
Ca	cancer or carcinoma	O.S.	left eye
CHF	congestive heart failure	O.U.	both eyes
CVA	cerebral vascular accident (stroke)	osteo	bone
DX	diagnosis	psych	related to psychology
Fx	fracture	pneumo	lung
gastric	stomach	resp	respirations
G.I.	gastrointestinal	Rt	right
G.U.	genitourinary	R.B.C.	red blood cell
H.O.H.	hard of hearing	staph	staphylococcus
Lt	left	S.O.B.	short of breath
M.I.	myocardial infarction (heart attack)	W.B.C.	white blood cell
N/V	nausea/vomiting		

Related to Measurements

amt.	amount	ht	height
approx.	approximately	kg	kilogram
C	centigrade or Celsius	lb	pound
cc	cubic centimeters	L	liter
dr	dram	min	minim
F	Fahrenheit	mg	milligram
g	gram	no	number
gr	grain	oz	ounce
gtt	drop	ss	one-half

(continued)

Related to Measurements

tbsp	tablespoon		wt	weight
tsp	teaspoon		I, II, III, IV	one, two, three, four

Related to Treatment

B/p	blood pressure		Sub-Q	subcutaneous (injection just into the superficial layers of skin)
cap	capsule			
cath	catheter or catheterization		PT	physical therapy
C/S	culture and sensitivity (laboratory procedure)		R	rectal
			ROM	range of motion
drsg.	dressing		Rx	prescription
EEG	electroencephalogram (brain wave tracing)		S/A	sugar/acetone (test of urine)
			supp	suppository
EKG or ECG	electrocardiogram (tracing of heart function)		SSE	soap suds enema
			tab	tablet
Foley	type of urinary catheter		TPR	temperature, pulse, respiration
H_2O	water		TWE	tap water enema
H_2O_2	hydrogen peroxide		U/A	urinalysis (laboratory procedure)
O_2	oxygen		UNG	ointment
IM	intramuscular (injection into the muscle)		V/S	vital signs (temperature, pulse, respiration, blood pressure)
IV	intravenous (injection within the vein)			

Related to Resident Orders/Activity

ADL	activities of daily living		C/O	complains of
ad lib	as desired		Dr.	doctor
amb	ambulate		pt	patient
assist	assistance		I&O	intake and output
BM	bowel movement		NPO	nothing by mouth
BR	bathroom		PCP	patient care plan
BRP	bathroom privileges		W/C	wheelchair

Figure 4–1 Commonly used abbreviations. (Source: From *Being a Long-Term Care Nursing Assistant* [5th ed., p. 107], by C. Will-Black and J. Eighmy, 2002, Upper Saddle River, NJ: Prentice Hall. Reprinted by permission.)

DIRECTIONS A brief description of a resident is given followed by 10 questions related to the resident. Each question has four possible answers. Read each question and all answer choices carefully. Choose the one best answer.

Mrs. Mary Taylor is 87 years old. She has CHF, arthritis, and a pressure sore on her left elbow. Her call signal is on.

1. You answer her call signal promptly. She is vomiting and crying. Her skin feels warm to you. She tells you that she has a headache. An example of a subjective observation is:
   A. vomiting
   B. crying
   C. warm skin
   D. headache

2. You report to the nurse immediately because:
   A. Mrs. Taylor needs to see the doctor
   B. Mrs. Taylor has a sudden change in condition
   C. the nurse needs to know why you are spending extra time with Mrs. Taylor
   D. Mrs. Taylor needs medication

3. When reporting Mrs. Taylor's condition to the nurse, you state:
   A. "Mrs. Taylor in room 43, bed 2 isn't feeling well. She is getting the flu."
   B. "Mrs. Taylor in room 43, bed 2 is vomiting. Her skin is warm, she is crying, and she says that she has a headache."
   C. "Mrs. Taylor has an upset stomach. Can you check her when you aren't busy?"
   D. "Mrs. Taylor in room 43, bed 2 has a temperature and upset stomach. She needs to get some rest."

4. In the afternoon, your assignment is to take Mrs. Taylor to PT in W/C. You will take her to:
   A. the party in the west corridor
   B. physical therapy with caution
   C. the podiatrist in a wheelchair
   D. physical therapy in a wheelchair

5. You record the care you gave Mrs. Taylor. Her chart is:
   A. confidential and can only be read by nurses and doctors
   B. an account of Mrs. Taylor's personal history
   C. used by nursing staff only
   D. a legal document that can be used in a court of law

6. You should record the care you gave to Mrs. Taylor:
   A. before you start your shift
   B. at the end of your shift
   C. throughout your shift, when the care is provided
   D. only if you have time

7. When recording information about Mrs. Taylor, you should:
   A. include her name, room number, and physician's name
   B. document your subjective observations

C. leave empty lines in case you forget something

D. use ditto marks to save time and be more efficient

8. You make a mistake when recording. You should:

A. erase the error and start again

B. use correction fluid, then sign your name and title

C. draw a single line through it, write "error," and sign your name and title

D. black out the error with a felt-tipped pen

9. You go to record the care you gave Mrs. Taylor and find that another CNA

has done some of the recording for you. You should:

A. thank her for helping you

B. tell the nurse

C. sign the entries if they are accurate

D. tell the other CNA to never do that again

10. At the end of your shift you should report observations and care given to:

A. the CNAs on the next shift

B. your supervising nurse

C. the nurse from the next shift

D. the director of nursing

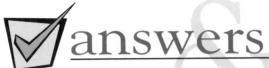

answers & rationales

1.
D. Subjective observations involve information that a resident tells you. It is impossible for someone else to know if a person's head hurts or not.

2.
B. A sudden change in condition requires immediate attention by the nurse. Report to the nurse immediately.

3.
B. Give the nurse an accurate report. Report all objective and subjective data without giving your opinion or assumptions. The report should describe objectively what the nursing assistant sees and touches and subjectively what the resident tells the nursing assistant.

4.
D. PT means physical therapy; W/C means wheelchair.

5.
D. The resident's chart is a permanent legal record that can be presented in a court of law as evidence of the resident's care and treatment.

6.
C. Record the care you give to a resident as soon as care is provided. It is easier to maintain accuracy if you document immediately.

7.
A. Before documenting, always be certain that a page contains the resident's name, room number, and doctor's name. Legally, each page of documentation must include the identifying information.

8.
C. Correct an error by drawing a single line through it, writing "error," and signing your name and title. It is important to keep an accurate record of all care. Legally, any entry made in a legal document must remain readable. Never scratch over or white out mistakes.

9.
B. Tell the nurse immediately if documentation is invalid. Nursing assistants can legally record only care that they have given. No nursing assistant should ever record for another nursing assistant.

10.
B. The nursing assistant reports to the supervising nurse. Following the proper chain of command assures proper flow of information.

CHAPTER

5

Infection Control

chapter outline

I. CHAIN OF INFECTION

Infection—the invasion and growth of pathogens in the body

A. Infection control:
1. is the responsibility of all staff
2. reduces the risk of infection for residents, visitors, employees, and their families
3. is outlined in the facility's policies and procedures

Pathogens—disease-causing microorganisms

B. Infection is caused by pathogens that multiply in places that are:
1. warm
2. dark
3. moist

C. Pathogens are passed from person to person through the chain of infection, which includes:
1. *The causative agent*—the pathogen that causes infection:
   a. bacteria
   b. viruses
   c. fungi
   d. protozoa
2. *The reservoir of the agent*—the place where the pathogen is able to live and reproduce, including:
   a. humans
   b. animals
   c. objects
   d. the environment
3. *The portal of exit*—how the pathogens leave the reservoir:
   a. urine
   b. **feces**
   c. **saliva**
   d. tears
   e. drainage from wounds
   f. blood
   g. fluids from the respiratory or reproductive tracts
4. *The route of transmission*—how the pathogen gets from the reservoir to the new host:
   a. contact transmission:
      • direct contact—body to body
      • indirect contact—contaminated object to body
   b. droplet transmission:
      • coughing
      • sneezing
      • talking

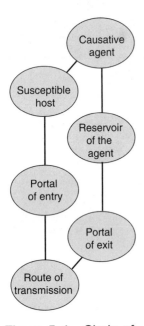

Figure 5–1 Chain of infection. (Source: From *The Nursing Assistant* [3rd ed., p. 53], by J. Pulliam, 2002, Upper Saddle River, NJ: Prentice Hall. Reprinted by permission.)

Feces (stool, bowel movement)—solid waste products eliminated by the body

Saliva—thin, clear liquid produced by salivary glands in the mouth

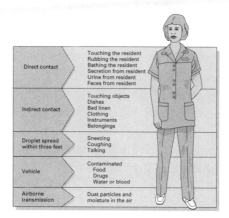

Direct contact	Touching the resident Rubbing the resident Bathing the resident Secretion from resident Urine from resident Feces from resident
Indirect contact	Touching objects Dishes Bed linen Clothing Instruments Belongings
Droplet spread within three feet	Sneezing Coughing Talking
Vehicle	Contaminated Food Drugs Water or blood
Airborne transmission	Dust particles and moisture in the air

Figure 5–2 Conditions that promote bacterial growth. (Source: From *Being a Long-Term Care Nursing Assistant* [5th ed., p. 44], by C. Will-Black and J. Eighmy, 2002, Upper Saddle River, NJ: Prentice Hall. Reprinted by permission.)

    c. airborne transmission:
- dust
- moisture in the air

5. *The portal of entry*—how the pathogen enters the body:
    a. cuts or breaks in skin or **mucous membranes**
    b. the respiratory tract
    c. the gastrointestinal tract
    d. the reproductive or urinary tracts
    e. the circulatory system
    f. passage from mother to fetus

> **Mucous membrane**—tissue lining many passages such as mouth, respiratory, digestive, and reproductive tracts

6. *The susceptible host*—the person who does not resist the pathogen, especially those who are:
    a. very young
    b. elderly
    c. debilitated
    d. very ill

D. The body has natural defenses to help prevent infection.

1. The skin is a barrier that keeps pathogens out (skin is the first line of defense against infection).
2. Mucous membranes secrete mucus that traps and kills pathogens.
3. **Cilia** in the respiratory tract move pathogens out of the body.
4. Coughing and sneezing get rid of pathogens.
5. Tears wash away and kill pathogens.
6. Stomach acid kills pathogens.
7. Phagocytes (special blood cells) trap pathogens.
8. Fever kills pathogens that cannot tolerate heat.

> **Cilia**—tiny hairs in respiratory tract

9. Inflammation brings blood and other substances to the source of infection.

10. The immune response creates proteins that can kill pathogens.

E. Signs of infection include:

1. reddening or increased heat in an area of inflammation
2. drainage or pus from a wound or from the eyes, ears, or nose
3. swelling
4. pain and tenderness
5. a change in the smell of drainage
6. fever
7. fatigue
8. loss of appetite, nausea, or vomiting
9. a rash

II. MEDICAL ASEPSIS

Medical asepsis—practices and procedures that foster a clean environment by eliminating pathogens

A. Terminology of medical asepsis includes the words:

1. *sterile*—free from all microorganisms
2. *clean*—not contaminated with pathogens
3. *contaminated*—having pathogens
4. *dirty*—contaminated with pathogens
5. *disinfection*—use of chemicals to kill or slow the growth of microorganisms

B. Follow these aseptic practices:

1. Use gloves if contact with bodily fluids is possible.
2. Wash your hands:
   a. before and after giving resident care
   b. before handling food
   c. after using the toilet
   d. after sneezing, coughing, or blowing your nose
   e. before and after eating
3. Cover your nose and mouth when coughing or sneezing.
4. Stay home if you have a fever, cold, or diarrhea.
5. Report open sores on your body or a resident's body to the nurse.
6. Dispose of tissues properly.
7. Use a resident's personal items only for that resident.
8. Carry items held away from your uniform.
9. Don't put linen on the floor.
10. Don't shake linen.
11. Don't place soiled items on the overbed table, bedside stand, or near the head of the bed, including:
    a. bedpans
    b. urinals
    c. soiled linen

12. Wipe stethoscope earpieces and diaphragm with alcohol before and after use.
13. Take dirty or contaminated items to the dirty utility room.
14. Wash and dry soiled mattresses when changing the bed.

C. Handwashing is the most important way to prevent the spread of pathogens. Wash your hands:

1. before and after eating
2. after using the bathroom
3. after combing your hair
4. before and after using gloves
5. after handling contact lenses, using lip balm, or applying makeup
6. after coughing, sneezing, or blowing your nose
7. after smoking
8. before and after giving care to each resident
9. after handling soiled equipment

D. Wash your hands effectively. See Procedure 5-1 in Appendix A.

1. Stand away from the sink so your uniform does not touch it.
2. Turn the water on with a paper towel and adjust the water to a comfortable temperature.
3. Discard the paper towel.
4. Hold your hands down and wet hands and 1–3 inches of wrists.
5. Apply soap and lather hands and wrists.
6. Rub all surfaces of hands and wrists, creating friction, for 15–20 seconds.
7. Clean your nails by gently rubbing them against the palm of your other hand.
8. Rinse your hands from wrists to fingertips under running water, holding your fingertips down.
9. Dry your hands thoroughly with a clean paper towel.
10. Discard the towel.
11. Turn off the faucet with a clean, dry paper towel and discard the towel without touching your other hand or the waste container.
12. If you touch the sink at any time during the procedure, rewash your hands.

E. Use antiseptic gels for hand hygiene. See Procedure 5-2 in Appendix A.

1. Use gels:
   a. before and between resident procedures
   b. after removing gloves
2. Wash your hands with soap and water if hands are visibly contaminated.

Why?
— The sink is contaminated and will contaminate your uniform.
— Using a paper towel to turn on the faucet reduces the amount of pathogens on the faucet.

Why?
— Skin may chap if left damp.
— The paper towel becomes contaminated when it touches the faucet. Transferring the paper towel from one hand to the other after it touches the faucet will contaminate your hand.

Why?
Antiseptic gels do not remove body fluids or dirt from the hands.

F. When using gloves:

1. Wash your hands before and after use.
2. Check the gloves for tears or holes.
3. Long fingernails and jewelry can damage gloves and increase the chance for contamination.
4. Change gloves for each resident and each task.
5. Never wear gloves outside the resident's room.
6. Use gloves that are not irritating to your hands.

G. Remove gloves properly. See Procedure 5-3 in Appendix A.

1. Grasp one glove one inch below the cuff.
2. Pull the glove off the hand, turning it inside out.
3. Hold the removed glove in the gloved hand.
4. Place the first two fingers of the ungloved hand inside the cuff of the glove.
5. Pull the glove off, turning it inside out as you remove it.
6. Discard gloves immediately.
7. Wash your hands.

H. When handling linen:

1. Wash your hands before touching clean linen.
2. Store clean linen in areas designated for clean linen.
3. Carry linens away from your body.
4. Take only the necessary amount of clean linen into the room.
5. Do not use linen that has fallen on the floor.
6. Do not shake or fluff linens.
7. Place soiled linen in covered containers, never on the floor.
8. Close soiled linen containers tightly.
9. Wash your hands after handling soiled linen.

III. STANDARD PRECAUTIONS

A. Standard precautions:

1. are infection control guidelines developed by the **CDC**
2. apply to all residents
3. are directed primarily at blood and body fluid transmission of diseases
4. are designed to reduce the risk of transmission of bloodborne and other pathogens in health care facilities

B. To comply with standard precautions:

1. Wash your hands after accidental contact with blood, body fluids, secretions, excretions, nonintact skin, or mucous membranes.

Why?
Damaged gloves let pathogens into and out of the gloves and do not protect you or the resident.

Why?
Gloves that are worn outside the resident's room contaminate any surfaces, equipment, supplies, or people touched by you.

Why?
When gloves are inside out and one inside the other, pathogens are contained.

Why?
— Your uniform is considered dirty and will contaminate clean linen.
— Items placed on the floor are a safety hazard for staff and other residents.

CDC—Centers for Disease Control, Atlanta, GA

2. Wash your hands before applying gloves and after removing gloves.
3. Wear gloves when you may come into contact with any body fluids, including:
    a. secretions
    b. excretions
    c. nonintact skin
    d. mucous membranes
4. Wear a gown when your uniform may come into contact with body fluids.
5. Wear a mask, face shield, and protective eyewear when contact with body fluids is possible.
6. Prevent soiled equipment and supplies from coming in contact with skin, mucous membranes, or clothing.
7. Clean and disinfect soiled equipment according to facility policy.
8. Treat all soiled linen as infectious.
9. Carefully dispose of sharp objects in the proper container.

IV. BLOODBORNE PATHOGEN STANDARD

A. The bloodborne pathogen standard was developed by OSHA to help protect health care workers who come into contact with blood or other infectious materials.

OSHA—Occupational Safety and Health Administration

B. Employers must:
1. establish an **exposure** control plan that includes:
    a. identification of workers at risk of contact with infectious material
    b. methods to protect employees from bloodborne pathogens
    c. procedures for use of protective equipment such as gloves, gowns, and masks
    d. educational programs for new employees and annual training for all employees
    e. proper disposal of needles and sharp objects
2. offer hepatitis B vaccine, at no cost, to employees who are at risk of exposure

Exposure—unprotected contact with pathogens or material that may be contaminated, such as medical instruments or body fluids

C. Employees are responsible for protecting themselves by:
1. attending training sessions
2. following standard precautions
3. reporting any exposure to the nurse immediately

Biohazardous waste—waste material that has been contaminated with blood, body fluids, or body substances that may cause infection

D. Requirements for handling biohazardous waste include:

1. placing contaminated material in a container separate from the regular trash
2. labeling bags, boxes, or containers that contain infectious substances as *biohazardous*

E. Some infectious diseases include:

1. *tuberculosis (TB)*—an infectious disease that commonly attacks the lungs, usually spread by contact with the **sputum** of an infected person
2. *AIDS (acquired immune deficiency syndrome)*—a condition in which the body's immune system is damaged by attack from the HIV virus, usually spread by contact with the blood of an infected person
3. *hepatitis B*—a viral disease that causes inflammation of the liver, usually spread by contact with the blood of an infected person
4. *scabies*—a disease caused by mites that burrow under the skin, usually spread by skin-to-skin contact with an infected person or by contact with infected surfaces

Sputum—waste material coughed up from the lungs or trachea

V. TRANSMISSION-BASED PRECAUTIONS

A. Transmission-based precautions (isolation) are a group of infection control methods based on the way a particular disease is spread.

B. Contact precautions:

1. Visitors should report to the nurses' station before entering the room.
2. *Resident placement*—private room if possible
3. *Gloves*—wear gloves when entering the room and for all resident care
4. *Gown*—wear a gown if clothing may come into contact with the resident or contaminated items or surfaces
5. *Masks and eyewear*—wear a mask and eyewear if you may come in contact with body fluids
6. *Handwashing*—wash hands after removing gloves and avoid touching any surface in the room
7. *Transport*—limit the movement and transport of the resident
8. Always follow standard precautions.

Why?
All surfaces in an isolation room can be considered contaminated.

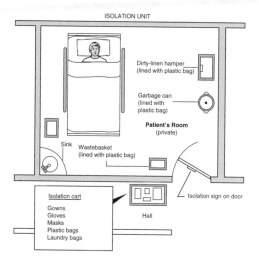

Figure 5–3 Besides the bed, the layout of an isolation unit includes a soiled-linen hamper, a garbage can, and a wastebasket, all lined with plastic bags; a sink with running water; and an isolation cart outside the door. This cart contains personal protective equipment for use in the room. (Source: From *The Nursing Assistant* [3rd ed., p. 67], by J. Pulliam, 2002, Upper Saddle River, NJ: Prentice Hall. Reprinted by permission.)

C. Droplet precautions:

1. Visitors should report to the nurses' station before entering the room.
2. *Resident placement*—private room if possible
3. *Gloves*—must be worn when in contact with blood and body fluids
4. *Gown*—must be worn during procedures or situations where there will be exposure to body fluids, blood, draining wounds, or mucous membranes
5. *Masks and eyewear*—in addition to standard precautions, wear mask when working within three feet of resident
6. *Handwashing*—hands must be washed before gloving and after gloves are removed
7. *Transport*—limit the movement and transport of the resident. If transport is necessary, mask the resident to minimize dispersal of droplets
8. *Resident care equipment*—clean and disinfect common use equipment
9. Always follow standard precautions.

D. Airborne precautions:

1. Visitors must report to the nurses' station before entering the room.
2. *Resident placement*—private room. Keep negative air pressure in relation to the surrounding areas. Keep door closed at all times.

Why?
Wearing a mask will filter airborne microorganisms preventing you from inhaling microorganisms or body fluids that may be in the air in the resident's room and prevent the resident from inhaling pathogens you may introduce into the air.

3. *Gloves*—must be worn when in contact with blood and body fluids

4. *Gown or apron*—must be worn during procedures or situations where there will be exposure to body fluids, blood, draining wounds, or mucous membranes

5. *Masks and eyewear*—must be worn if there is a possibility of exposure to airborne pathogens or body fluid splashes

6. *Handwashing*—hands must be washed before gloving and after gloves are removed. Skin surfaces must be washed immediately and thoroughly when contaminated with body fluids or blood

7. *Transport*—limit the movement and transport of the resident. If transport is necessary, mask the resident

8. *Resident care equipment*—clean and disinfect common use equipment

9. Always follow standard precautions.

E. The N-95 respirator is a more complex device worn when there is a chance of exposure to highly contagious microorganisms including tuberculosis.

F. Use personal protective equipment, including gloves, gown, and mask, when indicated. Use the equipment correctly to protect yourself and the resident. See Procedure 5-4 in Appendix A.

G. When handling infectious waste:

1. Place linen, trash, and other waste in appropriate bags.

2. Close bag tightly before taking it out of the room.

3. Store filled bags in a locked room labeled with a biohazard sign.

H. The resident's self-image may be affected because of isolation.

1. Be kind, patient, and respectful.

2. Answer the call signal promptly.

3. Check the resident frequently.

4. Talk to the resident frequently.

5. Encourage residents to talk about their feelings.

6. Help family and visitors understand the need for transmission-based precautions.

7. Be certain the resident has access to diversions.

DIRECTIONS

A brief description of a resident is given followed by 10 questions related to the resident. Each question has four possible answers. Read each question and all answer choices carefully. Choose the one best answer.

Mrs. Kara Phillips is 78 years old. She has tested positive for tuberculosis.

1. The doctor orders transmission-based precautions for Mrs. Phillips because she:
   A. has a contagious disease
   B. does not walk
   C. cannot communicate
   D. is very demanding

2. Because Mrs. Phillips has TB, she should:
   A. be isolated in a private room
   B. have the curtain pulled between her and her roommate
   C. be moved to a TB sanitarium
   D. receive no visitors until she is well

3. Before entering Mrs. Phillips's room, you should put on a:
   A. paper mask
   B. face shield
   C. N-95 respirator
   D. sterile surgical gown

4. You may be more susceptible to infection and communicable disease if you:
   A. are tired or stressed
   B. exercise every day
   C. eat a well-balanced diet
   D. stay in Mrs. Phillips's room too long

5. If you shake the linen while changing Mrs. Phillips's bed, you will:
   A. make the bed quicker
   B. spread microorganisms
   C. eliminate wrinkles in the sheets
   D. prevent infection

6. You accidentally drop the bedspread on the floor. The bedspread is then considered:
   A. dirty
   B. disinfected
   C. sterile
   D. clean

7. The best way to prevent the spread of infection and disease is to:
   A. cover your mouth when you cough
   B. stay at home if you do not feel well
   C. touch residents only when wearing gloves
   D. wash your hands frequently

8. Your body's primary defense against infection is your:
   A. heart
   B. hair
   C. lungs
   D. skin

9. You have a phone call at the nurse's station. If you wear contaminated gloves in public areas and touch telephones, doors, or elevator buttons, you:
   A. should tell housekeeping to clean the contaminated areas
   B. put everyone at risk for infection
   C. know that pathogens die quickly on surfaces so there is no danger
   D. should take off the gloves and put them in your pocket

10. Because Mrs. Phillips is on transmission-based precautions, she can:

    A. become lonely and depressed

    B. take too much of your time

    C. demand that you stay with her

    D. report you to the supervisor if you leave her room

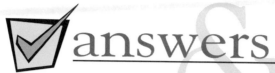

answers & rationales

1.

A. Transmission-based precautions are ordered for residents who have a contagious disease. Residents with a contagious disease are isolated because they could infect others.

2.

A. Moving a resident with a communicable disease to a private room reduces the risk of infecting others. The pathogens that cause TB are carried in small droplets that remain suspended in the air after being exhaled and may be inhaled by others.

3.

C. An N-95 respirator mask must be worn by everyone entering the room of an isolated resident who has tuberculosis. The mask protects against known or suspected pulmonary tuberculosis.

4.

D. Emotional stress and fatigue may make a person more susceptible to infection and communicable disease.

5.

B. Avoid shaking or flapping bed linens to prevent spreading the microorganisms.

6.

A. If linen falls on to the floor, it is considered dirty because the floor is dirty and contaminated with pathogens.

7.

D. Frequent handwashing is the most important way to prevent the spread of infection. Antiseptic gels used between handwashing also reduce pathogens.

8.

D. Skin is the first line of defense against infection.

9.

B. Touching telephones, doors, or elevator buttons with contaminated gloves puts everyone at risk for infection. Pathogens transfer from the gloves to other surfaces.

10.

A. A resident in isolation may become lonely and depressed. Remember that it is the pathogen, not the resident that is being isolated. Give care with kindness and respect.

Body Mechanics and Alignment

6

chapter outline

I. BODY MECHANICS

A. Correct body mechanics means using the body safely and efficiently.

B. Use correct body mechanics to:
1. protect the resident from injury
2. protect yourself from injury
3. maximize strength
4. minimize fatigue
5. conserve energy
6. avoid back strain

C. Use correct body mechanics when:
1. sitting
2. standing
3. walking
4. working
5. lifting
6. moving objects

Body mechanics—the use of the body to produce motion

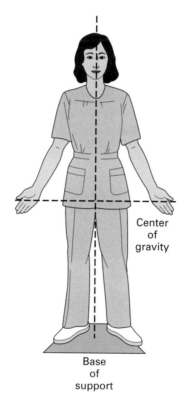

Center
of
gravity

Base
of
support

Figure 6–1 The line of gravity passes through the center of gravity and the base of support. (Source: From *Being a Long-Term Care Nursing Assistant* [5th ed., p. 36], by C. Will-Black and J. Eighmy, 2002, Upper Saddle River, NJ: Prentice Hall. Reprinted by permission.)

Fatigue—a feeling of tiredness or weariness

Center of gravity—place where the bulk of an object or person is centered

Base of support—foundation of an object or person

Why?
— A good base of support improves balance.
— Bending the knees reduces strain on the back.

Why?
— The large muscles of the legs and arms are designed to support weight.
— Twisting puts extreme stress on the spine.

Why?
— Keeping a back support tightened constantly can weaken back muscles.
— Elevating the work surface allows you to perform procedures with good posture and body alignment which reduces stress to your back, joints, and muscles.

Body alignment—placing the body parts in correct anatomical position

D. To prevent fatigue and back strain:
1. Change your position frequently.
2. Stretch and relax occasionally.
3. Use correct body mechanics.

E. Terms related to body mechanics:
1. *Center of gravity*—the pelvis
2. *Base of support*—the feet

F. Principles of correct body mechanics include:
1. Maintain a wide base of support by standing with your feet 8 to 12 inches apart.
2. Bend at your knees (squat), not at your waist or hips.
3. Keep your back straight.
4. Keep your knees bent.
5. Keep your weight balanced evenly on both feet.
6. Use the large muscles of your legs and arms.
7. Stand close to the object when lifting.
8. Turn your whole body at once; don't twist.
9. Turn or pivot with your feet.
10. Use smooth, coordinated movements.
11. Push or pull an object rather than lift it if possible.
12. Lift heavy objects with both hands.
13. Support heavy objects you are carrying with your arms.
14. Put your elbows close to your body.
15. If you use a back support, tighten it immediately before lifting and loosen it immediately after.
16. Keep beds and other surfaces at a comfortable working height.
17. Plan ahead and get help if needed.
18. Always count "one, two, three" when working with another person (resident or staff) so you work together.

II. BODY ALIGNMENT

A. For good posture, keep:
1. head up, eyes straight ahead
2. neck straight
3. back straight
4. chest out
5. abdomen in
6. arms relaxed at sides
7. knees slightly relaxed
8. feet straight, toes forward

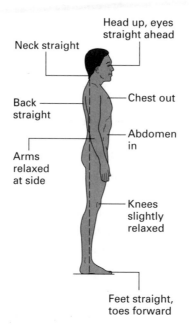

Figure 6–2 Body alignment. (Source: From *Being a Long-Term Care Nursing Assistant* [5th ed., p. 231], by C. Will-Black and J. Eighmy, 2002, Upper Saddle River, NJ: Prentice Hall. Reprinted by permission.)

B. Check the resident for good body alignment:
1. before and after changing the resident's position
2. before and after transferring the resident
3. when the resident is seated in a chair
4. when the resident is lying in the bed

C. For proper body alignment, the resident's:
1. ears should be above the shoulders
2. shoulders should be above the hips
3. arms should be at the sides
4. legs should be straight and slightly apart if lying down or at a 90° angle to the torso if sitting up
5. feet should be flat on the floor when sitting

DIRECTIONS
A brief description of a resident is given followed by 10 questions related to the resident. Each question has four possible answers. Read each question and all answer choices carefully. Choose the one best answer.

Mr. Frank Pierce is 68 years old. He has had a stroke and is weak on his left side.

1. Every time you need to move a resident, you should ask yourself:
   A. Is this a convenient time to move him?
   B. Does he really need to be moved?
   C. Can I do this alone or do I need help?
   D. Should I let him do the move himself?

2. You assist Mr. Pierce to a chair. To keep him and you safe, you must:
   A. get permission from the nurse
   B. move him quickly
   C. have him in good body alignment
   D. use correct body mechanics

3. When helping Mr. Pierce move, you create a good base of support to:
   A. help you maintain good balance
   B. keep Mr. Pierce upright if he begins to fall
   C. help you twist when you move him
   D. help Mr. Pierce be dependent

4. You want Mr. Pierce to help himself move as much as possible. You should:
   A. tell him to move when he is ready
   B. count to three so he knows exactly when to help
   C. let go of him during the move to see if he is able to move alone
   D. move him quickly to reduce stress

5. When helping Mr. Pierce stand up, you should:
   A. stand close to him
   B. keep him far away from you
   C. grab him under the armpits
   D. pull him up by his arms

6. After helping Mr. Pierce sit in the chair, you check for:
   A. bruises
   B. proper body alignment
   C. signs of distress
   D. good base of support

7. Mr. Pierce should be seated with his back straight against the back of the chair and:
   A. his hands in his lap
   B. his arms straight at his sides
   C. his feet flat on the floor or on a stool
   D. his legs straight

8. Mr. Pierce drops his book on the floor. You should:
   A. pick it up by bending at the waist
   B. tell him that it is contaminated
   C. pick it up by bending at the knees
   D. tell him to pick it up himself for exercise

9. You straighten Mr. Pierce's bed. You should:
   A. elevate the bed to a working height
   B. put the bed in the lowest position for his safety
   C. always change the sheets to eliminate pathogens
   D. ask Mr. Pierce to help you so he gets exercise

10. If you use a back support when moving, you should:

    A. have the support tightened at all times

    B. tighten it immediately before lifting and loosen it immediately after

    C. use it only for lifting heavy objects never when moving residents

    D. clean it with alcohol after each use

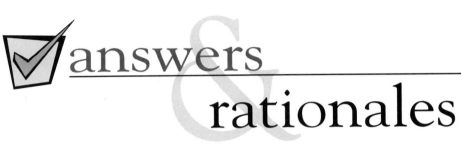

answers & rationales

1.

C. When moving residents, consider the safety of both the resident and you. If the resident is unable to help during the move or is difficult to move, ask other staff for help. Safety is the first consideration for the resident and you.

2.

D. Correct body mechanics protect both the nursing assistant and the resident from injury. Correct body mechanics saves energy, prevents fatigue, and promotes safety.

3.

A. The nursing assistant creates a good base of support to maintain good balance. A person's base of support is at the feet and is the foundation on which the body rests. Feet should be spread apart approximately 18 inches to improve balance and stability.

4.

B. Always count to three before moving a resident. Letting the resident know the exact moment the move will begin allows the resident to assist as much as possible.

5.

A. When helping the resident stand up, stand close to him. Correct body mechanics include standing close to the person or object you are moving. Keeping the resident close distributes weight and improves your balance.

6.

B. After a move, check the resident for correct body alignment. Proper body alignment promotes comfort and reduce stress on the musculoskeletal system.

7.

C. When a resident is sitting in a chair, his feet should be flat on the floor or a stool to promote stability and comfort.

8.

C. Pick up an object from the floor by bending at the knees. Bending at the knees protects the back from strain and injury. Using leg muscles reduces strain on the back.

9.

A. Elevate adjustable beds to a working height (approximately waist high) before performing care. Elevating the bed prevents the need to stretch and reach, and decreases stress on back and joints.

10.

B. If you use a back support you must tighten it immediately before lifting and loosen it after use. Keeping the back support tightened, over time, may decrease muscle strength and result in a greater chance of injury.

7 Safety

chapter outline

I. CAUSES OF ACCIDENTS

A. The reasons elderly people have more accidents than any other age group except children include:

1. physical changes of aging:
   a. slower blood circulation, which results in dizziness when changing position
   b. weak muscles and stiff joints
   c. brittle bones
   d. vision and hearing loss
   e. decreased sense of touch
   f. slower reflexes
2. disease processes, including:
   a. arthritis
   b. stroke
   c. Parkinson's disease
3. mental impairment:
   a. any decrease in awareness
   b. Alzheimer's disease
   c. chronic brain syndrome
   d. confusion
   e. disorientation
4. life changes and losses:
   a. admission to facility
   b. unfamiliar environment
   c. depression
   d. any type of loss
5. medications:
   a. may have a stronger effect than in younger people
   b. effects may last longer
   c. may cause confusion or drowsiness
   d. may result in drug interactions because of taking multiple medications

B. Injuries may result from:

1. staff carelessness or negligence:
   a. failure to correctly identify the resident
   b. delay in answering the call signal
   c. incorrect moving or lifting
   d. failure to lock the brakes on equipment with wheels
   e. failure to clean up spills
   f. failure to place call signal within reach

2. falls caused by:
    a. wet, slippery floors
    b. improper footwear
    c. poor lighting
    d. clutter
    e. staff carelessness or negligence
3. burns from:
    a. careless smoking
    b. hot water and other liquids
    c. procedures involving heat or cold
    d. decreased sensitivity to heat
    e. negligence
4. poisoning by ingestion of a **toxic** substance:
    a. caused by poor vision or confusion
    b. includes cleaning solutions and disinfectants

Toxic—poisonous

5. suffocation caused by:
    a. choking
    b. drowning
    c. smoke inhalation
    d. electrical shock

II. ACCIDENT PREVENTION

A. To prevent accidents:

1. Correctly identify the resident.
2. Follow the nurse's instructions when providing care.
3. Be aware of special needs such as:
    a. no weight bearing
    b. keep head of bed elevated at all times
    c. do not position resident on left side
    d. out of bed with assistance only
    e. needs eyeglasses/hearing aid
4. Ask questions if you do not understand.
5. Perform only procedures that you are trained to do.
6. Use gloves if there is a possibility of coming in contact with body fluids.
7. Follow infection control policies to prevent the spread of infection.
8. Use proper body mechanics.
9. Get help when necessary.
10. Elevate the bed to a **working height** when performing procedures.
11. Use handrails on stairways.

Working height—the height that allows you to perform procedures with the least amount of strain or bending. The mattress should be level with your waist.

B. Falls are the most common type of accident in health care facilities.

1. To prevent falls when walking:
   a. Clean up spills immediately.
   b. Keep hallways and rooms free of clutter.
   c. Provide adequate lighting.
   d. Make sure the resident is wearing proper footwear:
      - nonskid soles
      - low heels
      - shoes that fit properly and are in good repair
      - shoelaces tied or buckles fastened
      - closed heel and toe
   e. Assist resident to use cane or walker when needed.
   f. Encourage residents to use safety bars and rails when walking in hallways.
   g. Walk on the right side in hallways and stairs.
2. To prevent falls when the resident is in bed:
   a. Answer call signals promptly.
   b. Keep the call signal in reach on the resident's unaffected side even if the resident is confused or unconscious.
   c. Put water and the TV control within resident's reach.
   d. Position the resident in proper body alignment.
   e. Raise side rails when bed is elevated to a working height.
   f. Return bed to the lowest position after completing a procedure.
   g. Place bed **gatch** in.
   h. Keep side rails up only if ordered by the physician.
3. To prevent falls by residents with special needs:
   a. Report to the nurse immediately if a resident is:
      - dizzy
      - unsteady
      - exhibiting aggressive behavior
   b. Closely monitor residents who wander.
4. To prevent falls and injuries during transfer and transport:
   a. When transferring a resident, lock the brakes on wheelchairs, beds, stretchers, and commodes.
   b. Move residents and equipment carefully around corners and through swinging doors.
   c. Be careful of the resident's feet when transporting in wheelchair.
   d. Get help if needed.

C. To prevent burns:

1. Cool hot food by stirring before feeding a resident.
2. Warn residents who feed themselves if food is hot.

Gatch—handle or crank used to raise and lower the bed, head of bed, or foot of bed

Why?
Place bed gatch in to avoid tripping or banging shin.

3. Test or have the resident test the water temperature before showers or baths.
4. Report water temperatures that seem too hot in residents' rooms, showers, or bathing areas.
5. Protect residents from overexposure to sunlight.
6. Monitor residents who smoke according to the facility policy.
7. Perform heat treatments according to procedure and monitor the resident closely.

D. To prevent poisoning:
1. Never use a substance that has no label.
2. Store all medicines and toxic substances in a locked cabinet when not in use.
3. Know what items residents are not allowed to keep in their rooms.
4. Never leave a medication or toxic substance unattended.

E. To prevent choking or suffocation:
1. Never leave a resident unattended in a bathtub.
2. Report to the nurse immediately if a resident has difficulty chewing or swallowing.
3. Know the signs of an obstructed airway and how to do the Heimlich maneuver.
4. Know how to administer CPR and first aid.
5. Frequently check residents who are restrained.
6. Check that the resident's pillow is not too soft.

F. Note proper use and condition of equipment:
1. Never use electrical equipment near water or where oxygen is being administered.
2. Dispose of sharp objects in special containers according to facility policy.
3. Report safety hazards and damaged equipment to the nurse immediately.
4. Use equipment according to the manufacturer's directions.

G. Incidents involving residents, visitors, or employees must be reported immediately.

Incident—an event that is not part of the facility's routine

1. Incidents may be:
   a. accidents
   b. errors in performing resident care
2. Written documentation of an incident includes:
   a. persons involved
   b. date
   c. time
   d. location of incident

e. witnesses

f. injuries, if any

Restraint—a device that restricts a person's freedom of movement

III. RESTRAINTS (PROTECTIVE DEVICES)

A. Federal and state laws regulate the use of restraints.

B. Restraints:

1. may be used for the safety of the resident
2. may never be used for the convenience of the staff
3. require a doctor's order

C. Using restraints without a doctor's order may be considered:

1. false imprisonment
2. abuse
3. violation of resident's rights

D. Physical effects of being restrained include:

1. skin breakdown
2. constipation
3. pneumonia
4. blood clots
5. muscle weakness
6. loss of mobility

E. Psychological effects of being restrained include:

1. loss of dignity
2. loss of independence
3. loss of control
4. loss of self-esteem
5. confusion
6. disorientation
7. anxiety
8. frustration
9. anger
10. combativeness
11. decrease in communication
12. decrease in social activity

F. As an alternative to restraints:

1. Interrupt behavior that might lead to the need for restraints.
2. Use music to calm the resident.
3. Use TV and radio for diversion.
4. Encourage activities as an outlet for energy.
5. Closely observe the confused resident.

6. Allow the resident to walk in safe areas.
7. Encourage family participation.
8. Use pillows, padding, and other equipment for support.
9. Answer a call signal immediately.
10. Take the resident to the bathroom frequently.
11. Let the resident stay up later.
12. Offer fluids routinely.
13. Respond immediately to door alarms.
14. Use reality orientation techniques.
15. Ambulate the resident frequently.
16. Provide activities the resident can do with the hands.
17. Offer snacks.

G. Types of restraints:

1. *soft belt restraints*—used to prevent falling out of wheelchair or bed

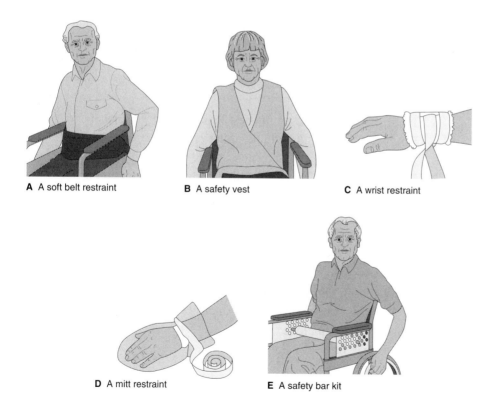

A A soft belt restraint   **B** A safety vest   **C** A wrist restraint

D A mitt restraint   **E** A safety bar kit

Figure 7–1 Types of restraints. (Source: From *The Long-Term Care Nursing Assistant* [2nd ed., p. 69], by P. Grubbs and B. Blasband, 2002, Upper Saddle River, NJ: Prentice Hall. Reprinted by permission.)

2. *safety vests*—used to prevent falling out of chair or bed; have more support than belt
3. *wrist restraints*—used to prevent the resident from removing dressings or pulling out tubes
4. *mitt restraints*—used to restrict finger movement without preventing movement of the hand or arm
5. *safety bars on wheelchairs*—used to prevent resident from falling

H. When applying restraints:

1. Use a restraint only when necessary and only with a doctor's order.
2. Use restorative techniques first (activities, recreation).
3. Understand that a geri-chair is considered a restraint.
4. Never restrain a resident in a chair without wheels.
5. Apply restraints only if you have been trained to do so.
6. Approach the resident calmly.
7. Use the correct size and type of restraint.
8. Explain what you are doing and why.
9. Be certain that the resident is properly aligned and comfortable.
10. Apply the restraint according to the manufacturer's directions.
11. Pad bony prominences under the restraint if necessary.
12. Tie a knot that can be released quickly.
13. Tie the restraint to the moveable part of the bed frame, never on the side rail.
14. Tie the restraint on the nonmoveable part of the wheelchair.
15. Do not restrain a resident to the toilet or bedside commode.
16. Allow as much movement as possible.
17. Check that the resident can breathe easily and circulation is not impaired.
18. Check that restraint is not too tight by putting your fingers between the restraint and the resident.
19. Place the call signal within the resident's reach.

I. When a resident is restrained:

1. Visually check the resident's safety every 30 minutes.
2. Check wrist restraints every 15 minutes for signs of circulation problems, which include:
   a. cold, pale, or bluish skin
   b. absence of a pulse
   c. complaint of pain
   d. numbness
   e. tingling
   f. chafing or indentation of skin
3. Remove the restraint every 2 hours; provide exercise, skin care, toileting, and reposition.

Why?
—If a restraint is applied in any other way than according to the manufacturer's directions and a resident is injured, the staff and facility are liable, not the manufacturer.
—Padding bony prominences prevents the restraint from rubbing against or exerting pressure on the skin and causing bruising or pressure sores.

4. Observe for complications such as skin irritation, injury, circulatory impairment, increased anxiety.
5. Observe for comfort and body alignment.
6. Reassure the resident frequently.
7. Keep the call signal within reach.
8. Make sure the restraint is clean and undamaged.
9. Document the type of restraint used, the times of application and removal, the reason for application, the resident's skin condition, any complications, and the resident's response.

J. Restraint alternatives:
1. wedge or saddle cushion
2. self-releasing belt
3. chair and bed alarms

IV. FIRE SAFETY

A. Fire safety features in a facility include:
1. fire exits
2. closed stairwells
3. smoke detectors
4. sprinkler systems
5. automatic fire door closers

B. Elements of a fire are:
1. fuel
2. oxygen
3. a spark

C. Causes of fires include:
1. improper use of matches or cigarettes
2. defective electrical equipment
3. overloaded circuits and plugs that are not properly grounded
4. paper or cloth clutter
5. improper trash disposal
6. defects in heating systems
7. **spontaneous combustion**
8. cooking materials
9. flammable liquids
10. oxygen equipment

Spontaneous combustion— ignition of burnable materials caused by a chemical reaction

D. To prevent fires:
1. Dispose of waste material correctly.
2. Store flammable liquids properly.
3. Check electrical equipment and report hazards.
4. Observe all rules for oxygen safety.

5. Obey "no smoking" signs.

6. Extinguish smoking materials carefully.

E. If a fire occurs:

1. Do not panic, run, or scream.

2. Reassure residents and visitors.

3. Use the RACE system:

    a. **R**emove residents from immediate vicinity.

    b. **A**ctivate the alarm.

    c. **C**ontain the fire and smoke by closing doors.

    d. **E**xtinguish a small fire.

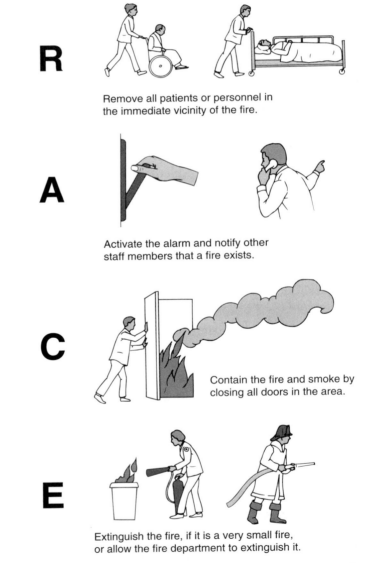

R Remove all patients or personnel in the immediate vicinity of the fire.

A Activate the alarm and notify other staff members that a fire exists.

C Contain the fire and smoke by closing all doors in the area.

E Extinguish the fire, if it is a very small fire, or allow the fire department to extinguish it.

Figure 7–2 The RACE system. (Source: From *The Long-Term Care Nursing Assistant* [2nd ed., p. 71], by P. Grubbs and B. Blasband, 2002, Upper Saddle River, NJ: Prentice Hall. Reprinted by permission.)

4. If there is smoke:
   a. Drop to your knees on the floor.
   b. Cover your mouth and nose.
   c. Crawl to the exit.
5. Use stairways instead of elevators.
6. If your clothing catches on fire,
   a. stop
   b. drop
   c. roll

F. To be prepared for a fire:

1. Know what types of fire extinguishers are available and how to use them.
2. Participate in facility fire drills.
3. Know the facility fire emergency plan.
4. Know the floor plan of the facility.
5. Know the exit routes.
6. Know the location of fire alarms and extinguishing devices.
7. Know how to report a fire.
8. Know how to use the fire extinguisher. Remember the PASS system:
   a. **P**ull the safety pin.
   b. **A**im toward the base of the fire.
   c. **S**queeze the trigger handle.
   d. **S**weep from side to side.
9. Keep fire exits clear of obstacles.

G. Use oxygen equipment safely:

1. Post "no smoking, oxygen in use" signs on the resident's door and at the bedside.
2. Check with the nurse before using electrical equipment around oxygen, including:
   a. electric razors
   b. fans
   c. radios
   d. TV sets
3. Never use flammable liquids near oxygen, including:
   a. alcohol
   b. nail polish remover
   c. paint thinner
4. Be certain oxygen cylinders are secured with a chain to prevent falling.
5. Use cotton blankets and clothing instead of wool or synthetic fabrics to reduce static electricity.

V. DISASTER PLANS

A. Disasters include:

1. floods
2. earthquakes
3. hurricanes
4. tornadoes
5. explosions
6. airplane or train crashes
7. riots

B. In a disaster:

1. Stay calm.
2. Remove residents from immediate danger.
3. Follow the directions of the nurse.
4. Help remove resident records and keep them safe.
5. Be supportive and help calm residents in the evacuation area.

DIRECTIONS A brief description of a resident is given followed by 10 questions related to the resident. Each question has four possible answers. Read each question and all answer choices carefully. Choose the best answer.

Mrs. Mary Fillmore is 81 years old. She has Alzheimer's disease and chronic obstructive pulmonary disease (COPD).

1. Mrs. Fillmore is confused and wanders. You must monitor her:
   A. as much as possible
   B. if she is more confused than usual
   C. when she gets near a door
   D. at all times

2. You assist Mrs. Fillmore to shower. The water temperature seems too hot. You should:
   A. leave Mrs. Fillmore and get maintenance to check the temperature
   B. ask Mrs. Fillmore if she minds the hot water
   C. regulate the water to a cooler temperature
   D. take Mrs. Fillmore to a different unit to shower

3. You wash Mrs. Fillmore's hair. You blow dry her hair:
   A. in her room
   B. in the shower room
   C. in the bathroom
   D. once a week

4. You bring Mrs. Fillmore her lunch. The soup is very hot. To cool it you should:
   A. blow on it to cool it
   B. stir it
   C. have Mrs. Fillmore test it with her finger to see if it is too hot
   D. feed her the soup last so it has time to cool

5. The nurse tells you to help Mrs. Fillmore into her wheelchair. To prevent an accident, you should:
   A. lock the brakes on the wheelchair before transferring her
   B. tell Mrs. Fillmore to help you or you may drop her
   C. place the wheelchair behind you so it is not in your way
   D. ask two other nursing assistants to help you lift her into the wheelchair

6. Mrs. Fillmore has a doctor's order for a lap restraint while she is in the wheelchair. Restraints should be applied:
   A. in the best way you think will keep the resident safe
   B. tightly so the resident cannot escape
   C. loosely so the resident is comfortable
   D. according to the manufacturer's directions

7. Mrs. Fillmore smokes. The nurse tells you to take her for a cigarette. You should:
   A. refuse because you do not smoke
   B. give her a cigarette, and check on her frequently
   C. take her to a smoking area and stay with her while she smokes
   D. ask other smoking residents to watch her so you can go get your work done

8. In the afternoon, you take Mrs. Fillmore outside for an activity. You should:

    A. be certain it is at least 80°F

    B. make her use an assistive device

    C. protect her from overexposure to sunlight

    D. ask her if she wants a cigarette

9. As you take Mrs. Fillmore back to her room, you notice that someone has left cleaning fluid on the counter at the nurse's station. You should:

    A. call housekeeping and tell them that their cleaning fluid is at the nurse's station

    B. tell the administrator that you found a problem

    C. put the cleaning fluid in a locked cabinet immediately

    D. take Mrs. Fillmore back to her room and then go back and remove the cleaning fluid

10. While walking past the laundry, you see smoke coming out of one of the machines. The first thing you should do is:

    A. activate the alarm

    B. extinguish the fire

    C. close the doors and windows

    D. remove residents from the immediate vicinity

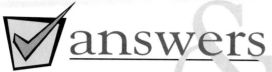

answers & rationales

1.

D. Residents who wander must be monitored at all times Confused residents are at greater risk for accidents.

2.

C. Prevent burns by checking the water temperature before assisting the residents in the shower. If the water seems too hot for the resident, regulate it to a cooler temperature. Report any problems to the nurse after you complete the care for the resident.

3.

A. Dry the resident's hair in the resident's room. Electrical equipment is only used away from water. Using electrical appliances near water may cause accidental electrocution.

4.

B. Stir hot foods to cool them. Blowing on food spreads pathogens. Having a resident test hot food with her finger may cause burns. The resident should be fed foods according to their preference.

5.

A. To prevent an accident, lock the brakes on a wheelchair before transferring the resident. If the brakes are not locked, the wheelchair could roll away when the resident touches it and cause a fall.

6.

D. Follow the manufacturer's guidelines when applying any type of restraint. If a resident in a restraint is injured because the restraint is not applied according to manufacturer's guidelines, the person who incorrectly applied the restraint may be liable.

7.

C. Supervise the resident. Many residents have a decreased awareness of pain and hot or cold; they may burn themselves before they react to a problem.

8.

C. Protect the resident from overexposure to sunlight. Older residents have more sensitive skin. Sunburn may occur quickly with older, thinning skin.

9.

C. If you notice an unsafe situation, handle it immediately. One of the nursing assistant's responsibilities is to keep residents safe. Toxic substances may cause injury, illness, or even death. Remove the substance and place it in a secure place away from residents. Then, report the situation to the nurse. All toxic substances must be kept in a locked cabinet.

10.

D. If you find a fire, first remove residents who are in immediate danger. Activate the alarm, contain the fire, and extinguish the fire if possible.

Emergencies

chapter outline

I. TYPES OF EMERGENCIES

A. If you are the first to discover an emergency:
1. Call for the nurse immediately and stay with the resident.
2. Stay calm and reassure the resident frequently.
3. Use standard precautions.
4. Follow the policies and procedures of the facility.
5. Do not do anything that you have not been trained to do.
6. Do not move an injured person.
7. Be sure the environment is safe.
8. Observe for life-threatening conditions:
   a. **cardiac arrest**
   b. **respiratory arrest**
   c. smoke inhalation
   d. electric shock
   e. **hemorrhage**
   f. stroke
   g. seizure
9. Monitor:
   a. consciousness
   b. pulse
   c. respirations
10. Observe for signs of **shock** due to drop in **blood pressure**:
    a. rapid pulse and respirations
    b. blue color of skin, lips, and nails
    c. cool, damp skin
    d. perspiration
    e. thirst
    f. dilated pupils
    g. nausea and vomiting

B. If the resident is in shock:
1. Call for help.
2. Keep resident calm.
3. Keep resident warm.
4. Keep resident lying flat.
5. Elevate resident's feet if there is no leg or head injury or breathing difficulties.
6. Turn resident on the side if he or she is vomiting or bleeding from the mouth.

C. If resident is hemorrhaging:
1. Call for help.
2. Put direct pressure on the wound with a sterile pad, clean dressing, or piece of cloth.

Why?
Moving an injured person may make the injury worse and cause further injuries.

Cardiac arrest—absence of heartbeats

Respiratory arrest—absence of breathing

Hemorrhage—severe bleeding

Shock—a condition that occurs when not enough blood is getting to vital parts of the body

Blood pressure—the force of the blood against the walls of a blood vessel

Why?
— Elevating the feet increases blood flow and volume to vital areas (brain, heart).
— Positioning the resident on the side prevents the resident from choking by allowing secretions to drain out of the mouth instead of down the throat.

Why?

— Applying pressure to the artery supplying blood will reduce flow of blood to the point of hemorrhage.

— Elevating a bleeding limb will reduce the amount of blood in the limb and slow hemorrhaging.

3. Follow standard precautions.
4. Do not remove the original dressing.
5. If hemorrhage continues, apply pressure with your fingers to the artery supplying blood to the area of injury.
6. Elevate a bleeding limb.
7. Keep the resident warm.

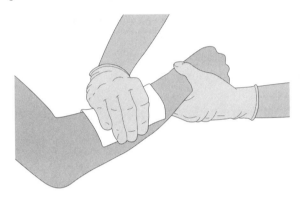

Figure 8–1 Apply direct pressure to stop hemorrhage. (Source: From *The Long-Term Care Nursing Assistant* [2nd ed., p. 83], by P. Grubbs and B. Blasband, 2000, Upper Saddle River, NJ: Prentice Hall. Reprinted by permission.)

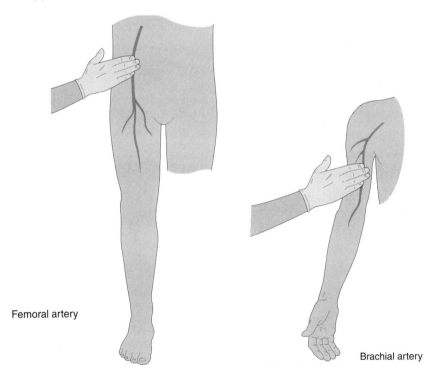

Femoral artery

Brachial artery

Figure 8–2 Pressure points may be used, in addition to the use of direct pressure, to stop hemorrhage. (Source: From *The Long-Term Care Nursing Assistant* [2nd ed., p. 84], by P. Grubbs and B. Blasband, 2000, Upper Saddle River, NJ: Prentice Hall. Reprinted by permission.)

D. If resident is having a seizure:

1. Call for help.
2. Loosen resident's clothing, especially around neck.
3. Remove objects that may cause injuries.
4. Do not restrain the resident.
5. Do not put anything in the resident's mouth.
6. Note length of seizure and body parts involved.
7. After the seizure, turn the resident onto his or her side.

E. If a resident falls:

1. Call for help.
2. Remove the object that caused the fall.
3. Do not move the resident.
4. Speak calmly to the resident.

F. If a resident is burned:

1. Call for help.
2. Observe for signs of shock, including:
   a. dilated pupils
   b. shallow, irregular, or labored respirations
   c. rapid, weak pulse
   d. cold, moist skin
   e. complaint of nausea and thirst
   f. restless or anxious behavior
3. Leave clothing in place if it is stuck to the burned area.

G. If a resident is poisoned:

1. Call for help.
2. Check mouth for signs of burns.
3. Check breath for odor.
4. Look for container.
5. Keep resident warm and comfortable.

II. EMERGENCY PREPARATION

A. Courses in first aid and CPR are offered through the:

1. American Red Cross
2. National Safety Council
3. American Heart Association

B. If a resident is choking:

1. Call for help.
2. Check if the resident:
   a. can breathe, talk, or cough
   b. is grabbing the throat with hands (universal sign for choking)

Seizure (convulsion)—sudden spasm of muscles caused by abnormal brain activity

Why?
— Loose clothing reduces chance of injury by strangulation.
— Turning the resident allows saliva to drain from the mouth and prevents choking.

Why?
— Inability to talk or cough identifies a blocked airway.

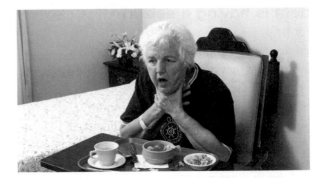

Figure 8–3   The universal sign of choking. (Source: From *The Long-Term Care Nursing Assistant* [2nd ed., p. 78], by P. Grubbs and B. Blasband, 2000, Upper Saddle River, NJ: Prentice Hall. Reprinted by permission.)

Cyanosis—blue or gray color of the skin, lips, and nail beds, indicating lack of oxygen

Unconscious—unaware of the surrounding environment and unable to respond to the spoken word

3. Check for complete or severe obstruction of airway:
   a. no air movement
   b. no chest movement
   c. no speech
   d. **cyanosis**
   e. weak cough
4. Begin the Heimlich maneuver if air exchange is absent:
   a. Stand behind the resident.
   b. Wrap your arms around the resident's waist.
   c. Place the thumb of your fist against the resident's abdomen an inch or two above the navel.
   d. Keep your fist away from the rib cage.
   e. Wrap your other hand around your fist.
   f. Squeeze inward and upward until the obstruction is cleared.
   g. If resident is **unconscious,** lower resident to the floor on his or her back.
   h. Tilt resident's head back and check the mouth for any visible objects.

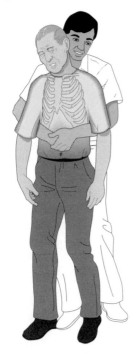

Figure 8–4   The Heimlich maneuver is the immediate first aid procedure to remove an airway obstruction. (Source: From *The Long-Term Care Nursing Assistant* [2nd ed., p. 79], by P. Grubbs and B. Blasband, 2000, Upper Saddle River, NJ: Prentice Hall. Reprinted by permission.)

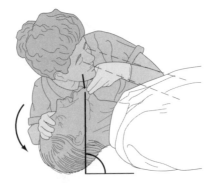

Figure 8–5   Use the head tilt/chin lift method to open the airway. Look, listen, and feel. (Source: From *The Long-Term Care Nursing Assistant* [2nd ed., p. 80], by P. Grubbs and B. Blasband, 2000, Upper Saddle River, NJ: Prentice Hall. Reprinted by permission.)

i. Perform finger sweep:
   • Open resident's mouth and hold lower jaw and tongue to keep the mouth open.
   • Put the forefinger of your other hand in mouth and sweep your finger from cheek to cheek.
   • Bend your finger and attempt to hook object in airway and pull it up into the mouth.
j. Straddle the resident.
k. Place the heel of one hand above the navel and the other hand on top of the first hand.

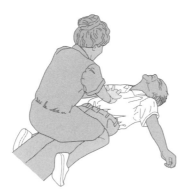

Figure 8–6 Place the heel of one hand on the abdomen slightly above the navel, at the midline. Place your other hand on top of the first hand and give up to five abdominal thrusts. (Source: From *The Long-Term Care Nursing Assistant* [2nd ed., p. 80], by P. Grubbs and B. Blasband, 2000, Upper Saddle River, NJ: Prentice Hall. Reprinted by permission.)

l. Keep your elbows straight and give three to five quick upward and inward thrusts.
m. Repeat the finger sweep followed by three to five thrusts until the airway is cleared or the nurse arrives.

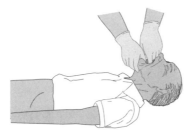

Figure 8–7 Perform a finger sweep and remove any objects. (Source: From *The Long-Term Care Nursing Assistant* [2nd ed., p. 80], by P. Grubbs and B. Blasband, 2000, Upper Saddle River, NJ: Prentice Hall. Reprinted by permission.)

n. Follow the supervising nurse's directions regarding resident care.
o. Assist nurse with documentation according to facility policy.
p. Check resident frequently for any signs of distress.

CPR—cardiopulmonary resuscitation, an emergency procedure used to reestablish effective circulation and respiration to prevent brain damage

C. See Procedure 8–1 in Appendix A.

D. If the resident is in cardiac and respiratory arrest:

1. Perform **CPR** only if you have been trained by a qualified instructor.
2. If the resident has a DNR (do not resuscitate) order, never perform CPR without the nurse's instruction.
3. The ABCs of CPR are:
   a. Airway—check it and keep the airway open.
   b. Breathing—get oxygen into the lungs by mouth-to-barrier breathing.
   c. Circulation—keep oxygenated blood circulating by performing chest compressions.

DIRECTIONS A brief description of a resident is given followed by 10 questions related to the resident. Each question has four possible answers. Read each question and all answer choices carefully. Choose the one best answer.

Mr. Thomas Hill is 81 years old. He is recovering from a stroke (cerebral vascular accident, or CVA).

1. Mr. Hill is eating in the dining room. He grabs his throat with his hands. You should:
   A. call for help and check if he can talk or cough; if he cannot, begin the Heimlich maneuver
   B. check his pulse and respirations; if they are absent, begin the Heimlich maneuver
   C. begin the Heimlich maneuver immediately and report to the nurse when Mr. Hill is feeling better
   D. loosen the clothing around Mr. Hill's neck and start CPR

2. When doing the Heimlich maneuver, you squeeze inward and upward:
   A. 15 times and then check Mr. Hill's pulse
   B. five times and then do a finger sweep
   C. gently to prevent injury
   D. until the obstruction is cleared

3. Later in the day, you find Mr. Hill on the floor next to his bed. He has fallen and is yelling. The first thing you do is:
   A. tell him to be quiet
   B. call for help
   C. help him up
   D. check if he is breathing

4. Mr. Hill has a deep cut on his forehead and is bleeding. You should put on gloves and:
   A. apply a tourniquet
   B. wrap a towel around his head

C. apply direct pressure with the palm of your hand
   D. lie him flat on his back

5. Mr. Hill has a seizure. You should call for help and:
   A. put a tongue blade in his mouth
   B. hold him down so he doesn't hurt herself
   C. remove his clothes so they don't restrict his movements
   D. remove objects that may injure him and loosen the clothes around his neck

6. After the seizure has stopped, you turn Mr. Hill onto his side to:
   A. prevent him choking on saliva or vomit
   B. keep him comfortable
   C. take pressure off the spinal cord
   D. check for incontinence

7. You report the seizure to the nurse when she arrives. She will want to know:
   A. if Mr. Hill said anything during the seizure
   B. the length of the seizure and the body parts involved
   C. what you did to cause the seizure
   D. if you needed to do CPR during the seizure

8. When responding to any emergency, you should:
   A. remain calm and do not move the resident
   B. yell at the resident to lie still

C. leave the resident and get help immediately

D. ask another resident to get help

9. The nurse tells you to call 911 (an outside emergency service). You should:

A. refuse because talking with other medical people is her job

B. ask a nurse from another unit to make the call

C. call 911 and calmly provide the information they need

D. tell another CNA to make the call because you need to stay with Mr. Hill

10. Mr. Hill has a DNR order. If he stops breathing, you will:

A. begin CPR

B. do the Heimlich maneuver

C. take no resuscitative measures

D. leave the room

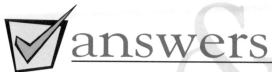

answers & rationales

1.

A. Grabbing the throat is the universal sign of choking. In emergency situations, immediately call for help. Check if the resident is able to talk or cough and if not, begin the Heimlich maneuver.

2.

D. The Heimlich maneuver is done to clear an obstructed airway. When doing the Heimlich maneuver, squeeze inward and upward until the obstruction is cleared.

3.

B. The first step the nursing assistant does in an emergency is call for help. In an emergency you want to have help as soon as possible. Stay with the resident. Do not move the resident until instructed by the nurse.

4.

C. If a resident is bleeding, call for help, put on gloves, and apply direct pressure over the wound with the palm of your hand. The most important action is to stop the bleeding.

5.

D. If a resident has a seizure, call for help immediately. Move furniture and equipment away from the resident and loosen any clothing around the neck.

6.

A. Turn the resident on his side after a seizure to reduce the risk of his choking on his own vomit or saliva.

7.

B. Report the seizure to the nurse. Observe the length of the seizure and the body parts involved. Use objective reporting skills and report everything you saw and heard.

8.

A. When responding to an emergency remain calm, provide reassurance, and not move the resident. Moving the resident may cause further injury.

9.

C. Follow the nurses instructions and call 911. Give the address of the facility, the phone number you are calling from, and a description of the emergency. Staying calm enables you to think more clearly.

10.

C. If a resident with a DNR order stops breathing, take no resucitative measures. A DNR order has been agreed upon by the resident and his doctors. It represents an informed decision and must be respected by the members of the health care team.

II

The Resident

9 Resident Rights

chapter outline

I. QUALITY OF LIFE

A. The Omnibus Budget Reconciliation Act (OBRA) is the federal law stating that long-term care facilities must provide care and services that either maintain or improve each resident's quality of life, health, and safety.

B. Quality of life includes everything that makes life worth living.

1. The individual is the best person to define his or her own quality of life.
2. The resident's quality of life is maintained when residents' rights are respected.

II. RESIDENTS' RIGHTS

A. Residents must be informed of their rights verbally and in writing in a language that they understand.

B. Residents' rights include the:

1. right to civil and religious liberties
   a. Encourage residents to vote in elections.
   b. Transport residents to religious services.
   c. Respect residents' religious beliefs.
   d. Treat residents' religious articles with respect.
   e. Learn the rules and rituals of different religions.
   f. Assist residents to social activities of their choice.
   g. Respect all residents and provide quality care without **discrimination** due to age, sex, religion, race, ethnic origin, or physical handicap.

2. right to file complaints without fear
   a. Assist residents to contact the appropriate person with complaints.
   b. Report residents' complaints to the nurse.
   c. Treat residents with respect and understanding.
   d. Maintain confidentiality by not discussing complaints with others.

3. right to be informed of their rights and the rules of the facility upon admission
   a. Review the facility bill of rights with new residents if directed by the nurse.
   b. Answer questions about rights.

4. right to inspect their records
   a. Report to the nurse if residents request to see their medical records.
   b. Follow the directions of the nurse while records are being viewed.

Discriminate—to show partiality or prejudice, to make distinctions in treatment

5. right to be informed of their medical condition and treatment and to take part in care planning
   a. Remind residents of care plan meetings.
   b. Transport residents to meetings.
6. right to refuse medical treatment
   a. Explain the importance of following the doctor's orders.
   b. Do not force medical treatments on residents.
   c. Never verbally abuse residents who refuse treatment.
   d. Encourage residents to attend care plan meetings.
7. right to information from agencies of inspection
   a. Give residents telephone numbers of agencies of inspection.
   b. Assist residents to contact agencies of inspection if requested.
   c. Get copy of inspection report for residents if requested.
8. right to be informed of responsibility for charges and services
9. right to manage their own financial affairs
10. right to receive appropriate health care
    a. Assist the nurse with medical procedures as instructed.
    b. Observe residents for physical or emotional changes and report your observations to the nurse.
    c. Offer residents choices whenever possible.
    d. Accurately take and document vital signs.
    e. Accurately measure intake, output, and weight.
    f. Encourage residents to participate in care.

> **Why?**
> Doctors and nurses make decisions about treatments and medications based on your measurements of the resident's vital signs and weight. If measurements are not accurate, the resident could be receiving incorrect care and medications.

11. right to be free from unnecessary physical restraints and drugs
    a. Use restraints only if ordered by the doctor and only to protect the resident from harm.
    b. Examples of restraints include:
       • vests, belts, mitts, and so on
       • side rails on the bed
       • geri-chairs
       • top sheets tucked under the sides of the mattress to keep the resident in bed
       • locked doors to keep residents in their rooms
       • certain medications
    c. Violation of this right is considered **false imprisonment.**
12. right to be free from physical, verbal, mental, or sexual abuse
    a. Physical abuse is causing injury to a person and includes:
       • false imprisonment
       • **battery** (hitting, pinching, twisting, grabbing, squeezing)
    b. Verbal abuse is yelling at or threatening a resident, including:
       • **slander**
       • **libel**
       • gossip

> **False imprisonment**—keeping or restraining a person without proper consent
>
> **Battery**—touching another person's body without permission
>
> **Slander**—making false statements that damage another person's reputation
>
> **Libel**—false statements made in writing

Assault—a threat to do bodily harm

Neglect—failure to provide the care that a nursing assistant should be reasonably expected to provide, which causes harm to a resident or the resident's property

Ombudsman—an impartial person who investigates complaints and acts as an advocate for residents and/or families

c. Mental abuse is causing residents to be afraid or feel bad about themselves and includes:
- belittling
- **assault**
- body language
- facial expression
- gestures
- **neglect**

d. Sexual abuse means causing another person to engage in unwanted sexual acts by force or threat.

e. *No one* may abuse, neglect, or mistreat a resident, whether facility staff, volunteers, family, friends, legal guardians, or other residents.

f. Report suspected abuse to the nurse immediately.

g. Report suspected abuse to an **ombudsman** if necessary.

h. Abandonment is the act of leaving, walking off the premises, deserting, or neglecting a resident.

i. Violations of residents' rights, including assault, battery, false imprisonment, negligence, theft, slander, or libel may be punishable by law.

13. right to personal privacy and confidentiality of information

a. Provide for privacy during procedures:
- Knock before entering the room.
- Shut the door.
- Close window curtains.
- Pull the bed drape.
- Keep the resident covered.
- Do not expose any more of the body than is necessary to perform the procedure.
- Never perform procedures in public areas, including the dining room, hallways, and any other common rooms.

b. Follow HIPAA regulations and do not discuss residents' medical information, behaviors, or conversations:
- in public areas of the facility such as hallways and common rooms
- with other residents, visitors, or families
- outside of the facility
- with other staff except the nurse

c. Keep medical records including charts and flowsheets secured and out of view.

d. Violation of this right is **invasion of privacy.**

14. right to be treated courteously, fairly, and with dignity

a. Address residents by their name and title (Mr. Jones, Mrs. Smith) unless requested by the resident to do otherwise.

Invasion of privacy—legal term used to describe circumstances when personal information is exposed publicly that violates an individual's right to privacy

   b. Speak to residents as adults.
   c. Do not use terms like "honey," "sweetie," and so on.
15. right to send and promptly receive mail that is unopened
   a. Bring mail unopened to the resident.
   b. If the resident has difficulty opening or reading mail, ask permission from the resident before you help.
   c. Keep all information confidential.
16. right to have private communication with any person of their choice
   a. Provide privacy for residents and visitors.
   b. Leave the room if the resident receives a phone call.
   c. Do not repeat any conversation you hear.
17. right to receive visitors at any reasonable hour
   a. Know the facility policies regarding visiting hours.
   b. Notify the nurse if visitors have special requests for visiting.
18. right to immediate access to family and friends
   a. Postpone routine care if the resident has visitors.
   b. Notify the resident immediately when visitors arrive.
19. right to choose a personal physician
20. right to have access to private use of a telephone
   a. Assist residents to use the phone.
   b. Leave the room if the resident has a phone call.
   c. Do not repeat any conversation you hear.
21. right to participate in social, religious, and group activities of their choice
   a. Let the resident choose the activity to attend.
   b. Assist the resident with grooming to improve self-esteem.
   c. Help residents to be on time for activities.
22. right to retain and use personal possessions and clothing as space permits
   a. Help residents place their possessions where they desire.
   b. Treat residents' property with care.
   c. Help mark resident's clothing according to facility policy.
   d. Assist with completing and updating inventory lists.
   e. Assist with investigations of lost, stolen, or damaged personal property.
   f. Observe and report any suspected theft to the nurse immediately.
   g. Violation of this right is **theft.**
23. right to equal care and practices regardless of source of payment
   a. Do not discuss residents' finances.
   b. Provide quality care for all residents.

Why?
Using generic names indicates lack of respect for and lack of interest in residents as individuals; for confused residents who depend on hearing their names as a form of reality orientation, using generic names can cause increased confusion and frustration.

Theft—the act of taking something from someone unlawfully; taking and removing personal property without the owner's consent

24. right to privacy during visits with a spouse and to share a room when a married couple resides in the same facility
   a. Knock before entering a room.
   b. Close the door if residents require privacy.

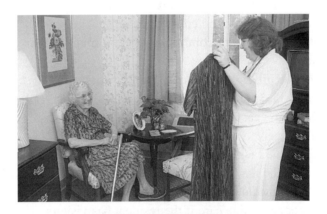

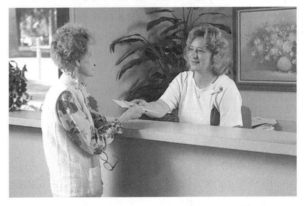

Figure 9–1 Residents' rights. (Source: From *Being a Long-Term Care Nursing Assistant* [5th ed., p. 10], by C. Will-Black and J. Eighmy, 2002, Upper Saddle River, NJ: Prentice Hall. Reprinted by permission.)

C. Protect yourself against legal actions.
1. Understand and protect residents' rights.
2. Use equipment according to manufacturer's guidelines only.
3. Document care you provide promptly and accurately.
4. Observe and report changes in a resident's condition promptly.
5. Ask for help when necessary.
6. Provide care according to the approved plan of care.
7. Give the resident choices.
8. Report any suspected abuse, neglect, or misappropriation of residents' belongings or funds.

III. ADVANCE DIRECTIVES

A. The Patient Self-Determination Act (PSDA) requires all health care facilities and agencies to notify residents of their right to consent to or refuse any medical treatment.

B. An advance directive protects the resident's right to make choices about care and treatment.

1. An advance directive is a legally binding document prepared when the resident has the ability to determine and express his or her wishes about care.
2. It takes effect when the resident is no longer able to state his or her wishes.
3. Facilities are required to provide advance directive information at admission.
4. Residents cannot be forced to prepare an advance directive if they do not choose to do so.
5. An advance directive may not be upheld in all states.
6. Types of advance directives include:
   a. *living will*—a document outlining the resident's wishes regarding prolonging life when terminally ill and indicating whether food or fluids are to be given or withheld
   b. *power of attorney for health care*—gives legal control of medical care decisions to another person chosen by the resident before the resident can no longer make decisions

C. A will is a written document that states how a person wants his or her property divided after death.

1. Notify the nurse if a resident wants to change a will.
2. If possible, do not witness the signing of a new will.
3. Never repeat information you may hear regarding a resident's will.

DIRECTIONS A brief description of a resident is given followed by 10 questions related to the resident. Each question has four possible answers. Read each question and all answer choices carefully. Choose the one best answer.

Mrs. Anna McDonald is a new resident. She is 89 years old, has Parkinson's disease, and is visually impaired.

1. Mrs. McDonald is unpacking her possessions. She has pictures, clothes, a table, a lamp, and a box of books. You should:
   A. decide what she can keep and ask her family to take the rest home
   B. treat her possessions with care and place them where she wants them
   C. tell her family to help because you have medical things to do
   D. tell Mrs. McDonald to select her three favorite things

2. You must take Mrs. McDonald's vital signs. Her roommate is in the room. You should:
   A. encourage the roommate to participate
   B. ask the roommate to leave
   C. pull the curtain between the beds
   D. do nothing since privacy only matters if you will be exposing her body

3. Mrs. McDonald's roommate asks you to help her to the bathroom. She is assigned to a different nursing assistant today. You should:
   A. help her to the bathroom as she requests
   B. tell her to call for her assigned nursing assistant
   C. ask Mrs. McDonald if you can help her roommate
   D. tell the nurse that the other nursing assistant did not do her job

4. Mrs. McDonald's son tells her that she is in the nursing home because she was such a bother for him. She puts her head down and does not look at him. This may be:
   A. physical abuse
   B. verbal abuse
   C. just a part of their relationship
   D. none of your business

5. Mrs. McDonald will only answer questions and does not talk with you. You notice bruises on both of her arms. You should:
   A. call the police and report the son
   B. demand that the son leave
   C. say nothing and wait to see if he tries to hurt her again
   D. report the possibility of abuse to the nurse immediately

6. The nurse comes to assess Mrs. McDonald. She has a chart with her and asks you to return it to the nurse's station. You should:
   A. tell the nurse that you are not allowed to touch the charts
   B. take the chart to the nurse's station and put it in the chart rack
   C. leave the chart in the hallway until you have time to take it to the nurse's station
   D. refuse to leave Mrs. McDonald until her son is out of the facility

7. In Mrs. McDonald's chart is a document that lists what care she wants at the end of her life. This is an example of:

A. an advance directive

B. a codicil to a will

C. alternative therapies

D. a planned death

8. You return to Mrs. McDonald's room to take her to the dining room for lunch. She says that she wants to eat in her room. You should:

A. reassure her that no one in the facility will ever hurt her and she is safe in the dining room

B. explain that she must eat in the dining room because it will meet her social needs

C. tell her that she must eat in the dining room or you will call her son

D. respect her right to make choices and report to the nurse

9. Mrs. McDonald lived in your neighborhood for years. Most of your family and friends know her. You should:

A. refuse to take care of her because you know her

B. tell your family and friends that her son was abusing her

C. answer their questions about her health and behavior

D. never discuss her personal information because it is unethical

10. If you tell your family, friends, and coworkers that Mrs. McDonald's son has been abusing her and an investigation proves that you are wrong, you are guilty of:

A. assault

B. defamation of character

C. libel

D. false imprisonment

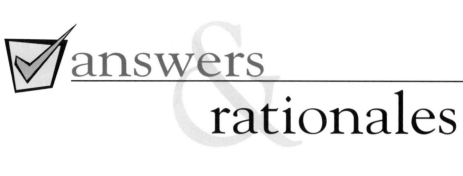

answers & rationales

1.

B. Treat residents' belongings with care and respect. Place the belongings where the resident wants them. Federal regulations guarantee the resident the right to retain and use personal possessions and clothing as space permits. The items the residents bring are usually very meaningful to them.

2.

C. Pull the curtain between the beds whenever you are performing personal care. A resident is guaranteed the right to personal privacy. By drawing the curtain, you have created a more comfortable setting for the resident.

3.

A. Assisting any resident in need whether or not you are assigned to that resident is an example of ethical behavior. A resident has the right to be assisted as soon as possible, and to be treated courteously, fairly, and with dignity.

4.

B. Verbal abuse includes threats, curses, or anything said that makes the resident feel bad or that lowers his or her self-esteem. All health care workers are responsible for ensuring that the resident is protected against abuse. If abuse is suspected, report to the nurse immediately.

5.

D. As a nursing assistant, you may be the first person to discover that a resident is being abused. The resident may appear to be afraid. Report suspected abuse to the nurse. It is your legal duty to report resident abuse. If you fail to report abuse, you are just as guilty as the abuser and can be held legally responsible.

6.

B. Return the chart to the nurse's station as the nurse requests. Put the chart in the chart rack or designated area that is not accessible to visitors. Information about residents must be kept confidential. All records should be handled carefully.

7.

A. The advance directive is a written document describing the individual's choices related to his or her medical treatment. It identifies someone to make treatment decisions for the resident if he or she is unable to do so.

8.

D. A resident has the right to make choices about his or her care and daily activities. If the resident wants to eat in her room, report the information to the nurse.

9.

D. Never discuss personal information about a resident with your family and friends. A resident has the right to confidentiality of information.

10.

B. Defamation of character means making false or damaging statements about another person, which injures his or her reputation. You may be legally liable for spreading false information about a person.

CHAPTER

10

Fostering Independence

chapter outline

I. INDEPENDENCE

Independence—being able to care for yourself and being in control of your life

A. Independence may mean something different to each resident, including being able to:

1. independently perform ADLs
2. make decisions about life

B. When the need for independence is not met, a resident may become:

1. angry
2. depressed
3. demanding

C. A holistic approach to resident care means:

1. meeting all of the resident's needs, including:
   a. physical needs
   b. psychological needs
   c. social and financial needs
   d. spiritual needs
2. encouraging residents to do as much as possible for themselves

D. The MDS is an assessment tool used to assess and identify residents' needs.

1. It is completed when the resident is admitted.
2. It is updated as the resident's needs change.
3. It includes observations made by the nursing assistant and reported to the nurse.

II. REHABILITATION

Rehabilitation—a type of health care that helps a resident regain the highest possible state of function

Impairment—a limitation caused by disease, injury, or a birth defect

Disability—a decrease in the ability to carry out daily activities

A. Rehabilitation may be needed by residents with:

1. an **impairment**
2. a **disability**

B. Rehabilitation:

1. promotes independence
2. focuses on how the resident can use his or her abilities
3. improves productivity
4. improves function and strength through therapy

C. The rehabilitation team includes all members of the health care team, including:

1. *physical therapist*—helps the resident strengthen muscles and regain physical independence by:
   a. evaluating and assisting the resident to regain muscle strength and **mobility**

Mobility—the ability to move

b. measuring, fitting, and teaching the resident to use a **prosthesis**

c. teaching the resident to use canes, crutches, braces, or walkers

Prosthesis—artificial body part

2. *occupational therapist*—helps the resident learn to independently perform activities of daily living, including:

a. changing position, reaching, holding, turning, or maintaining balance

b. relearning previous skills and developing new skills

c. functioning with limitations

d. using **adaptive equipment** to enhance function

Adaptive equipment (assistive devices, self-help devices)—equipment that is used to help the resident adjust to a disability and function as independently as possible

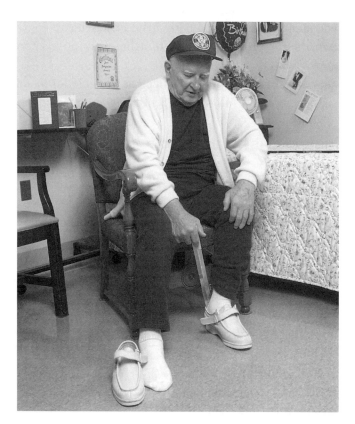

Figure 10–1   Encourage the use of adaptive equipment. (Source: From *The Long-Term Care Nursing Assistant* [2nd ed., p. 36], by P. Grubbs and B. Blasband, 2000, Upper Saddle River, NJ: Prentice Hall. Reprinted by permission.)

3. *speech therapist*—helps residents improve speech and communication by:

a. assessing and planning treatment of residents with speech impairments

b. evaluating swallowing disorders

c. treating residents with hearing losses

d. developing alternative methods of communication for residents who are aphasic

4. *social worker*—helps the resident and the family accept and adjust to life changes by:
   a. helping them identify and cope with their feelings
   b. addressing financial needs
   c. providing information about community resources
5. *activity director*—plans and implements programs to foster socialization and improve self-esteem by:
   a. offering daily activities and special events
   b. identifying activities that will be of interest to residents
   c. encouraging residents to participate in activities
6. *nursing staff*—provide direct care using restorative approaches that:
   a. encourage residents to do as much as possible for themselves
   b. support residents' efforts by identifying and praising all accomplishments

D. The nursing assistant's role in rehabilitation includes:

1. helping the resident with exercises
2. maintaining a safe environment
3. offering psychological support
4. observing and reporting the resident's progress
5. listening to the resident
6. maintaining a positive attitude
7. encouraging the resident to be independent
8. **motivating** the resident to achieve the highest possible level of function

Motivation—reason, desire, need, or purpose that causes a person to do something

E. The nursing assistant should observe and report:

1. signs of pain:
   a. crying, yelling, moaning
   b. facial expression including grimacing
   c. withdrawing from touch
   d. stiffening or tensing up
   e. loss of appetite
   f. fatigue
   g. withdrawal from social situations
   h. restlessness
2. signs of being tired:
   a. loss of interest
   b. refusal to participate
   c. lack of cooperation
   d. inability to face task
   e. yawning
3. signs of improvement

4. signs of depression, including:
   a. **pessimism**
   b. unhappiness
   c. feelings of hopelessness
   d. low self-esteem
   e. withdrawal or isolation
   f. **apathy**
   g. loss of appetite or excessive appetite
   h. constant fatigue
   i. excessive irritability
   j. recurring thoughts of suicide or death

Pessimism—a tendency to see or anticipate the worst

Apathy—loss of interest

III. RESTORATIVE CARE

A. Principles of restorative care include:
1. Treat the whole person by:
   a. being aware of cultural differences
   b. respecting spirituality
   c. approaching each resident as an individual
   d. identifying and meeting all needs
2. Assist rehabilitation to:
   a. prevent **complications**
   b. improve resident's self-esteem
   c. prevent depression
3. Stress ability, not disability, because most residents:
   a. will respond to a positive attitude
   b. will try to meet your expectations
4. Encourage physical and social activity to:
   a. strengthen the mind and body
   b. improve circulation, digestion, elimination, and mobility
   c. prevent complications
   d. increase mental **acuity**
   e. prevent depression

Restorative care—the care that is given to assist the resident to maintain the highest level of function and independence

Complication—an additional problem that results from disease or other condition

Acuity—sharpness, keenness of perception

B. To promote restorative care, the health care team works to:
1. set realistic goals with each resident
2. prevent complications from inactivity
3. increase residents' mobility
4. help residents improve levels of independence and self-care abilities

C. Guidelines for restorative care include:
1. Understand the resident's abilities and disabilities.
2. Be aware of the resident's fears.

3. Encourage the use of adaptive equipment.
4. Encourage the resident to make decisions.
5. Foster family involvement in the resident's care.
6. Keep directions simple—one step at a time.
7. Be consistent and do procedures the same way every time.
8. Arrange furniture and belongings for the resident's convenience.
9. Allow the resident to be independent, giving as little assistance as possible.
10. Be patient and don't rush the resident.
11. Allow the resident to try, but don't allow him or her to become frustrated.
12. Watch for signs of fatigue.
13. Never scold or humiliate the resident.
14. Praise even small accomplishments.
15. Approach the resident with empathy.

IV. RESTORATIVE PROGRAMS

A. Restorative programs help residents who have difficulty performing activities of daily living.

B. Personal hygiene and grooming programs:

1. help residents perform hygiene and grooming skills independently
2. improve residents' well-being, quality of life, and self-esteem
   a. Encourage residents to select their own clothing and dress themselves if possible.
      - Provide privacy.
      - Dress the weak part of the body first.
      - Undress the weak part of the body last.
   b. Encourage residents to use a mirror after dressing.
   c. Use adaptive equipment to promote independence, including:
      - electric or suction toothbrushes
      - long-handled combs, brushes, and sponges
      - long-handled shoehorns
      - buttonhooks
      - sock pullers
      - zipper pullers

C. Restorative dining programs:

1. help residents who have difficulty feeding themselves
2. make eating more enjoyable for residents
3. use adaptive equipment to promote independence

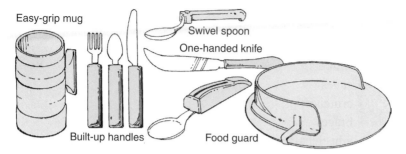

Figure 10–2 Assistive eating devices include: mugs designed for easy gripping, silverware with built-up or curved handles, and plates with a food guard attached so patients can push food against it. (Source: From *The Nursing Assistant* [3rd ed., p. 284], by J. Pulliam, 2002, Upper Saddle River, NJ: Prentice Hall. Reprinted by permission.)

D. Ambulation programs:

Ambulate—to walk

1. help residents maintain mobility and independence
2. The goal is to increase or maintain the resident's ability to walk.
   a. Have the resident walk with as little assistance as possible.

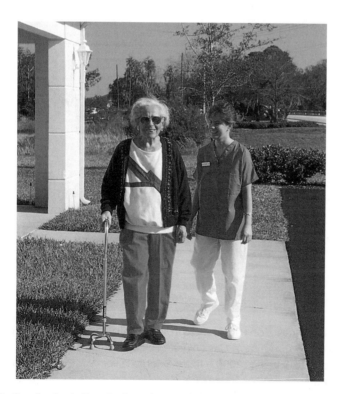

Figure 10–3 Ambulation helps the resident to maintain independence. (Source: From *The Long-Term Care Nursing Assistant* [2nd ed., p. 38], by P. Grubbs and B. Blasband, 2000, Upper Saddle River, NJ: Prentice Hall. Reprinted by permission.)

b. Use adaptive equipment, including:
- walkers
- canes
- crutches
- braces
- wheelchairs
- prostheses
- **orthotics**

Orthotic—an appliance used to support, align, prevent, or correct deformities

Why?
Residents who lose control of bowel and bladder may develop physical, emotional, and social problems.

E. Bowel and bladder programs:
1. help residents regain control of bowel and bladder functions
2. help residents to follow the program consistently
3. offer positive reinforcement for success

F. Range of motion exercise programs:
1. help residents with limited mobility
2. benefit all body systems
3. keep residents more alert
4. promote a positive attitude
5. help reduce stress

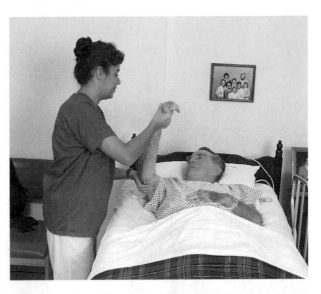

Figure 10–4 Range-of-motion exercises help to prevent complications. (Source: From *The Long-Term Care Nursing Assistant* [2nd ed., p. 38], by P. Grubbs and B. Blasband, 2000, Upper Saddle River, NJ: Prentice Hall. Reprinted by permission.)

6. improve appetite
7. improve sleep patterns
8. maintain muscle strength
9. prevent joints from stiffening

G. Promote wellness for all residents.

1. Restorative measures that increase self-esteem and independence also increase wellness.

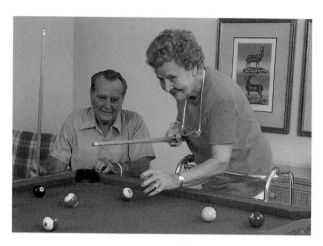

Figure 10–5   Wellness is living life to the fullest. (Source: From *The Long-Term Care Nursing Assistant* [2nd ed., p. 38], by P. Grubbs and B. Blasband, 2000, Upper Saddle River, NJ: Prentice Hall. Reprinted by permission.)

2. Help the resident to attain wellness by:
   a. learning the warning signs of disease
   b. ensuring personal hygiene
   c. using safety measures
   d. following infection control policies
   e. assisting with nutrition and fluids
   f. encouraging rest, relaxation, and sleep
   g. providing continuity of care

DIRECTIONS

A brief description of a resident is given followed by 10 questions related to the resident. Each question has four possible answers. Read each question and all answer choices carefully. Choose the one best answer.

Mr. Felipe Cruz is 68 years old. He is diabetic, has had his left leg amputated, and is in the facility for rehabilitation.

1. The goal of Mr. Cruz's rehabilitation program is to help him:
   A. become healthy and strong
   B. regain the highest possible state of function
   C. become just as independent as he was before the surgery
   D. accept his limitations and live a less productive life

2. Mr. Cruz has a prosthesis to help him walk, which is:
   A. a cane
   B. an artificial leg
   C. a walker
   D. a brace

3. Other types of prostheses include:
   A. canes and crutches
   B. walkers and wheelchairs
   C. braces, elastic stockings, and ace bandages
   D. a glass eye, dentures, or artificial breast

4. Because Mr. Cruz has a prosthesis, you should take special care of his:
   A. skin, especially the bony areas
   B. hands, which may become calloused
   C. joints by doing frequent range of motion exercises to improve his strength
   D. gums, which may be irritated when eating

5. You help create a restorative environment for Mr. Cruz by:
   A. doing everything for him
   B. pushing him past his ability
   C. keeping his bed lowered with the wheels locked
   D. putting his possessions just beyond his reach

6. Mr. Cruz uses a walker to help him:
   A. walk more quickly
   B. improve balance and support while walking
   C. transfer from the bed to the chair
   D. with range of motion

7. You watch Mr. Cruz struggle to walk. You understand that:
   A. his ability to function will decline without repetition and practice
   B. you should stop him because he may get hurt
   C. he should be walking with the physical therapist only
   D. his family should be there to help him

8. Mr. Cruz uses a long-handled shoehorn to help him dress, which is considered to be:
   A. a prosthetic device
   B. an orthotic device
   C. an unnecessary device
   D. a self-help or assistive device

9. You help to motivate Mr. Cruz during rehabilitation by:
   A. rewarding him with presents
   B. giving him frequent encouragement and praise
   C. constantly telling him that he could be doing better if he just tried harder
   D. refusing to take him to his favorite activity unless he does more for himself

10. As a member of the health care team, your role in Mr. Cruz's rehabilitation includes:
    A. observing and reporting his condition and progress to the nurse
    B. deciding how much he should do for himself
    C. feeling sorry for him when he struggles
    D. telling him what he must be able to do if he wants to go home

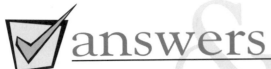

answers

& rationales

1.

B. Rehabilitation programs are individually designed to help the resident regain the highest possible state of function.

2.

B. A prosthesis is any device that replaces a missing body part. An artificial leg is a prosthesis.

3.

D. Dentures, an artificial breast, and a glass eye replace missing body parts and are prostheses.

4.

A. Take special care of skin that comes into contact with a prosthesis. The skin can become irritated, dried, and cracked, which will cause pain and possible infection.

5.

C. The nursing assistant helps create a restorative environment by keeping the bed close to the floor with the wheels locked, which helps the resident safely get in and out of bed independently.

6.

B. To assist the resident to walk safely, walkers provide balance and support.

7.

A. Repetition and practice improve the resident's ability to function. Residents should be encouraged to do as much as possible independently.

8.

D. Assistive devices help residents perform an activity more easily, efficiently, and independently. A long-handled shoehorn is an example of an assistive device.

9.

B. The nursing assistant can help motivate residents during rehabilitation by offering frequent encouragement and praise.

10.

A. Part of the role of the nursing assistant in rehabilitation is to assist the nurse by observing and reporting the condition and progress of the resident. Information provided by the nursing assistant is shared with the healthcare team. The resident's healthcare plan may be altered to reflect the changed needs of the resident based on the observations reported by the nursing assistant.

11 The Residents Family

chapter outline

I. ROLE OF THE FAMILY

A. The resident's well-being is improved when he or she has the support and love of family members.

B. A positive relationship between facility staff and family benefits the resident.

1. When the resident is admitted:
   a. Answer questions as completely as possible or refer them to the nurse.
   b. Be courteous if you need to ask family members to leave during the admission procedure.
   c. Explain procedures such as:
      • visiting hours
      • the resident's routines
      • procedures for taking the resident off the unit
   d. Tour the facility with the resident and family.
   e. Introduce the resident and family to staff, roommates, and neighbors.
2. During admission, families may experience many feelings of:
   a. grief
   b. guilt
   c. relief
   d. worry
   e. nervousness
   f. sadness
   g. anger
3. If the resident has no relatives:
   a. Close friends may be as important as family to the resident.
   b. Treat close friends with respect and courtesy.

C. Encourage residents and families to participate in health care planning.

1. Listen to the family's suggestions about the resident's:
   a. care needs
   b. cultural needs
   c. food preferences
   d. favorite activities
2. Keep residents and families informed of the date, time, and location of health care planning meetings.

D. Family members may not be allowed to:

1. remove any facility property
2. bring food, beverages, or smoking materials to the resident without checking with the nurse
3. provide nursing services for the resident

E. Develop a trusting relationship with the resident's family and friends through communication.

1. The nursing assistant is the staff person who usually spends more time with the resident and the resident's family and friends.
2. To develop relationships:
   a. Let the family and visitors know that you care.
   b. Develop trust.
   c. Listen if the family member is angry.
   d. Do not become defensive if you are criticized by family or visitors.
   e. Be pleasant, polite, and considerate.
   f. Be aware of your body language.
3. When communicating with visitors:
   a. Be helpful and friendly.
   b. Maintain confidentiality.
   c. Identify the visitor's anxieties and fears.
   d. Never argue with visitors.
   e. Listen to what is being said.
   f. Be courteous and have empathy.
   g. Treat visitors as guests.
   h. Refer questions about medications or treatments to the nurse.
   i. Ask if you can help.

Why?
Listening can help the person who is angry because expressing negative feelings in words helps the person work through the feelings.

F. A visit from family or friends meets the resident's social needs.

1. Visits from family and friends can:
   a. relax the resident's tensions
   b. ease the resident's feelings of loneliness and isolation
   c. reduce the resident's fears
2. Prepare residents for visits by:
   a. helping the resident dress and groom
   b. reminding confused residents of the visit
   c. reminding residents with memory loss of family members' names
   d. bringing extra chairs into the room
3. Encourage families to visit by:
   a. greeting family members and visitors warmly and courteously
   b. encouraging residents to describe what they have been doing
   c. trying not to interrupt the visit with routine care procedures
4. Report to the nurse if:
   a. the resident becomes anxious, upset, or tired during a visit
   b. visitors or family members tell you anything about the resident that may improve the resident's care
   c. visitors or family members make suggestions, complain, or comment about the resident or the facility

Why?
Surprises for a confused resident can be very upsetting. By reminding the resident of a scheduled visit, you will lessen the confusion.

5. Let family members and visitors know that you share their concern for the resident.

G. Avoid involvement in family disagreements.

1. Listen to the visitor or family member.
2. Don't take sides in quarrels.
3. Do not give confidential information about the resident to family or visitors.
4. Never discuss family members or visitors with anyone.
5. Do not become involved in family matters.

H. It is normal for family members or visitors to be worried and upset about the resident.

1. Families and visitors may have feelings of:
   a. helplessness
   b. anger
   c. guilt
2. Treat family members and visitors with empathy by being:
   a. patient
   b. courteous
   c. professional
3. If family members or visitors become verbally abusive or interfere with your work:
   a. Do not confront them.
   b. Do not become defensive.
   c. Be kind and concerned.

II. CULTURAL DIFFERENCES

A. Accept the differences between all residents.

1. Learn about other cultures.
2. Communicate with the resident and try to learn about cultural differences.
3. If communicating with a person who speaks English as a second language:
   a. Ask the person to repeat anything you do not understand.
   b. Choose words that can be clearly understood.
   c. Rephrase what you are saying if the person does not understand you.

B. Culture affects beliefs and customs about:

1. food
2. clothing
3. relationships
4. religion
5. health practices and health care
6. aging and the elderly
7. pain
8. death and dying

C. In many cultures, the family is the most important social group.

1. The extended family may be the center of concern.
2. The whole family may be involved with decision making.
3. Gender roles may differ.
4. Culture may be male or female oriented.

III. SPECIAL NEEDS OF FAMILIES OF DYING RESIDENTS

A. The family and the dying resident need time to:

1. share memories
2. discuss the future
3. make apologies
4. say goodbye

B. Anything you do for the family helps the resident.

1. Family members of a dying resident:
   a. may remain with the resident at all times
   b. usually do not want answers or advice, but want you to listen
   c. may be tired, sad, or tearful
2. To help the family, you should:
   a. Give support and be understanding.
   b. Show that you are concerned about them.
   c. Be available, courteous, and considerate.

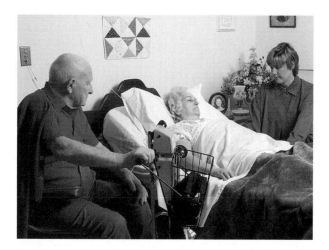

Figure 11–1   The presence of family and friends comforts the dying resident. (Source: From *The Long-Term Care Nursing Assistant* [2nd ed., p. 391], by P. Grubbs and B. Blasband, 2000, Upper Saddle River, NJ: Prentice Hall. Reprinted by permission.)

      d. Answer their questions but refer questions about the resident's condition to the nurse.

      e. Provide privacy for family visits.

C. Allow the family to be involved with the resident's care.

1. Make the family feel welcome.
2. Involving the family in the resident's care increases self-esteem and reduces feelings of helplessness.

D. Never impose your own beliefs on the resident and family.

E. After the resident's death, focus on the grieving family or friends.

1. Be available for the family.
2. Support the family by listening.

DIRECTIONS

A brief description of a resident is given followed by 10 questions related to the resident. Each question has four possible answers. Read each question and all answer choices carefully. Choose the one best answer.

Mr. Marco Gomez is 82 years old. You are assisting with his admission. He has been transferred to the facility by ambulance from the hospital. He is recovering from a fractured hip. Several of his family members are with him.

1. When Mr. Gomez is being admitted part of your responsibility is to:
   A. orient both Mr. Gomez and his family to the unit and facility
   B. explain Mr. Gomez's medical problems to his family
   C. tell Mr. Gomez about his roommate's medical status
   D. help Mr. Gomez walk around his room so you can assess him

2. Mr. Gomez asks to use the urinal. You should:
   A. give him the urinal and keep him covered
   B. politely ask his family to leave the room
   C. tell his family that they must wait in the hall
   D. ask Mr. Gomez if he wants his family to stay while he uses the urinal

3. Mr. Gomez's wife tells you that no one can take care of him as well as she did when he was at home. You should:
   A. tell her that he will have better care now
   B. ask her why he broke his hip if she was giving such good care
   C. listen to her with empathy
   D. ask Mr. Gomez if he would rather go home

4. To help Mr. Gomez adjust to the facility, you should:
   A. be patient and warm with him and his family members
   B. tell his family to leave as soon as possible
   C. ask his family not to visit for the first two weeks
   D. invite his family to stay with him 24 hours a day

5. You explain to Mr. Gomez and his family that adjustment to the facility:
   A. will only occur if they leave him alone
   B. will involve good days and bad days
   C. depends on how supportive his family is
   D. should take no more than three days

6. Mr. Gomez's wife and children are arguing about his care. You should:
   A. tell them that it is none of their concern any longer
   B. inform them that Mr. Gomez can decide about his own care
   C. tell the children that their mother decides what is to be done
   D. avoid becoming involved in family arguments

7. When Mr. Gomez's family members suggest how you should take care of him, you should:
   A. tell them that you know how to take care of him
   B. ask them to leave the room

C. listen to their suggestions

D. report them to the nurse

8. You want to establish a successful relationship with Mr. Gomez and his family. You should:

   A. tell them to be more like you

   B. teach them how to act around other residents

   C. point out the differences in cultures

   D. learn about their culture, beliefs, and customs

9. You use your knowledge of Mr. Gomez's culture to:

   A. increase your understanding of him and his family

B. judge him and his family

C. label them

D. make assumptions about them

10. You treat Mr. Gomez and his family as individuals. If you assume that every person from a culture is the same, you are:

    A. being realistic

    B. prejudiced

    C. stereotyping

    D. being judgmental

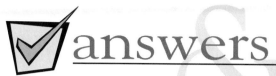

answers & rationales

1.

A. When admitting a new resident to the facility, part of the responsibility of the CNA is to orient the resident and family members to the unit and the facility. Introduce the resident to staff and other residents. Be professional and maintain confidentiality at all times.

2.

B. If the resident needs to use the urinal, preserve his right to privacy. Politely ask his visitors to leave the room. Be courteous and pleasant and tell the visitors that you will get them as soon as possible so they can continue their visit.

3.

C. Listen to what the family has to say and be empathetic. The family may experience feelings of nervousness, sadness, and anger when their loved one is being admitted to the facility. These feelings are common.

4.

A. To help a resident adjust to the facility, the CNA should be kind and patient with the resident and the family. During admission, the resident begins developing trust in the staff and the environment. Trust will minimize anxiety and fear.

5.

B. Be truthful and realistic when admitting a new resident. Explain that adjustment to the facility

takes time. The family should expect that the resident will have good days and bad days while getting used to the facility.

6.

D. If family members are arguing about the resident and his care, avoid becoming involved. The argument is not your concern and taking sides will result in offending someone. Leave the room if possible and report to the nurse.

7.

C. Always listen to suggestions from family members regarding care of the resident. Family members know the resident and the resident's preferences. When you listen, you help the family remain a part of the resident's care and you help the resident gain trust because you care about what he wants and likes.

8.

D. To establish a successful relationship with a resident and family of a different culture, ask questions and learn about that culture. Respect the resident's beliefs and customs.

9.

A. When you learn about, understand, and accept the resident's culture, you will better understand the resident, his family, and their needs. If you understand cultural differences you will be less likely to criticize, label, or judge the resident.

10.

C. If you assume that every person from a culture is the same, you are stereotyping. Treat each person as an individual. Being realistic means viewing things and people based on fact. Being prejudiced means being intolerant, disliking, or even hating persons of other races, creeds, religions, etc. just because they are different. Judgmental means assuming a person is or is not of value based on standards that you think are important.

12 Psychosocial Needs

chapter outline

Holistic care—providing for all of the resident's needs
Need—a requirement for survival

I. HOLISTIC CARE

A. Provide care for residents that meets all needs.

1. Physical needs must be met before any others. Physical needs include the need for:
   a. oxygen
   b. food
   c. water
   d. sleep
   e. sex
2. Psychosocial needs are met through interaction with others and include:
   a. emotional needs
   b. social needs
   c. spiritual needs

B. Quality of life depends on meeting all basic needs, including:

1. physical needs
2. safety and security needs
   a. feeling free from harm
   b. able to trust others
   c. able to trust the environment
3. love and belonging needs
   a. feeling like part of a group
   b. giving and receiving affection
   c. feeling connected with others
   d. having positive relationships
4. self-esteem needs
   a. feeling good about oneself
   b. feeling important and useful
   c. being needed by others
   d. being able to care for oneself

Self-actualization—the need to prove oneself

5. **self-actualization** needs
   a. accepting challenges
   b. meeting goals
   c. attaining spiritual fulfillment
   d. learning
   e. creating
   f. striving to achieve
   g. competing

C. All residents need:

1. to feel that they are loved
2. a sense of self-worth
3. a sense of achievement
4. recognition

II. MEETING CULTURAL, SPIRITUAL, AND RELIGIOUS NEEDS

A. To be comfortable with residents of different cultures, you should:

1. Learn about other cultures.
2. Identify your feelings.
3. Understand how your attitude affects residents.
4. Help residents feel accepted and comfortable.
5. Accept that cultural and religious beliefs affect attitude about health.
6. Observe for responses to pain that may be influenced by culture.
7. Develop methods of communicating with residents who speak a different language.
8. Note cultural differences in:
   a. body space requirements
   b. privacy issues
   c. family interactions
   d. levels of formality
9. Realize that hand gestures may have different meanings in different cultures.
10. Understand that you may seem strange to the resident.
11. Treat residents with empathy by understanding how you would feel if you were living in another culture.

Why?
A resident of a different culture who is comfortable in a facility has developed trust in the staff, confidence in medical treatment, and acceptance within the social structure. When comfortable, residents will be able to maintain independence and health.

B. Spirituality and religion have different meanings to different people.

1. When spiritual needs are met, the resident has:
   a. a sense of fulfillment
   b. joy
   c. emotional energy
2. Everyone expresses spirituality differently.
3. Respect all religious practices or the lack of religion.

III. MEETING PSYCHOSOCIAL NEEDS

A. Psychosocial changes affect the resident's needs.

1. Psychosocial changes that affect aging residents include:
   a. role changes
   b. retirement
   c. loss of income
   d. loss of spouse and friends
   e. loss of health
   f. loss of home
2. Emotional health is affected by psychosocial changes.

B. The ability to meet the resident's psychosocial needs is challenging because:

1. being in an unfamiliar environment increases the potential for unmet psychosocial needs
2. being separated from loved ones makes the resident feel unloved
3. being dependent on others affects self-esteem
4. sharing living quarters with many others makes it difficult to maintain privacy and individuality
5. moving a resident to a different room or changing roommates may cause disorientation

C. The nursing assistant should:

1. Help residents be independent and maintain or regain self-esteem.
2. Make residents feel safe and secure.
3. Be loving and caring.
4. Help residents accomplish their goals.
5. Report signs of unmet needs to the nurse.

D. Restorative methods used to meet the resident's psychosocial needs include:

1. helping residents regain independence
2. helping residents feel comfortable by addressing the residents' need for:

   a. safety and security
   - Follow safety rules.
   - Develop trusting relationships.
   - Keep your promises.
   - Show concern by communicating with and listening to the resident.
   - Help residents feel comfortable in their environment.
   - Speak well of other residents and staff.

   b. love and belonging
   - Care about the residents and their needs.
   - Take time to talk to the residents.
   - Encourage and praise the residents.
   - Listen attentively.
   - Use nonverbal skills, including a smile, a touch, or a hug.
   - Encourage residents to socialize with others.
   - Take residents to activities.
   - Clean residents' glasses and hearing aids.
   - Encourage residents to try new things.
   - Enjoy each resident's individuality.
   - Address residents by their proper name and title to show respect.
   - Ask the residents for their opinion.

Why?
— Carrying through with your promises increases the resident's ability to trust you, which increases the resident's sense of security.
— If you complain about the facility and other staff, the resident loses trust and may become fearful of others and the environment.

Why?
Cleaning the residents' glasses and hearing aids improves their sensory perception.

c. self-esteem
- Help residents with grooming.
- Give residents the opportunity to feel useful.
- Encourage independence.
- Treat residents as individuals.
- Recognize the residents' past and present accomplishments.
- Be positive.

d. self-actualization
- Help residents achieve goals such as walking, grooming, or eating without assistance.
- Encourage residents to participate in activities that they enjoy.
- Encourage residents to share memories.
- Foster spiritual expression and respect rituals, beliefs, and religious objects.
- Take residents to religious services if requested.
- Encourage residents to recognize purpose and direction in their life.

Why?
— Having a positive attitude helps residents feel good about the present and future. Negative or unkind reactions toward residents will lower their self-esteem.
— Sharing memories helps residents personally acknowledge and take pride in their past accomplishments.

IV. MEETING SPECIAL NEEDS

A. Sexuality is a part of the whole person.
1. Sexual fulfillment includes the need for:
   a. closeness
   b. love
   c. affection
2. Sexuality is an individual need.
3. Sexuality continues throughout life.
4. The need for a close relationship with another may increase with aging.
5. Staff who are uncomfortable with sexuality may create problems for residents.
   a. Manage your reactions to residents' behavior.
   b. Protect residents' privacy.
   c. Do not gossip about or judge residents.
   d. Accept residents as individuals.

B. Residents participating in rehabilitation programs need special encouragement to foster success.
1. Help residents to participate in and understand their care planning.
2. Help residents to participate in activities that provide sensory stimulation.
3. Encourage residents to socialize with family and friends.
4. Encourage residents to be accountable for their rehabilitation.
5. Protect residents' right to respect and dignity.
6. Help residents develop belief in their own ability to regain independence.

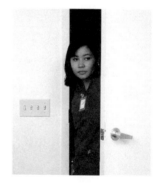

Figure 12–1 Consider the residents' right to privacy. (Source: From *Being a Long-Term Care Nursing Assistant* [5th ed., p. 391], by C. Will-Black and J. Eighmy, 2002, Upper Saddle River, NJ: Prentice Hall. Reprinted by permission.)

C. The resident in isolation precautions is removed from others and is more dependent on you for fulfillment of emotional needs.

1. Communicate with residents frequently.
2. Encourage residents to identify fears and concerns.
3. Observe for signs of depression.
4. Encourage self-care and independence.
5. Observe for signs of decreased self-esteem that may indicate feelings of:
   a. rejection
   b. fear
   c. feeling dirty
6. Encourage other staff members to visit residents.

D. Report to the nurse if the resident's behavior changes, including signs of:

1. depression
2. anger
   a. clenched fist
   b. clenched teeth
   c. loud speech
   d. rigid posture
3. withdrawal
   a. refusal to participate in activities
   b. lack of interest in relationships with others
   c. loss of appetite
   d. decreased desire to care for self

DIRECTIONS
A brief description of a resident is given followed by 10 questions related to the resident. Each question has four possible answers. Read each question and all answer choices carefully. Choose the one best answer.

Mr. Michael Wong is 88 years old. He has congestive heart failure (CHF) and arthritis.

1. Mr. Wong's friend tells you that Mr. Wong was a stubborn young man and is still stubborn. As people age, their personalities and behaviors:
   A. should change
   B. are consistent
   C. no longer matter
   D. must be controlled

2. Mr. Wong tells you that the things he was unable to accomplish in his life no longer bother him. Letting go of past disappointments and regrets:
   A. means that he is forgetful
   B. is a common developmental task for the elderly
   C. shows how the elderly lose their ability to function independently
   D. is a sign of weakness associated with aging

3. Because Mr. Wong no longer has the responsibility to provide for his family, he may have:
   A. low self-esteem
   B. improved self-esteem
   C. a feeling of independence
   D. a sense of relief

4. You help Mr. Wong feel that he has some control over his life by:
   A. giving him a choice between a morning or evening shower
   B. telling him which family member he should include at the care conference
   C. insisting that he attend Residents' Council
   D. giving him a copy of the state regulations and his rights as a resident

5. To help Mr. Wong improve his self-esteem, you can:
   A. encourage him to improve his independence with ADLs
   B. give him medications that make him feel better
   C. let him help provide care for his roommate
   D. tell him that he is the best resident in the facility

6. Mr. Wong is afraid to be alone. To help reassure him of his safety, you should:
   A. keep his door locked
   B. tell him not to worry because you are in control
   C. encourage him to be in a room with a lot of other residents
   D. listen to him and encourage him to discuss his concerns

7. A nonverbal way you show Mr. Wong that you care about him is by:
   A. answering questions quickly
   B. smiling and touch
   C. continuing to do your work while he is trying to talk with you
   D. saying, "OK," "sure," and "I agree" at the right times

8. Mr. Wong has no family that visits. To improve his sense of belonging, you should:
   A. tell him that you feel sorry for him
   B. keep him away from residents who have visitors
   C. encourage him to attend social group activities
   D. make other residents accept him into their group

9. You help Mr. Wong shave, put on aftershave lotion, and select clothing that looks good on him. A positive self-image enhances his:
   A. sexual identity

B. sense of security
C. ability to trust you
D. ability to recuperate

10. Mr. Wong tells you that he will die soon. He asks you to pray with him. You should:
    A. respect his wishes
    B. refuse and try to convert him to your faith
    C. tell him that he is healthy and will live a long time
    D. ask him why he thinks that he is going to die

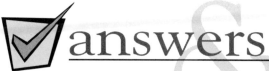

answers & rationales

1.
B. As a person ages, personality and tendency toward certain behaviors are consistent.

2.
B. Accepting things that cannot be changed and letting go of past disappointments and regrets is a common developmental task for the resident who is elderly. The resident can then begin focusing on the present.

3.
A. The resident may develop low self-esteem and a poor sense of self-worth if he feels that he has no important role to play and no responsibilities that make him feel important in other people's lives.

4.
A. You give control to residents when you give them choices. The more choices they make, the more they feel in control of their lives. Letting the resident choose when to take a shower gives the resident a sense of control.

5.
A. Encouraging the resident to be independent and to care for himself improves self-esteem. Self-esteem is a person's sense of his or her own worth and dignity (self-respect). The nursing assistant should encourage each resident to do as much as possible.

6.
D. Encourage residents to talk about their fears. Listen to the residents and develop a relationship based on caring and trust.

7.
B. To nonverbally show a resident that you care, smile, use touch, a hug, or a pat on the shoulder. Pay attention to the resident. Take time to listen.

8.
C. If a resident does not have family that visit, encourage the resident to attend social activities in the facility. Social programs help the resident maintain a sense of belonging.

9.
A. A positive self-image enhances the resident's sexual identity. Encourage and assist the resident with personal grooming. Compliment residents when they look good.

10.
A. Respect the resident's wishes whenever possible. Even if the resident is of a different faith, pray with the resident, if possible, and respect his or her beliefs. Do not impose your religious views on the resident.

The Environment

chapter outline

I. RESIDENT'S UNIT

A. Residents' rooms are their homes. You are the guest.

B. Maintain a restorative environment that encourages independence.

1. Keep furniture, equipment, and personal items in places that are:
   a. convenient for the resident
   b. safe for the resident
2. Provide lighting by:
   a. having switches or controls within the resident's reach
   b. using the type of lighting that best meets the need of the individual resident

Resident's unit—the room or area that contains the resident's furniture and belongings

Why?
Feeling safe and secure promotes independence.

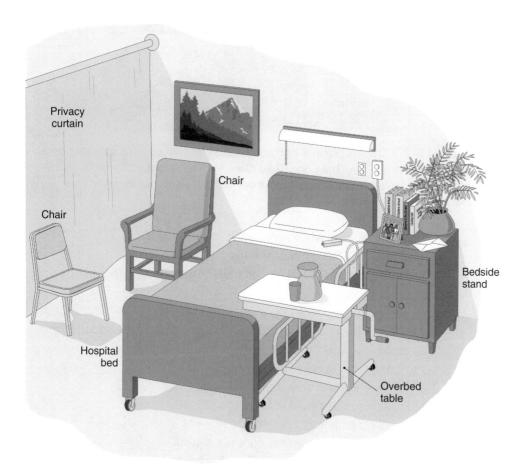

Figure 13–1   Furniture is provided in each unit to meet the resident's basic needs. (Source: From *The Long-Term Care Nursing Assistant* [2nd ed., p. 183], by P. Grubbs and B. Blasband, 2000, Upper Saddle River, NJ: Prentice Hall. Reprinted by permission.)

3. Provide for safety by:
   a. placing the call signal within the resident's reach on the unaffected side even if the resident is confused or comatose
   b. positioning the bed close to the floor so getting in and out is easy and safe
   c. locking the wheels on the bed
   d. checking the condition of emergency signal and safety bars in the bathroom

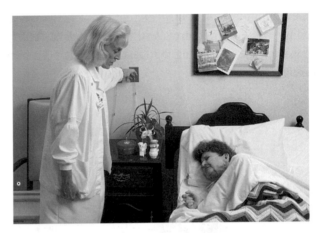

Figure 13–2 The call signal allows the resident to call for assistance as needed. (Source: From *The Long-Term Care Nursing Assistant* [2nd ed., p. 184], by P. Grubbs and B. Blasband, 2000, Upper Saddle River, NJ: Prentice Hall. Reprinted by permission.)

Why?
— Privacy increases feelings of self-worth.
— A closed door lets others know that the resident needs privacy.
— Keeping residents covered lets them know that you respect them and honor their dignity as human beings.
— A calm atmosphere promotes safety and security.

4. Maintain privacy when performing procedures by:
   a. closing window drapes or blinds
   b. pulling curtains between bed units if the resident does not have a private room
   c. closing the resident's door
   d. keeping the resident covered and exposing only the smallest area of the body necessary to perform a procedure
5. Provide a calm atmosphere by:
   a. keeping the area free from loud noise
   b. speaking in a normal tone, not loudly
   c. handling equipment quietly
   d. checking that equipment does not squeak
6. Control the climate to ensure that the resident is comfortable.
   a. Let the resident determine the room's temperature (it should be approximately 70°F).
   b. Older residents may require a higher room temperature.

    c. Open or close windows as the resident wishes.

    d. Remove wastes quickly to control odor.

7. Keep the room clean and neat.

    a. Remove meal trays, dishes, and crumbs to control pests.

    b. Use infection control procedures to prevent the spread of infection.

    c. Clean up spills immediately to maintain safety.

    d. Report problems with the environment to the nurse immediately.

Why?
Keeping the room clean helps keep the resident healthy and free from disease, which makes it easier for the resident to maintain independence.

8. Ensure that the room is comfortable and homelike.

    a. Encourage residents to display personal items.

    b. Handle residents' personal items carefully.

    c. Show interest in residents' personal items.

    d. Be sure residents have fresh water, cups, and straws if necessary.

    e. Keep personal items clean and in good condition.

    f. Put frequently used items within easy reach.

    g. Leave the resident's belongings where he or she wants them.

Why?
A homelike room increases a sense of belonging.

C. A restorative environment:

1. improves self-esteem, motivation, and independence

    a. The resident with high self-esteem feels motivated.

    b. Motivated residents strive for independence.

    c. Being independent improves self-esteem.

2. protects dignity and privacy

3. maintains the resident's individual identity

II. FURNITURE AND EQUIPMENT

A. Standard furniture and equipment found in the resident's room includes:

1. bed

    a. electric or manual (operated with a gatch)

    b. may have side rails to be used if the bed is elevated to working height, but requires a doctor's order if used to restrict the resident's movements

    c. with wheels that lock for safety

Why?
Side rails prevent the resident from falling off the bed when it is elevated to a working height.

2. overbed table

    a. has wheels and adjusts to various heights

    b. is considered a clean surface and used for meals, personal care and grooming, treatments, and procedures

    c. Do not place contaminated linens or equipment on the overbed table.

3. bedside stand
   a. used for storage of personal care equipment, including washbasin, bedpan, toothbrush, toothpaste, hairbrush, hearing aid, and eyeglasses
   b. a place for the resident to display personal mementos or pictures
4. call signal
   a. used to signal the need for assistance
   b. may activate light, bell, or intercom at nurse's station
   c. must be placed within the resident's reach on the unaffected side
   d. should be promptly answered
5. chairs for use by residents or visitors
6. bathrooms located in the room or between two rooms

Why?
A prompt response to call signals helps the resident trust that someone will come when help is needed.

Emesis—vomitus

B. Equipment in the resident's room includes:

1. **emesis** basin—kidney-shaped pan into which the resident spits or vomits

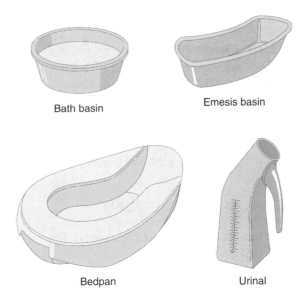

Bath basin

Emesis basin

Bedpan

Urinal

Figure 13–3 Examples of standard equipment that will be in the resident's unit. (Source: From *The Long-Term Care Nursing Assistant* [2nd ed., p. 184], by P. Grubbs and B. Blasband, 2000, Upper Saddle River, NJ: Prentice Hall. Reprinted by permission.)

2. *urinal*—container that male residents use when urinating
3. *bath basin*—larger basin used for bathing
4. *standard bedpan*—used for urination or defecation if resident is unable to go into the bathroom
5. *fracture pan*—type of bedpan with a flat end that keeps the hips in better alignment

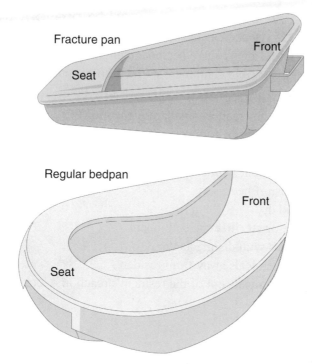

Figure 13–4 A fracture pan and a regular bedpan. (Source: From *The Long-Term Care Nursing Assistant* [2nd ed., p. 334], by P. Grubbs and B. Blasband, 2000, Upper Saddle River, NJ: Prentice Hall. Reprinted by permission.)

C. Special equipment in the resident's room may be used for:
1. oxygen administration
2. tube feedings
3. IV infusion

D. Personal assistive equipment includes:
1. *wheelchairs*—may belong to facility or individual
2. *canes, walkers, crutches*—usually belong to individual resident
3. Do not use one resident's personal equipment for another resident.

III. CARE AND USE OF EQUIPMENT

A. Use equipment correctly to prevent infection and injury to the resident and yourself.
1. Always follow manufacturers' instructions.
2. To prevent accidents, do not take shortcuts.
3. Ask the nurse if you have not been trained to use a piece of equipment.

Why?
Sharing equipment increases the risk of spreading infection, violates the residents' right to have their personal items for their own exclusive use, and shows disrespect for the residents' property.

B. Disposable equipment is used to prevent the spread of microorganisms.

1. Do not let residents share personal equipment.
2. Discard disposable equipment in the proper container.

C. Clean nondisposable equipment before reuse.

1. Wear gloves and follow standard precautions.
2. Rinse equipment in cold water first to remove body wastes, food, or other material.
3. Wash equipment with soap and hot water.
4. Use a brush if necessary.
5. Rinse and dry.
6. **Disinfect** or **sterilize** the equipment.
7. Be cautious with disinfectants:
   a. Keep chemicals away from residents.
   b. Store chemicals out of the resident's reach in a locked cabinet.

Why?
— Cleaning reduces the number of microorganisms on equipment and improves infection control.
— Hot water causes body wastes, food, or other material to become thick, hard, and difficult to remove.

Disinfect—use of chemicals to destroy most pathogens
Sterile—free of all microorganisms

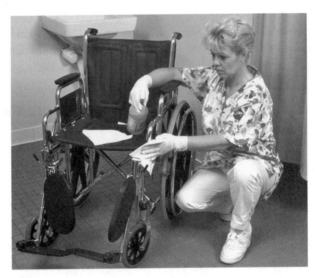

Figure 13–5 Disinfectants are used to destroy pathogens. (Source: From *The Long-Term Care Nursing Assistant* [2nd ed., p. 185], by P. Grubbs and B. Blasband, 2000, Upper Saddle River, NJ: Prentice Hall. Reprinted by permission.)

D. If equipment is defective or damaged:

1. Never attempt to use it.
2. Never attempt to fix it.
3. Report defects to the nurse immediately.

IV. BEDMAKING

A. Provide for safety when making a bed.

1. Use correct body mechanics:
   a. Raise the bed to a working height.
   b. Stand with your feet apart and your back straight.
   c. Bend at your knees, not waist.
   d. Avoid twisting motions by turning your whole body.
   e. Make one side of the bed before beginning the other to save time and energy.
2. Maintain proper body alignment for the resident:
   a. Help the resident feel more comfortable.
   b. Use pillows, pads, and other special equipment to support the body and prevent bony areas from rubbing together.
3. Protect the resident's skin and prevent **pressure sores:**
   a. Avoid anything that might cause pressure on the resident's skin.
   b. Keep linen free of wrinkles, small objects, or crumbs.
   c. Change a wet or dirty bed immediately.
   d. If protective pads are used, change them as soon as they are wet or dirty and do not use excessive padding.
   e. If a plastic sheet is used, be certain the plastic never touches the resident's skin by covering it with a cotton sheet.
4. Use furniture and equipment safely:
   a. Return the bed to its lowest position.
   b. Lock the wheels on the bed.
   c. Position gatch handles out of the way.
   d. Put the call signal within the resident's reach.

B. Follow standard precautions and rules of asepsis when making a bed.

1. Wash your hands:
   a. before you begin
   b. before handling clean linen
   c. after handling soiled linen
   d. before leaving the room
2. Use gloves if linen is contaminated with body fluids.
3. When handling clean linen:
   a. Place clean linen on the overbed table or another clean surface.
   b. Do not place clean linen on another resident's bed or furniture.
   c. Carry clean linen away from your uniform.
   d. Do not shake clean linen.
   e. Wash your hands before handling clean linen.
   f. Keep the clean-linen cart covered.
   g. Keep the clean-linen cart away from used-linen hampers, housekeeping carts, and trash containers.

Pressure sores (bed sores; decubitus ulcers)—breakdown of tissue that occurs when blood flow is interrupted

Why?
— Soiled linen against the resident's skin can cause skin rashes, breakdown, and eventually pressure sores.
— Excessive padding can cause pressure and skin irritation.
— Plastic on skin causes perspiration, does not allow the skin to breathe, and can result in skin irritation.
— Placing the bed in the lowest position with the wheels locked allows the resident to safely get into and out of bed independently.

Why?
Shaking clean linen will contaminate the linen with pathogens in the air.

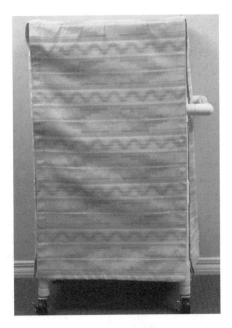

Figure 13–6 Keep the linen cart covered. (Source: From *The Long-Term Care Nursing Assistant* [2nd ed., p. 191], by P. Grubbs and B. Blasband, 2000, Upper Saddle River, NJ: Prentice Hall. Reprinted by permission.)

Why?
Unused linen in the resident's room is considered contaminated and must be placed in the used-linen hamper. It may not be used for another resident.

   h. Take only the linen you need into the room.

   i. Clean linen that touches the floor is contaminated and must be put into the used-linen hamper.

4. When handling dirty (used) linen:

   a. Wear gloves.

   b. Do not shake dirty linen.

   c. Hold dirty linen away from your uniform.

   d. Fold dirty linen away from you with the side that touched the resident on the inside.

   e. Never place dirty linen on the overbed table, bedside stand, or the floor.

   f. Use bags if provided or take dirty linen directly to the dirty linen hamper.

   g. Wash your hands after handling dirty linen.

   h. Keep the dirty linen hamper away from food and medicine carts and clean linen storage.

   i. Do not take hallway linen hampers into resident rooms.

   j. Keep linen hampers covered.

   k. Empty dirty linen hampers regularly.

C. When preparing to make a bed:

1. Collect linen in the order of use:
   a. mattress pad
   b. bottom sheet

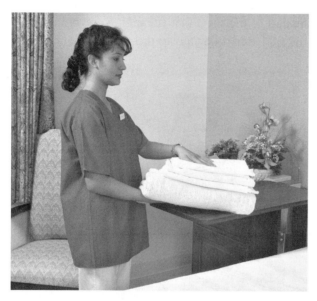

Figure 13–7 Stack the linen in the order that it will be used. (Source: From *The Long-Term Care Nursing Assistant* [2nd ed., p. 192], by P. Grubbs and B. Blasband, 2000, Upper Saddle River, NJ: Prentice Hall. Reprinted by permission.)

   c. draw sheet
   d. top sheet
   e. blanket
   f. bedspread
   g. pillowcase
2. Carry linen away from your uniform.
3. Place linen on a clean surface, turning the stack over so that it is in the order of use.

D. Remove (strip) dirty linen from unoccupied beds:

1. Check linen for personal items, including jewelry, glasses, or dentures.
2. Raise the bed to a working height.
3. Loosen the linen.
4. Roll the linen away from you with the side that touched the resident inside the roll.
5. Roll linen from head to foot of the bed (cleanest to dirtiest).
6. Immediately place dirty linen in a bag or dirty linen hamper.
7. If linen was soiled or wet, wipe the mattress with disinfectant before putting on the clean linen.

Stripping a bed—removing linen from the bed

8. Tell the nurse if the mattress is damaged.
9. Slide the mattress to the head of the bed.

E. To make a mitered corner:

1. Grasp the edge of the sheet 10–12 inches from the corner and place it on top of the mattress.
2. Tuck the part of the sheet that is hanging down under the mattress.
3. Bring the folded part down over the edge of the mattress.

Why?
The purpose of mitering corners is to keep the top linen on the bed, prevent the corners of the linen from becoming contaminated by touching the floor, and allow the top linen to be opened like an envelope so the resident can safely get into or out of the bed without his or her feet becoming tangled in the sheets.

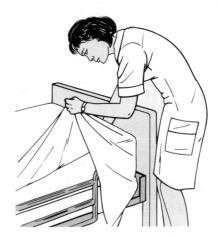

Figure 13–8 Miter the top corner. (Source: From *Being a Nursing Assistant* [9th ed., p. 216], by F. Wolgin, 2005, Upper Saddle River, NJ: Prentice Hall. Reprinted by permission.)

F. To make an unoccupied bed:

1. Strip the bed.
2. Put a mattress pad on the bed.
3. Place the bottom sheet on the bed.
   a. If a flat sheet is used:
      • Put the narrow hem at the bottom of the bed.
      • Tuck the sheet under the top of the mattress.
      • Make a mitered corner.
      • Tuck the sheet under the mattress along the side.
   b. If a fitted sheet is used, pull the fitted corners over the top and bottom of the mattress on one side.
4. If a draw sheet is used:
   a. Place it on top of the sheet about 12 inches from the top edge of the mattress.
   b. Tuck the draw sheet under the mattress on one side.
5. Place the top sheet on the center of the bed.
6. Unfold the sheet with as little movement as possible.

Why?
Place linen on the bed, never shake it, to prevent the spread of microorganisms into the air.

7. Center the top sheet so that the wide hem is even with the top of the mattress and the stitched or seamed side is up.
8. Place the blanket over the top sheet:
   a. The top edge of the blanket should be 6–8 inches below the top edge of the top sheet.
   b. Fold the top sheet down over the top of the blanket to make a cuff.
9. Tuck the bottom linen and the blanket under the foot of the bed, make a mitered corner, and make a toe pleat.
10. Move to the other side of the bed.
11. Unfold and secure clean bottom and top linen.
12. Place the pillow on the bed and put on the pillowcase:
    a. Grasp the clean pillowcase at the center of the seamed end.
    b. Turn the pillowcase back over that hand.

Why?
Toe pleats provide additional room for the resident's feet and prevent pressure on the toes that could cause skin breakdown.

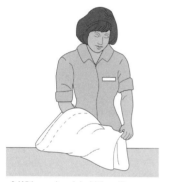

A With one hand, hold the pillowcase at the center of the seamed end.

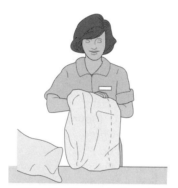

B Turn the pillowcase back over that hand with your free hand.

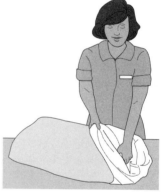

C Grasp the pillow at the center of one end with the hand that is inside the pillowcase.

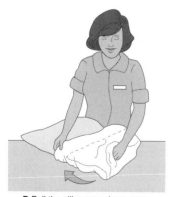

D Pull the pillowcase down over the pillow with your free hand.

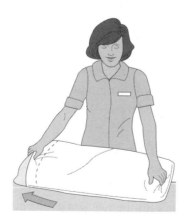

E Straighten the pillowcase.

Figure 13–9 The Nursing assistant is putting the pillow into the pillowcase. (Source: From *The Long-Term Care Nursing Assistant* [2nd ed., p. 198], by P. Grubbs and B. Blasband, 2000, Upper Saddle River, NJ: Prentice Hall. Reprinted by permission.)

c. Grasp the pillow at the center with the hand that is inside the pillowcase.

d. Pull the pillowcase down over the pillow with your free hand.

e. Line up the seams of the pillowcase with the edges of the pillow.

f. Make sure that the corners of the pillow are in the corners of the pillowcase.

g. Fold the extra material of the pillowcase under the pillow.

13. Place the pillow on the bed so that the open edge is facing away from the door.

14. For an **open bed:**

a. Fanfold the top linen toward the foot of the bed.

b. Be certain that the cuff edge is closest to the head of the bed so the resident who returns to the bed can easily get covered.

Open bed—a bed made with the linen turned down for residents who will return to bed after being up for a short while

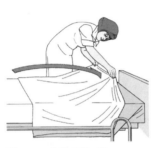

Figure 13–10 (Source: From *The Nursing Assistant* [3rd ed., p. 201], by J. Pulliam, 2002, Upper Saddle River, NJ: Prentice Hall. Reprinted by permission.)

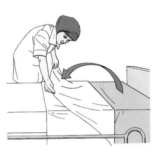

Figure 13–11 (Source: From *The Nursing Assistant* [3rd ed., p. 201], by J. Pulliam, 2002, Upper Saddle River, NJ: Prentice Hall. Reprinted by permission.)

Closed bed—a fully made bed with blanket and bedspread made for a resident who is up for the day or made when the bed will not be in use

15. For a **closed bed:**

a. Place the bedspread over the blanket and the pillow.

b. Tuck the bedspread along the lower edge of the pillow and along the top of the pillow.

16. See Procedure 13–1 in Appendix A for steps in making an unoccupied bed.

Occupied bed—a bed with the resident in it because of inability to get out of bed

G. To make an occupied bed:

1. Explain the procedure to the resident.

2. Place the clean linen in the order of use on a clean surface.

3. Provide for the resident's privacy by pulling the curtain around the bed, closing the door and window drapes.

Why?
Side rails protect the resident from falling when the bed is elevated.

4. Put up side rails, raise the bed to a working height, and lock the wheels.

5. Lower the head of the bed to a comfortable level for the resident.
6. Lower the side rail on the side of the bed nearest you.
7. Loosen the top linen at the foot of the bed.
8. Remove the blanket.
9. Drape the resident with a bath blanket:
   a. Unfold the bath blanket over the top sheet.
   b. Ask the resident to hold the top of the bath blanket or tuck the top edge under the resident's shoulders to keep it in place.
   c. Roll the sheet under the bath blanket to the foot of the bed and remove it.
10. Turn the resident away from you toward the side rail on the far side of the bed.
11. Loosen the bottom linen, roll it toward the resident, and tuck it under the resident's body.
12. Put the mattress pad on the bed.
13. Place the bottom sheet on the bed.
    a. If a flat sheet is used:
       • Put the narrow hem at the bottom of the bed.
       • Tuck the sheet under the top of the mattress.
       • Make a mitered corner.
       • Tuck the sheet under the mattress along the side.
    b. If a fitted sheet is used, pull the fitted corners over the top and bottom of the mattress on one side.
14. If a draw sheet is used, place it on top of the sheet about 12 inches from the top edge of the mattress and tuck it under the mattress on one side.
15. Fold the clean linen toward the resident next to the used linen.
16. Raise the side rail on the side near you.
17. Ask the resident to turn onto his or her back and adjust the pillow.
18. Move to the other side of the bed, lower the side rail, and help the resident to turn toward the side rail on the far side of the bed.
19. Loosen the used bottom linen.
20. Roll linen from the head to the foot of the bed, remove it, and place it with other used linen.
21. Unfold clean bottom linen from beneath the resident, tucking it under the mattress while pulling it snug.
22. Assist the resident into a comfortable position.
23. Put the top sheet over the bath blanket and unfold it with as little movement as possible.
24. Unfold the top sheet with the wide hem toward the head of the bed.
25. Place the blanket over the top sheet about 6–8 inches below the top edge of the top sheet and fold the top sheet down over it to form a cuff.

Why?
— Loosening the linen over the resident's feet provides extra room and prevents pressure on the toes.

26. Ask the resident to hold the top linen, roll the bath blanket from the head to the foot of the bed, and remove it.
27. Tuck the top linen under the bottom of the mattress and make mitered corners.
28. Raise the side rail.
29. Loosen the top linen over the resident's feet.
30. Put a clean case on the pillow:
    a. Grasp the clean pillowcase at the center of the seamed end.
    b. Turn the pillowcase back over that hand.
    c. Grasp the pillow at the center with the hand that is inside the pillowcase.
    d. Pull the pillowcase down over the pillow with your free hand.
    e. Line up the seams of the pillowcase with the edges of the pillow.
    f. Make sure that the corners of the pillow are in the corners of the pillowcase.
    g. Fold the extra material of the pillowcase under the pillow.
31. Place the pillow under the resident's head with the open edge facing away from the door.
32. Return the bed to its lowest position and lower the side rails.
33. Open the curtain, window drapes, and door.
34. Dispose of linen in the used linen hamper.
35. Be certain that the resident is comfortable, in proper body alignment, and has the call signal.
36. See Procedure 13–2 in Appendix A for steps in making an occupied bed.

Why?
— A doctor's order is needed to leave side rails up when procedures are finished and the bed is in its lowest position.

DIRECTIONS
A brief description of a resident is given followed by 10 questions related to the resident. Each question has four possible answers. Read each question and all answer choices carefully. Choose the one best answer.

Mrs. Sarah Cole is being admitted to the facility. She is 76 years old and has Alzheimer's disease and coronary artery disease.

1. Mrs. Cole's family is with her during her admission to the facility. Families often experience feelings of:
   A. hostility or frustration
   B. power or aggression
   C. panic or anxiety
   D. grief, guilt, or relief

2. The resident environment should look:
   A. clinical
   B. coordinated
   C. homelike
   D. modern

3. Mrs. Cole has brought several very expensive items with her. Her valuables should be:
   A. kept in a locked box in her room
   B. placed in the facility safe or sent home with relatives
   C. never taken out of the room
   D. hidden in the room

4. Upon admission, you complete a personal-effects inventory list for Mrs. Cole that includes:
   A. all of Mrs. Cole's belongings at the time of admission
   B. clothing and jewelry only
   C. furniture and bedding only
   D. all of her legal papers signed at the time of admission

5. The personal-effects inventory list is kept:
   A. in Mrs. Cole's health record
   B. in Mrs. Cole's dresser drawer
   C. at her daughter's home
   D. in the administrator's office

6. Mrs. Cole is right-handed. Her bedside stand and call signal should be:
   A. on her right side
   B. on her left side
   C. wherever the facility wants it
   D. where it will be convenient for you

7. Mrs. Cole is incontinent. When making her bed, you use a plastic sheet. You should:
   A. place it on top of the bedspread
   B. put it the full length of the mattress
   C. place it directly against her skin
   D. cover it completely with a cotton draw sheet

8. After you complete the procedure that you are doing for Mrs. Cole, you leave the bed at:
   A. its lowest horizontal position
   B. the highest position possible
   C. the height she desires
   D. the middle position

9. You place Mrs. Cole's pillow on the bed with:

    A. no pillowcase until bedtime
    B. the closed end of the pillowcase away from the door
    C. the open end of the pillowcase away from the door
    D. the pillow under the fitted sheet

10. To help Mrs. Cole feel comfortable in her room, she should be able to look around her room and:

    A. appreciate how well the facility has decorated it
    B. recognize familiar objects
    C. wish she were at home
    D. be grateful for having someplace to live

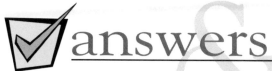# answers & rationales

1.

D. When a resident is first admitted to a facility, the family may experience many feelings, including grief, guilt, and relief.

2.

C. The resident's environment should be homelike. The resident's room should contain the resident's personal items, small pieces of furniture, pictures, and special mementos that are special to the resident. For many residents, the facility is their home.

3.

B. Residents and their families should be discouraged from bringing very valuable items to the facility. If the resident insists on keeping the items in the facility, they should be put into the facility safe.

4.

A. The resident's personal-effects inventory is completed upon admission and should include all belongings that were brought to the facility at the time of admission.

5.

A. The resident's completed personal-effects inventory list is put into the resident's health record (chart).

6.

A. The resident's bedside stand and call light should be placed for the convenience and ease of use of the resident. If the resident is right-handed, they should be placed on the right-hand side of the bed.

7.

D. When using a plastic draw sheet on the bed of an incontinent resident, cover it completely with a cotton draw sheet. The plastic should never touch the resident's skin because it can cause skin breakdown.

8.

A. After completing care for the resident, be certain that the bed is at its lowest height for the resident's safety.

9.

C. When making a bed, the pillow should be placed at the head of the bed with the open end of the pillowcase away from the door.

10.

B. The resident will feel most comfortable in the room if he or she recognizes familiar objects. A positive, restorative environment is familiar and homelike to the resident.

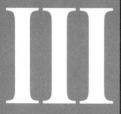

SECTION

III Body Structure and Function

14 The Human Body

chapter outline

I. ANATOMY AND PHYSIOLOGY

Anatomy—the study of body parts, how the body is made, and what it is made of

Physiology—the study of how the body functions, how all the body parts work independently and together

A. Basic anatomy and physiology help you understand:
1. how the body works
2. how and why illnesses occur
3. the impact of environment on health
4. the importance of performing procedures correctly
5. how to identify and accurately observe physical changes

B. Anatomical position shows the location of body parts.
1. In anatomical position the:
   a. body is standing, face forward
   b. arms are at sides with palms out
   c. right side is always on your left
2. Terms that describe the location of body parts include:
   a. *anterior*—toward the front
   b. *posterior*—toward the back
   c. *ventral*—on the abdominal side
   d. *dorsal*—on the back side
   e. *superior*—the upper portion (toward the head)
   f. *inferior*—the lower portion (toward the feet)
   g. *superficial*—on or near the surface
   h. *deep*—distant from the surface
3. Terms that describe posture include:
   a. *erect*—standing up

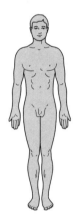

Figure 14–1 Anatomical position. (Source: From *Being a Long-Term Care Nursing Assistant* [5th ed., p. 136], by C. Will-Black and J. Eighmy, 2002, Upper Saddle River, NJ: Prentice Hall. Reprinted by permission.)

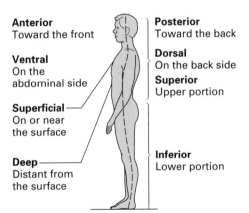

Anterior
Toward the front

Ventral
On the abdominal side

Superficial
On or near the surface

Deep
Distant from the surface

Posterior
Toward the back

Dorsal
On the back side

Superior
Upper portion

Inferior
Lower portion

Figure 14–2 Terms that describe where body parts are located.
(Source: From *Being a Long-Term Care Nursing Assistant* [5th ed., p. 136], by C. Will-Black and J. Eighmy, 2002, Upper Saddle River, NJ: Prentice Hall. Reprinted by permission.)

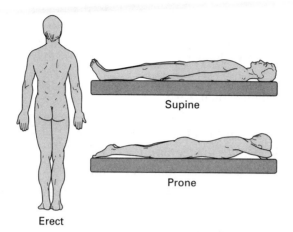

Figure 14–3 Terms that describe anatomical postures. (Source: From *Being a Long-Term Care Nursing Assistant* [5th ed., p. 136], by C. Will-Black and J. Eighmy, 2002, Upper Saddle River, NJ: Prentice Hall. Reprinted by permission.)

    b. *supine*—lying on the back

    c. *prone*—lying on the abdomen

II. COMPOSITION OF THE BODY

A. The cell is the building block of all living organisms.
1. Cells:
    a. use food for energy
    b. use oxygen to break down food and give off carbon dioxide

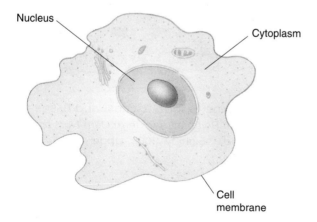

Figure 14–4 Structure of the cell. (Source: From *The Long-Term Care Nursing Assistant* [2nd ed., p. 128], by P. Grubbs and B. Blasband, 2000, Upper Saddle River, NJ: Prentice Hall. Reprinted by permission.)

       c. use water to transport substances

       d. grow and repair themselves

       e. reproduce by dividing

       f. die

    2. Cells have three main parts:

       a. *nucleus*—center of cell

       b. *cytoplasm*—material around the nucleus

       c. *cell membrane*—outer covering of the cell

    3. Groups of cells combine to form tissues.

B. Tissue is a group of similar cells that function alike.

    1. Types of tissue include

       a. *epithelial tissue*—protects, secrets, absorbs, and receives sensations

       b. *connective tissue*—holds other tissue together

       c. *muscle tissue*—makes body move by stretching and contracting

       d. *nerve tissue*—carries messages to and from the brain and regulates body functions

    2. Groups of tissues combine to form organs.

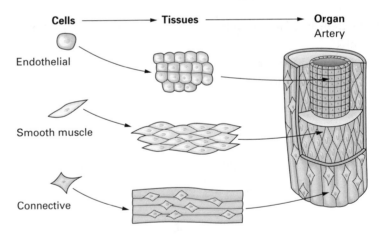

Figure 14–5 Cells combine to form tissues, and tissues combine to form organs. (Source: From *Being a Long-Term Care Nursing Assistant* [5th ed., p. 139], by C. Will-Black and J. Eighmy, 2002, Upper Saddle River, NJ: Prentice Hall. Reprinted by permission.)

C. An organ is made of several types of tissue that perform a certain function.

    1. Organs are usually located in body cavities.

    2. Groups of organs combine to form systems.

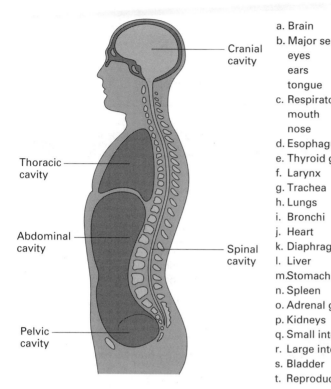

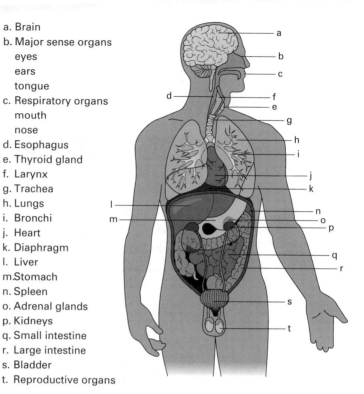

a. Brain
b. Major sense organs
   eyes
   ears
   tongue
c. Respiratory organs
   mouth
   nose
d. Esophagus
e. Thyroid gland
f. Larynx
g. Trachea
h. Lungs
i. Bronchi
j. Heart
k. Diaphragm
l. Liver
m. Stomach
n. Spleen
o. Adrenal glands
p. Kidneys
q. Small intestine
r. Large intestine
s. Bladder
t. Reproductive organs

Figure 14–6 Body cavities. (Source: From *Being a Long-Term Care Nursing Assistant* [5th ed., p. 139], by C. Will-Black and J. Eighmy, 2002, Upper Saddle River, NJ: Prentice Hall. Reprinted by permission.)

Figure 14–7 Location of important organs. (Source: From *Being a Long-Term Care Nursing Assistant* [5th ed., p. 139], by C. Will-Black and J. Eighmy, 2002, Upper Saddle River, NJ: Prentice Hall. Reprinted by permission.)

III. DISEASE

A. Disease is an abnormal change in an organ or system.

1. A sign is an indication of disease that is observed by others.
2. A symptom is an indication of disease that is felt by the individual.
3. Disease affects the body's **homeostasis.**

B. Disease may be

1. acute
   a. comes on suddenly
   b. is severe
   c. generally lasts a short time
2. chronic
   a. lasts over a period of time
   b. may recur often
3. genetic
   a. due to defective genes
   b. passed from one or both parents to a child

Homeostasis—the body's attempt to keep the internal environment in balance

C. A complication is an unexpected condition that makes a disease or illness worse.

D. The nursing assistant should:

1. observe residents closely for signs and symptoms of disease
2. immediately report to the nurse any observed signs or symptoms

GENERAL SIGNS AND SYMPTOMS OF DISEASE	
Complaints of weakness, dizziness, or headache.	Excessive thirst.
	Drowsiness.
Shortness of breath or rapid breathing.	Pus or unusual drainage.
Sweating, fever, or chills.	Urine with a dark color, strong odor, or blood or sediment in it.
Pain (complained of or observed).	
Nausea or vomiting.	Difficulty urinating; pain or burning or urinating.
Coughing.	
Blue color to the lips.	Urinating frequently in small amounts.

Figure 14–8   (Source: From *The Nursing Assistant* [3rd ed., p. 101], by J. Pulliam, 2002, Upper Saddle River, NJ: Prentice Hall. Reprinted by permission.)

DIRECTIONS

A brief description of a resident is given followed by 10 questions related to the resident. Each question has four possible answers. Read each question and all answer choices carefully. Choose the one best answer.

Mrs. Mary Gibson is 78 years old and recovering from a stroke. Earlier today she fell trying to get out of her chair. Since you were the first person to reach her, you will assist the nurse to fill out an incident report.

1. Most incident reports include a drawing of a human body:
   A. in color that includes all internal organs
   B. in anatomical position
   C. in Sims' position
   D. in prone position

2. When you entered Mrs. Gibson's room, she was lying on her back. You report to the nurse that she was:
   A. prone
   B. supine
   C. reclining
   D. erect

3. You noticed a bruise on Mrs. Gibson's shoulder blade. The injury is:
   A. dorsal
   B. ventral
   C. anterior
   D. inferior

4. Anatomically, Mrs. Gibson's shoulder blade is:
   A. superior to her feet
   B. inferior to her feet
   C. dorsal to her feet
   D. ventral to her feet

5. You discovered a superficial abrasion on Mrs. Gibson's elbow. An abrasion is:

A. on the surface of the body
B. deep into the body
C. not serious and should be ignored
D. serious and may cause her to hemorrhage

6. After falling, Mrs. Gibson's blood pressure is higher than usual. The injuries may have affected her body's:
   A. ability to produce blood
   B. homeostasis
   C. ability to heal properly
   D. core temperature

7. Mrs. Gibson tells you that she has pain in her arm and back. This is:
   A. subjective data
   B. irrelevant data
   C. assumed data
   D. objective data

8. The superficial abrasion, the bruise, and any other injuries you may have noted, are all:
   A. subjective data
   B. irrelevant data
   C. assumed data
   D. objective data

9. Mrs. Gibson just turned 78 years old yesterday. This is her:
   A. developmental age
   B. chronological age

C. approximate age

D. geriatric age

10. You go into Mrs. Gibson's room to ask her if she needs anything. She seems very angry and throws her book at you. You should:

A. pick up the book and throw it back at her

B. understand that she may be frustrated

C. inform her that she cannot treat you this way

D. tell her that no one will answer her call signal if she treats people this way

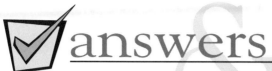
answers & rationales

1.

B. Most incident reports include a drawing of a human body in anatomical position, standing straight facing you, with palms out and feet together. This allows the person documenting the incident to mark the location of any injuries in a way that everyone will understand.

2.

B. If the resident is lying on her back, she is supine. Supine means lying flat on the back. Prone is lying on the abdomen. Lateral is lying on the side. Erect is standing upright.

3.

A. If a bruise is on the resident's shoulder blade it is dorsal, on the backside of the body. Ventral is on the abdominal side of the body. Anterior is toward the front of the body. Inferior is the lower portion of the body.

4.

A. Anatomically, the shoulder blade is superior to the feet. Superior means the upper portion. Inferior means the lower part of the body. Dorsal means on the backside of the body. Ventral means on the abdominal side of the body.

5.

A. If an abrasion is superficial, it is on or near the surface of the skin.

6.

B. Homeostasis is the body's attempt to keep the internal environment in balance. Illness, injury, and stress may affect the internal environment and cause changes in vital signs.

7.

A. If a resident tells you that she has pain, she is giving you subjective data. Subjective data is information stated by the resident about how he or she is feeling.

8.

D. Abrasions, bruises, and any other visible injuries are objective data. Objective data includes information you observe through the senses: sight, hearing, smell, and touch.

9.

B. Chronological age is a person's actual age in years and months.

10.

B. If the resident seems angry, understand that the resident may be experiencing frustration because of the loss of mobility and independence. The resident can become aggressive and use poor judgment because of the level of frustration. The resident may become aggressive toward the nursing assistant with no provocation.

Body Systems

chapter outline

I. HUMAN BODY

A. The human body is a combination of all body systems.

B. Body systems must work together.

1. The body is healthy if the systems work together.
2. A change in one system can affect the other systems and cause disease.

II. INTEGUMENTARY SYSTEM

A. Structure

1. *skin*—largest organ in the body
   a. *epidermis*—outer layer containing **melanin**
   b. *dermis*—inner layer containing blood vessels and nerve endings
   c. **subcutaneous** fatty tissue—provides insulation and protection
2. **appendages**
   a. nails
   b. hair
   c. sweat glands
   d. oil glands

Melanin—pigment that occurs in skin, hair, and parts of the eye that determine color

Subcutaneous—beneath the skin

Appendage—an extension of a body part

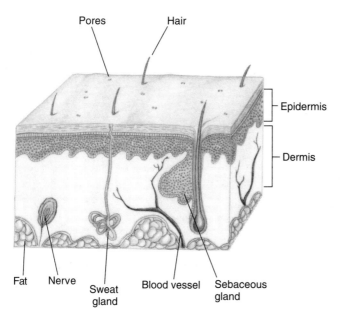

Figure 15.1   The layers of the skin. (Source: From *The Long-Term Care Nursing Assistant* [2nd ed., p. 132], by P. Grubbs and B. Blasband, 2000, Upper Saddle River, NJ: Prentice Hall. Reprinted by permission.)

B. Function

1. skin
   a. protects internal parts of the body
   b. is a barrier against germs
   c. affects water balance in the body
   d. helps maintain body temperature through perspiring
   e. helps eliminate waste products
   f. receives information about the environment—heat, cold, pressure, pain—from nerve endings
   g. stores fat and vitamins for energy
2. *nails*—protect tips of fingers and toes
3. *hair*—protects skin, nose, ears, and eyes
4. *sweat glands*—cool the body
5. *oil glands*—keep skin and hair moist and smooth

C. First signs of aging are often seen in the skin:

1. thinning hair and loss of hair color
2. dry, thin, fragile skin
3. wrinkles and liver spots
4. loss of fatty tissue
5. decrease of feeling
6. thick, hard nails

D. Common disorders:

1. skin **lesions**, including:
   a. blisters
   b. rashes
   c. whiteheads
   d. scabs
   e. scrapes
   f. athlete's foot
   g. **eczema**
   h. skin cancer
   i. **dermatitis**
   j. acne
   k. **impetigo**
   l. **shingles**
2. decubitus ulcers (pressure sores, bedsores)
   a. develop when pressure on one area of the body decreases circulation
   b. usually develop on residents who are bedridden and not turned routinely
3. burns
   a. destroy skin tissue
   b. allow the loss of fluids and chemicals

Lesion—localized abnormality of the skin, such as a wound, sore, or rash caused by injury or disease

Eczema—inflammation of the skin that causes itching and crusted sores

Dermatitis—acute or chronic inflammation of the skin

Impetigo—bacterial infection of the skin

Shingles—viral infection of the skin, usually occurring in adults

c. increase the chance of infection

d. are classified according to the depth of the burn

4. gangrene

a. death of tissue due to disease, injury, or blockage of blood supply

b. may result in **amputation**

Amputation—removal of a body part

E. Some responsibilities of the nursing assistant:

1. Keep the resident's skin clean and dry.

2. Protect the resident from injury to the skin.

3. Report changes in skin condition or color to the nurse, including:

a. *redness of skin*—indicates increased body temperature, prolonged pressure, infection, or injury

b. **cyanosis**—indicates decreased circulation, a life-threatening problem

Cyanosis—blue or gray color of skin, lips, and nail beds indicating lack of oxygen

c. *pale or white color*—indicates circulatory problems related to shock

III. MUSCULOSKELETAL SYSTEM

A. Structure

1. 206 bones in the human body

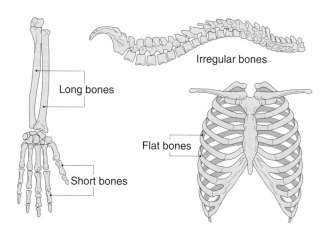

Figure 15–2 Types of bones. (Source: From *The Long-Term Care Nursing Assistant* [2nd ed., p. 133], by P. Grubbs and B. Blasband, 2000, Upper Saddle River, NJ: Prentice Hall. Reprinted by permission.)

2. Joints are composed of:

a. *ligament*—connects bone to bone

b. *tendon*—connects muscle to bone

c. *bursa*—small sac of fluid that lubricates joints

d. *cartilage*—provides padding between bones

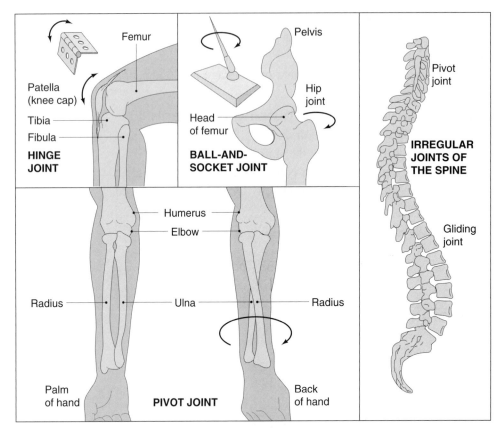

Figure 15–3 Types of joints. (Source: From *The Long-Term Care Nursing Assistant* [2nd ed., p. 133], by P. Grubbs and B. Blasband, 2000, Upper Saddle River, NJ: Prentice Hall. Reprinted by permission.)

  3. muscles
     a. *voluntary*—controlled by will (muscles in arms or legs)
     b. *involuntary*—work automatically (muscles used to breathe and digest food)
     c. *cardiac*—muscle that controls the heartbeat

B. Function
  1. produce movement
  2. protect vital organs
  3. provide support and framework for the body

C. Changes with aging
  1. muscle weakening and loss of muscle tone
  2. slowing of body movements
  3. stiff joints
  4. brittle bones
  5. changes in posture and loss of height

D. Related disorders

1. bursitis
   a. bursae in joints become inflamed
   b. causes pain
2. arthritis
   a. inflammation of one or more joints
   b. produces redness, stiffness, pain, and deformity
   c. *osteoarthritis*—common form that occurs with aging and affects weight-bearing joints such as knees, hips, fingers, and **vertebrae**
   d. *rheumatoid arthritis*—chronic form of arthritis that can occur at any age
3. **fractures**
   a. usually caused by falls and accidents
   b. common in people who have **osteoporosis**
   c. Common sites in older people include hip, shoulder, vertebrae.
   d. Signs and symptoms of fractures include pain, swelling, bruising, limitation of movement, bleeding, and color changes at fracture site.
   e. Signs of fractured hip include external rotation and shortening of the leg.

Vertebrae—bones of the spinal column

Fracture—any break or crack in a bone

Osteoporosis—loss of calcium in bones, resulting in extremely brittle bones

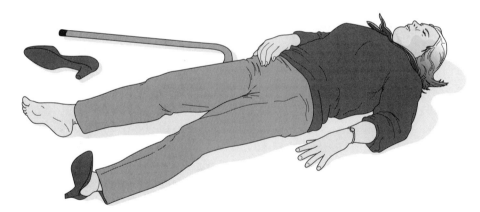

Figure 15–4   External (outward) rotation of the hip. (Source: From *Being a Long-Term Care Nursing Assistant* [5th ed., p. 200], by C. Will-Black and J. Eighmy, 2002, Upper Saddle River, NJ: Prentice Hall. Reprinted by permission.)

4. contracture
   a. permanent shortening of a muscle
   b. joints become frozen from inactivity
   c. can be prevented but cannot be reversed
   d. can limit movement and interfere with positioning and hygiene

E. Some responsibilities of the nursing assistant:

1. Provide care carefully to reduce joint pain.
2. Keep traffic patterns clear to prevent falls.

3. Frequently turn or change position of dependent residents.
4. Move residents carefully and with assistance when necessary.
5. Provide for the resident's safety by placing frequently used items within reach.
6. Provide range of motion exercises to maintain strength and prevent contractures.
7. For residents recovering from a fractured hip:
    a. Provide a straight-back chair with arm rests.
    b. Move the resident toward the strong side.
    c. Observe and report complaints of pain.
    d. Offer encouragement.
    e. Understand that the resident may be fearful of falling again.

IV. RESPIRATORY SYSTEM

A. Structure
1. nose
2. pharynx (throat)
3. larynx ("voice box" containing vocal chords)
4. trachea
5. **epiglottis**
6. bronchi
7. lungs
8. alveoli (small air sacs of the lungs)

Epiglottis—piece of cartilage covering the trachea that lifts when you breathe or talk and closes when you swallow to prevent food in the throat from entering the airway

B. Function
1. The respiratory system brings oxygen into the body and removes carbon dioxide from the body.
2. Respiration is the process of breathing.
    a. inhalation (breathing in)—**diaphragm** flattens, chest enlarges, and lungs expand and fill with oxygen
    b. exhalation (breathing out)—diaphragm expands, chest decreases, forcing air with carbon dioxide out of the lungs

Diaphragm—a muscle located immediately below the lungs that separates the chest cavity from the abdominal cavity

C. Changes with aging
1. The rib cage becomes more rigid.
2. Muscles weaken.
3. The lungs become less elastic.
4. The voice weakens.

D. Related disorders
1. upper respiratory infections (URI)
    a. inflammation of the nose, throat, and bronchi caused by bacteria or viruses
    b. Symptoms include fever, runny nose, sneezing, watery eyes.

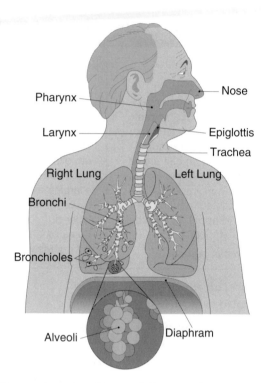

Figure 15–5 The major structures of the respiratory system. (Source: From *The Long-Term Care Nursing Assistant* [2nd ed., p. 134], by P. Grubbs and B. Blasband, 2000, Upper Saddle River, NJ: Prentice Hall. Reprinted by permission.)

2. pneumonia
   a. inflammation of the lungs caused by bacteria or viruses.
   b. Symptoms include fever, pain on breathing or coughing, rapid pulse.
3. chronic obstructive pulmonary disease (COPD)—disease that permanently affects air flow in the respiratory system
4. lung cancer
   a. one of the most common sites for cancer.
   b. Symptoms include persistent cough, coughing up blood, shortness of breath, wheezing, pain in the chest, weight loss.
5. tuberculosis (TB)
   a. An infectious disease transmitted through droplets released by sneezing and coughing.
   b. Organisms cause damage to lungs and other parts of the body.
   c. Symptoms include fatigue, weight loss, coughing up blood, night sweats, fever.

E. Some responsibilities of the nursing assistant:
1. Encourage the resident to rest between activities.
2. Avoid rushing the resident.

CHRONIC OBSTRUCTIVE PULMONARY DISEASE		
Chronic Bronchitis	**Emphysema**	**Asthma**
Cigarette smoking, repeated infections, or other chronic irritations of the respiratory tract cause chronic bronchitis, an inflammation of the air tubes (bronchi) in the lungs. Symptoms include a recurrent cough and excessive mucous secretions.	Emphysema is a disorder in which the alveoli can no longer expand and contract completely, and the normal exchange of oxygen and carbon dioxide cannot occur. People who smoke are at higher risk for developing emphysema. Signs and symptoms include a persistent cough, fatigue, loss of appetite, and the coughing up of mucus. Emphysema can be fatal.	Asthma causes spasms of the bronchial tube walls that cause the air passages to narrow. Excess mucus is produced and air passage linings swell. Asthma attacks, as they are commonly called, may be brought on by allergies or stress. The attacks result in difficulty breathing, wheezing, coughing, and sometimes blue-tinged skin if air flow is very restricted.

Figure 15–6 (Source: From *The Nursing Assistant* [3rd ed., p. 105], by J. Pulliam, 2002, Upper Saddle River, NJ: Prentice Hall. Reprinted by permission.)

3. Offer fluids frequently, which will keep passages moist and thin out secretions.
4. Assist with breathing exercises if instructed by the nurse.
5. Position the resident sitting up or leaning forward to help with breathing.
6. Report any changes in skin color, increase in respiratory rate, or persistent cough and mucus immediately.

V. CIRCULATORY SYSTEM

A. Structure
1. *heart*—pumps blood through blood vessels
   a. about the size of your fist
   b. composed of cardiac muscle
   c. located in the chest slightly left of the midline
   d. protected by the rib cage
   e. divided into four chambers
   f. two stages of cardiac cycle **diastole** and **systole**
2. *blood vessels*—tubes that carry blood throughout the body and include:
   a. *arteries*—carry blood away from the heart
   b. *veins*—carry blood back to the heart
   c. *capillaries*—connect arteries to veins
   d. *pulmonary artery*—carries blood from the heart to the lungs
3. *blood*—carries products to and from cells
   a. An adult has 4–6 quarts of blood in the body.
   b. composed of plasma and cells
   c. three main types of blood cells:
      • Red blood cells carry oxygen and give blood its color.

Diastole—stage of the cardiac cycle when the heart is resting and filling with blood

Systole—stage of the cardiac cycle when the heart is contracting and pumping out blood

- White blood cells fight disease and are part of the body's immune system.
- Platelets help blood to clot.

B. Function
1. transport food, water, and oxygen to the cells
2. transport waste products away from the cells
3. help regulate body temperature
4. protect the body against disease

C. Changes with aging
1. The heart pumps with less force.
2. The blood vessels become narrow.

D. Related disorders
1. *hypertension*—high blood pressure
   a. Affects one in four adults.
   b. Person may have no symptoms or may experience dizziness, headaches, and blurred vision.
   c. Occurs more frequently in people:
      - with family history of hypertension
      - who are overweight
      - who smoke
   d. Untreated, it can cause damage to the heart and blood vessels.
   e. It can lead to heart attack or stroke.
2. *arteriosclerosis*—group of disorders that causes thickening and hardening of the artery walls
   a. major cause of heart disease
   b. It can cause arteries to become clogged or completely blocked by fatty deposits and calcium.
   c. Contributing factors include:
      - stress
      - lack of exercise
      - genetic factors
      - diabetes
      - a diet high in cholesterol and fats
   d. It may lead to heart attack or stroke.
3. *angina pectoris*—chest pain caused by decreased blood supply to heart
   a. Brought on by physical exertion, overeating, or stress.
   b. It is a warning sign that a person is at risk for a heart attack.
4. *myocardial infarction (MI)*—heart attack
   a. leading cause of death in the United States
   b. It occurs when the coronary arteries that supply blood to the heart become blocked.

c. Part of the heart loses blood supply and tissue death occurs.
d. Signs and symptoms include:
- severe chest pain
- indigestion or nausea
- weak and irregular pulse
- perspiration
- dizziness
- pale or blue-tinged skin
- wet and clammy skin
- shortness of breath
5. congestive heart failure (CHF)
a. form of heart disease in which the heart is unable to pump enough blood
b. It occurs because of damage to the heart from myocardial infarction, from chronic hypertension, or from severely narrowed blood vessels.
c. Signs and symptoms include:
- difficulty breathing
- **edema**
- fluid in the lungs
- blue-tinged skin
- confusion
- irregular, rapid pulse

Edema—swelling of body tissue due to excessive accumulation of fluid

E. Some responsibilities of the nursing assistant:
1. Take blood pressure accurately and report it to the nurse.
2. Be certain that the resident is comfortable and relaxed, because stress can increase blood pressure.
3. Encourage the resident to reduce salt in the diet and avoid smoking.
4. If the resident has a **pacemaker,** report to the nurse incidents of hiccups, pain, or discoloration of skin around the pacemaker, or pulse rate below the preset rate.
5. Report dizziness, swelling, shortness of breath, or irregular heartbeat.

Pacemaker—small, battery-operated device that regulates heartbeat

VI. DIGESTIVE SYSTEM

A. Structure
1. **alimentary canal**
a. mouth
b. pharynx (throat)
c. esophagus, which moves food into the stomach through **peristalsis**
d. *stomach*—churns food into small pieces
e. *small intestine*—digests food particles, which are absorbed and released into the bloodstream

Alimentary canal—a long continuous tube from the mouth to the anus

Peristalsis—muscular contractions that move food through the digestive system

f. *large intestine (colon)*—removes water from the food

g. *rectum*—stores solid waste (feces) that remains after water is removed

h. *anus*—opening from the rectum through which feces are expelled from the body

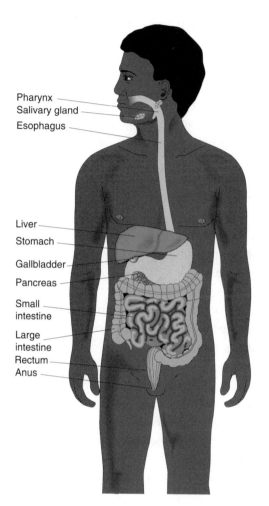

Figure 15–7   The digestive system. (Source: From *The Long-Term Care Nursing Assistant* [2nd ed., p. 137], by P. Grubbs and B. Blasband, 2000, Upper Saddle River, NJ: Prentice Hall. Reprinted by permission.)

2. accessory organs, including:

a. teeth

b. *tongue*—allows the food to be tasted and helps swallowing

c. *salivary glands*—produce chemicals that break down food

d. *liver*—produces digestive juices

e. *gallbladder*—stores digestive juices

f. *pancreas*—produces digestive juices

B. Function
1. prepares food for the body's use
2. eliminates solid wastes

C. Changes with aging
1. decrease in saliva and taste buds
2. decrease in digestive juices
3. difficulty in chewing and swallowing
4. slowed peristalsis
5. reduced absorption of vitamins and minerals

D. Related disorders
1. Common disorders are constipation and diarrhea.
2. Signs and symptoms of more serious disorders include:
   a. nausea
   b. vomiting
   c. blood in emesis or stools
   d. **flatus**
   e. pain in stomach
   f. difficulty swallowing
   g. poor appetite
3. cancers
   a. Cancer can occur anywhere along the alimentary canal.
   b. Colon cancer is the most common.
4. inflammations
   a. occur when organs become infected
   b. appendicitis, colitis, **diverticulitis, hepatitis**
5. ulcerations
   a. sore or breakdown of tissue
   b. occur anywhere in alimentary canal
   c. Symptoms include:
      • burning pain two hours after eating
      • passing black feces
      • watery, foul-smelling stools
6. gallbladder conditions
   a. due to inflammation or stones
   b. Symptoms include:
      • indigestion
      • pain
      • **jaundice**
7. hernias
   a. A portion of an organ protrudes through the wall of a cavity.
   b. Protruding tissue can become trapped and die because of decreased circulation to the area.

Flatus—intestinal gas

Diverticulitis—inflammation of the intestines

Hepatitis—inflammation of the liver

Jaundice—a yellow discoloration of the skin and whites of the eyes, a principal sign of many liver or gallbladder disorders

8. hemorrhoids
    a. enlarged veins in the anal area
    b. Sitting and moving are painful.
    c. Symptom is bright red blood in the stools.
9. cirrhosis
    a. severe disease of the liver
    b. Scar tissue replaces normal liver tissue.
    c. Jaundice is usually present.

E. Some responsibilities of the nursing assistant:

1. Provide care for residents with **ostomies.**
    a. Clean and protect skin around **stomas.**
    b. *colostomy*—a portion of large intestine is brought to the abdominal wall
    c. *ileostomy*—a portion of the ileum (lower part of the small intestine) is brought to the abdominal wall
    d. Observe resident for psychological effects of ostomy, which may include:
        • frustration and embarrassment from inability to control bowel function
        • worry about odor and leakage
        • worry that ostomy bag will show through clothing
    e. Observe resident for changes in color of stoma or irritation of skin around site.
2. Report change in stool consistency, bleeding, or unabsorbed medications.
3. Report changes in skin color.
4. Report any signs or symptoms of digestive distress to the nurse.

Ostomy—surgical procedure in which an artificial opening is created

Stoma—artificial opening of an internal organ on the surface of the body

VII. URINARY SYSTEM

A. Structure

1. *kidneys*—two bean-shaped organs located in the upper abdomen toward the back that filter blood and produce urine
2. *ureters*—tube leading from each kidney to the bladder
3. *bladder*—muscular sac that stores urine
4. *urethra*—tube leading from the bladder through the **urinary meatus** to eliminate urine from the body

Urinary meatus—external opening of the urethra

B. Function

1. Filter waste from the blood.
2. Eliminate liquid waste (urine) from the body.
3. Help maintain the body's fluid and chemical balance.

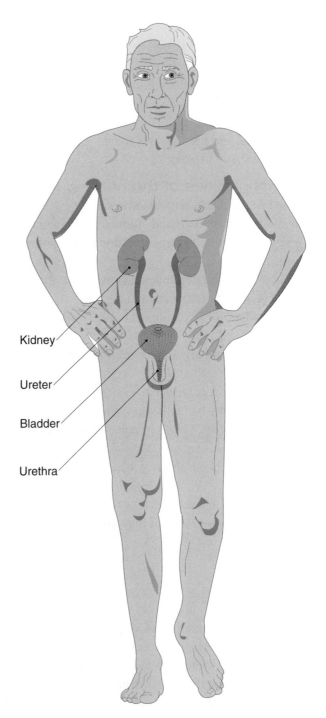

Kidney

Ureter

Bladder

Urethra

Figure 15–8 The urinary system. (Source: From *The Long-Term Care Nursing Assistant* [2nd ed., p. 138], by P. Grubbs and B. Blasband, 2000, Upper Saddle River, NJ: Prentice Hall. Reprinted by permission.)

C. Changes with aging
1. decrease in kidney filtration
2. decrease in bladder muscle tone

D. Related disorders
1. **incontinence**
   a. affects people of all ages
   b. caused by nerve damage, weakened muscles, medications, or urinary tract infections
2. urine retention
   a. occurs when blockage prevents urine from flowing
   b. Symptoms include difficulty passing urine, urinating in small amounts, constantly feeling the need to urinate.
3. urinary tract infection (UTI)
   a. Those most likely to develop infection are incontinent persons, older persons, and females.
   b. Signs and symptoms:
      • burning or stinging on urination
      • inability to hold urine
      • urine with abnormal appearance or foul odor
4. cystitis
   a. also known as bladder infection
   b. Signs and symptoms are frequent painful urination, blood in urine, bladder spasms.
5. renal calculi (kidney stones)
   a. If stones lodge in urinary passages, will cause sudden, intense pain.
   b. Stones can cause tissue damage.
6. nephritis
   a. an inflammation of the kidney that affects kidney cells, reducing the kidney's ability to produce urine
   b. can be life threatening
   c. Symptoms include hypertension and edema.

E. Some responsibilities of the nursing assistant:
1. Observe and report any unusual color, odor, amount, or clarity of urine.
2. Observe residents for signs of pain on urination.

VIII. NERVOUS SYSTEM

A. Structure
1. brain
   a. part of central nervous system
   b. divided into sections that each control specific functions
   c. The right side of the brain controls the left side of the body.

Incontinence—the inability to control bladder or bowel function

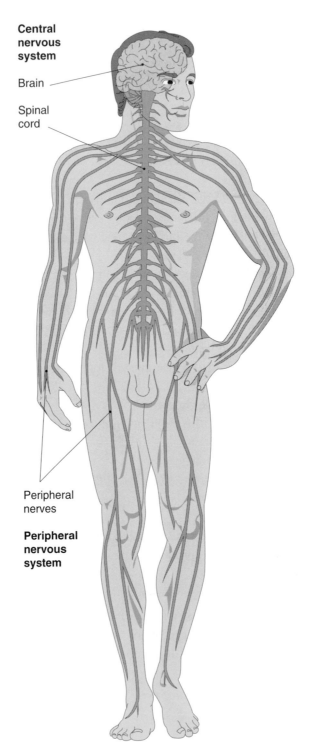

Figure 15–9 The nervous system. (Source: From *The Long-Term Care Nursing Assistant* [2nd ed., p. 139], by P. Grubbs and B. Blasband, 2000, Upper Saddle River, NJ: Prentice Hall. Reprinted by permission.)

      d. The left side of the brain controls the right side of the body.

      e. protected by skull

  2. spinal cord

      a. part of the central nervous system

      b. protected by the vertebral column

  3. nerves

      a. make up the peripheral nervous system

      b. *cranial nerves*—carry messages in and out of the brain

      c. *spinal nerves*—carry messages to and from the spinal cord

      d. *neurons (nerve cells)*—send messages throughout the body

B. Function

  1. Controls and coordinates the body's activities.

  2. As the communication center, receives information from the senses and transmits responses throughout the body.

C. Changes with aging

  1. decrease in nerve cells

  2. slowed message transmission

  3. slowed responses and reflexes

  4. decreased sensitivity of nerve endings

  5. short-term memory loss

D. Related disorders

  1. CVA (stroke)

      a. Blood flow to the brain is interrupted by **hemorrhage, thrombus, or embolus.**

      b. Signs and symptoms include:

        • seizures

        • loss of consciousness

        • difficulty breathing or swallowing

        • headaches

        • dizziness

        • nausea

        • weakness or paralysis in an extremity or on one side (hemiplegia)

        • incontinence

        • disorientation

        • inability to communicate (aphasia)

  2. Parkinson's disease

      a. Part of the brain slowly degenerates.

      b. Symptoms include:

        • a masklike facial expression

        • trembling

        • a shuffling walk

        • stooped posture

Hemorrhage—bleeding caused by rupture of a blood vessel

Thrombus—blood clot that forms in and blocks a blood vessel

Embolus—clot or other mass that travels through the bloodstream and eventually blocks a blood vessel

- stiff muscles
- slow movements
- slurred or monotone speech
- drooling

3. multiple sclerosis
   a. loss of the nerves' ability to function, usually occurring in young adulthood and progressing gradually
   b. Signs and symptoms include:
   - visual disturbances
   - weakness
   - fatigue, which can lead to blindness
   - contractures
   - paralysis of arms and legs
   - loss of bowel and bladder control
   - respiratory muscle weakness

4. epilepsy (seizure syndrome)
   a. electrical disturbance in the brain
   b. Seizures vary from momentary erratic behavior to convulsive uncontrolled movements, muscular rigidity, and loss of consciousness.

5. meningitis
   a. inflammation of the **meninges**
   b. Signs and symptoms include:
   - headaches
   - nausea
   - stiff neck
   - convulsions
   - chills
   - high temperature

Meninges—membranes that line and protect the brain and spinal cord

DIFFERENCES BETWEEN RIGHT AND LEFT BRAIN INJURIES	
Right Brain Injury (Left Paralysis)	**Left Brain Injury (Right Paralysis)**
Partial or complete paralysis of the left side of the face, arm, and leg.	Partial or complete paralysis of the right side of the face, arm, and leg.
Loss of sensation of pain, touch, and temperature on the left side.	Loss of sensation of pain, touch, and temperature on the right side.
Difficulty in judging size, distance, and rate of movement.	Aphasia (about 50 percent of left-handed people will have aphasia from a right brain injury).
May act impulsively and unsafely.	May act cautiously and slowly.

Figure 15–10   (Source: From *The Nursing Assistant* [3rd ed., p. 120], by P. Grubbs and B. Blasband, 2000, Upper Saddle River, NJ: Prentice Hall. Reprinted by permission.)

E. Some responsibilities of the nursing assistant:

1. Observe for signs and report to nurse any:
   a. labored breathing
   b. blue-tinged skin
   c. unconsciousness
   d. seizures
   e. muscle spasms
   f. airway obstructions
   g. fever
   h. loss of mental alertness
2. Assist with ADLs as necessary.
3. Assist with ambulation to prevent falls.
4. Perform range-of-motion exercises.
5. Be patient.

IX. ENDOCRINE SYSTEM

A. Structure

1. pituitary gland
   a. "master" gland that regulates other glands
   b. Hormones regulate growth, water balance, and reproduction.
2. thyroid gland
   a. located in the neck
   b. Hormones affect body growth and development and regulate metabolism.
3. parathyroid glands
   a. located on the back of the thyroid gland
   b. Hormones regulate calcium levels that affect nerve and muscle tissue.
4. thymus
   a. Hormones assist in the immune process and helps the body resist germs and disease.
   b. **"T-cells"** develop in the thymus.
5. pancreas
   a. Hormones necessary for metabolism of sugar.
   b. Islets of Langerhans are clusters of cells that produce insulin and glucagons that convert sugar to energy.
6. adrenal glands
   a. located on top of the kidneys
   b. Hormones control the body's response to stress (adrenalin), allowing the body to produce large amounts of energy in an emergency.
7. gonads
   a. Hormones affect development of male and female characteristics and control human reproduction.

T-cells—white blood cells that regulate the immune function

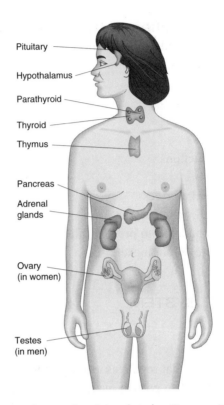

Figure 15–11 The major endocrine glands. (Source: From *The Long-Term Care Nursing Assistant* [2nd ed., p. 142], by P. Grubbs and B. Blasband, 2000, Upper Saddle River, NJ: Prentice Hall. Reprinted by permission.)

   b. *male*—testes produce testosterone
   c. *female*—ovaries produce estrogen and progesterone

B. Function
 1. Glands control and regulate body functions by secreting hormones directly into the bloodstream.
 2. Each gland produces a different hormone with specific purposes.

C. Changes with aging
 1. decrease in hormones
 2. reduced regulation of body activities

D. Related disorders
 1. thyroid disorders
  a. *hyperthyroidism*—secretion of too much thyroxin; signs and symptoms include:
- irritability
- restlessness
- nervousness
- rapid pulse

- increased appetite
- weight loss
  b. *hypothyroidism*—secretion of too little thyroxin; signs and symptoms include fatigue, weight gain
  c. *goiter*—lack of iodine in diet; may lead to enlarged thyroid gland
  2. pancreatic disorders
  a. *diabetes mellitus*—due to not enough insulin being produced; results in high levels of sugar in blood
    - Type I diabetes—insulin dependent; occurs in people under 40 years old; signs and symptoms include excessive thirst, frequent urination, hunger, and sugar in urine.
    - Type II diabetes—onset in people over 40; signs and symptoms may be similar to those of Type I but can also be less obvious and include fatigue, vision problems, tingling or pain in fingers and toes, and itching in pubic area.
    - A combination of diet, exercise, and drugs is used to control diabetes.
    - If uncontrolled, it can lead to thickening of blood vessels, circulation problems, blindness, and kidney disease.
  b. *hypoglycemia*—not enough sugar in the blood
  c. *hyperglycemia*—too much sugar in the blood

E. Some responsibilities of the nursing assistant:

1. Help visitors understand they should only bring in food that the resident on a special diet is permitted to have.
2. Observe and report to the nurse sores, cuts, or redness on the resident's feet.
3. Wash and dry the resident's skin carefully and completely.
4. Report the resident's need to have toenails clipped to the nurse, since a **podiatrist** or nurse should cut the nails.
5. Encourage the resident to be active.
6. Report changes in activity level, interest, or behavior to the nurse immediately.

Podiatrist—foot doctor

X. REPRODUCTIVE SYSTEM

A. Structure

1. female reproductive system
  a. *ovaries*—produce **ova** and create female hormones
  b. *fallopian tubes*—carry ova to uterus
  c. *uterus*—protects and nourishes fetus during pregnancy, expels fetus at childbirth

Ova—eggs, the female reproductive cells

Sperm—male reproductive cells

    d. *vagina*—passageway for birth of fetus and receptacle for penis during sexual intercourse
  2. male reproductive system
    a. *testes*—produce **sperm** and male hormones
    b. *scrotum*—two sacs located behind penis that contain the testes
    c. *penis*—releases semen that contains sperm during intercourse
    d. *seminal vesicles*—secrete fluids that become part of semen
    e. *prostate gland*—secretes fluids that become part of semen

B. Function
1. produce reproductive cells
2. secrete hormones that cause the development of sex characteristics

C. Changes with aging
1. menopause in women
2. drying and thinning of vaginal walls
3. enlargement of male prostate gland
4. change in male hormone levels

D. Related disorders
1. in females
  a. *menstrual irregularities*—excessive flow of blood or absence of flow
  b. *fungus infections*—producing thick, white, cheesy vaginal discharge, inflammation, and itching
  c. *hernias*—between wall of vagina and rectum or bladder and vagina
  d. benign and malignant tumors of uterus or ovaries
2. in males
  a. disorders of prostate gland, especially in older men; prostate enlarges, which causes narrowing of urethra and difficulty urinating
  b. cancer of testes

E. Some responsibilities of the nursing assistant:
1. Provide privacy for residents.
2. Observe and report any unusual discharge from the vagina or penis.
3. Report complaints of difficulty urinating.
4. Provide perineal care to prevent infection and odor.

XI. SPECIAL SENSES

A. Five senses:
1. sight
2. hearing
3. smell
4. taste
5. touch

B. Nerve endings transmit information to the brain from the:

1. eye—the sense organ for vision
   a. eyeball—globe-shaped part of eye composed of three layers:
      - sclera (white part of eye) and cornea (focuses light rays)
      - iris (colored part of eye), pupil (dark opening in center of iris that controls the amount of light entering the eye, and lens (located behind iris), which focuses light images onto retina
      - retina (inner layer of eyeball)
   b. Images are carried from the retina by the optic nerve to the brain.

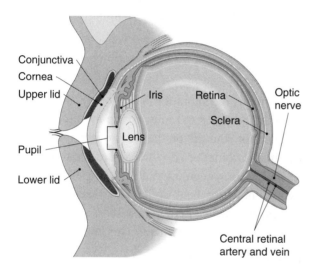

Figure 15–12 The structure of the eye. (Source: From *The Long-Term Care Nursing Assistant* [2nd ed., p. 140], by P. Grubbs and B. Blasband, 2000, Upper Saddle River, NJ: Prentice Hall. Reprinted by permission.)

2. *ear*—the sense organ for hearing and balance
   a. divided into three parts: outer ear, middle ear, and inner ear
   b. The tympanic membrane (eardrum) separates the outer and middle ear.
   c. Semicircular canals, located in the inner ear, contain nerve receptors for balance.
3. *nose*—contains receptors for smell
   a. Messages are sent to the brain by the olfactory nerve.
   b. Senses of smell and taste are closely related, yet smell is more accurate.

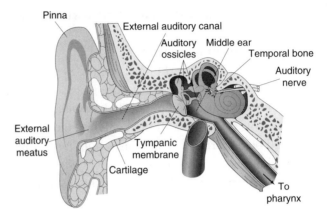

Figure 15–13   The structure of the ear. (Source: From *The Long-Term Care Nursing Assistant* [2nd ed., p. 141], by P. Grubbs and B. Blasband, 2000, Upper Saddle River, NJ: Prentice Hall. Reprinted by permission.)

4. *tongue*—contains receptors for taste
   a. Taste buds for sweet and salty are on the tip of the tongue.
   b. Taste buds for sour are on the sides of the tongue.
   c. Taste buds for bitter are on the back of the tongue.
   d. Taste buds help you enjoy food.
5. skin—senses pressure, heat, cold, pain, pleasure, and touch
   a. increases awareness of environment
   b. allows persons to protect themselves and stay comfortable

C. Changes with aging
1. decrease in vision
2. hearing loss
3. loss of ability to smell
4. changes in sense of balance
5. less distinctive sense of taste
6. diminished sense of touch

D. Related disorders
1. hearing loss
   a. range from slight hearing impairment to deafness
   b. A person may:
      • speak too loudly
      • ask to have things repeated
      • lean forward to hear
      • turn and cup the better ear
      • respond inappropriately to questions

2. vision problems
   a. myopia—nearsightedness
   b. hyperopia—farsightedness
   c. astigmatism—blurred vision
   d. glaucoma—increased pressure in the eye that damages the retina and optic nerve and may lead to blindness; signs and symptoms include:
      - blurred vision
      - tunnel vision
      - blue-green halos around lights
      - severe eye pain caused by its sudden onset
      - nausea
      - vomiting
   e. cataract—lens of eye becomes cloudy so light cannot enter eye, resulting in gradual blurring and dimming of vision

E. Some responsibilities of the nursing assistant:
1. Be patient during communication.
2. Be certain the resident's glasses are clean and hearing aid is working.
3. Describe food to enhance its smell.
4. Allow extra time when assisting residents with ADLs.
5. Check skin for bruising or injuries that may not be felt by the resident.

DIRECTIONS

A brief description of a resident is given followed by 10 questions related to the resident. Each question has four possible answers. Read each question and all answer choices carefully. Choose the one best answer.

Mr. Harmon Fox is 92 years old. He has multiple diagnoses, including chronic bronchitis, chronic hepatitis, osteoarthritis, and CVA.

1. Mr. Fox has chronic bronchitis and seems to be having more difficulty breathing. He is receiving oxygen. You should:
   A. quickly increase the oxygen he is receiving
   B. report to the nurse immediately
   C. be sure that the oxygen tubing is kinked
   D. start CPR

2. Mr. Fox has a history of chronic hepatitis, which is inflammation of the:
   A. liver
   B. heart
   C. lungs
   D. stomach

3. Mr. Fox has osteoarthritis, which commonly occurs with:
   A. bronchitis
   B. stroke
   C. hepatitis
   D. aging

4. Mr. Fox is paralyzed on the left side of his body because the stroke occurred on:
   A. the right side of the brain
   B. the base of the brain
   C. the left side of the brain
   D. the middle of the brain

5. Because of changes in mobility, Mr. Fox may experience common disorders of the digestive system, including:
   A. bursitis and arthritis
   B. constipation and diarrhea
   C. ulcers and cancer
   D. thrombus and embolus

6. Mr. Fox spilled coffee. The burn may make Mr. Fox:
   A. confused
   B. agitated
   C. susceptible to infection
   D. anorexic

7. You monitor Mr. Fox closely because he acts impulsively and unsafely due to his:
   A. osteoarthritis
   B. hepatitis
   C. dementia
   D. right-brain injury

8. Because of paralysis on the left side of his body, Mr. Fox has lost:
   A. all mobility for the rest of his life
   B. sensations of pain, touch, and temperature on the paralyzed side
   C. the ability to speak
   D. vision and hearing on the paralyzed side

9. Mr. Fox's left side is flaccid, which means:
   A. tense
   B. spastic
   C. limp and weak
   D. painful

10. You perform range-of-motion exercises with Mr. Fox to:

   A. strengthen muscles and prevent contractures

   B. improve his breathing

   C. increase pain and improve circulation

   D. maintain his dependence

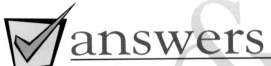

answers & rationales

1.

B. Report to the nurse immediately if a resident is having increased difficulty breathing. Do not change the rate of flow of oxygen. The nurse must assess the resident to determine the resident's needs. Never allow the oxygen tubing to become kinked because it will limit or eliminate the flow of oxygen to the resident. Never begin CPR on a person who is breathing and has a pulse.

2.

A. Hepatitis is an inflammation of the liver caused by a viral infection. Hepatitis B is a form of hepatitis that may be acquired by health care workers through contact with body fluids.

3.

D. Osteoarthritis is a common form of arthritis that occurs with aging as the cartilage in the joint wears down. Arthritis is the inflammation of one or more joints.

4.

A. Right-brain injury results in left-sided paralysis. Left-brain injury results in right-sided paralysis. Paralysis can be partial or complete on the face, arm, and leg.

5.

B. Changes in mobility may increase or decrease peristalsis and cause common disorders of the digestive system including constipation and diarrhea.

6.

C. Burns cause damage to the skin. The skin is the first line of defense against infection. Any breaks in the skin make a resident more susceptible to infection.

7.

D. Right-brain injury may affect the resident by causing him to act impulsively and unsafely. Monitor the resident closely to ensure his safety.

8.

B. Paralysis may cause the loss of the sensations of pain, touch, and temperature on the affected side of the body. The resident is then at higher risk for injury and infection because he can no longer identify when a problem in the affected part of the body exists.

9.

C. Flaccid means limp, weak, soft, and flabby. When the left side of the body is paralyzed after a stroke, the muscles become limp and weak because the person can no longer use them. Tense means stretched tightly. Spastic means having a sudden involuntary muscle movement.

10.

A. Range-of-motion exercises strengthen muscles and prevent contraction of muscles. Contractures are the permanent shortening of muscles. If contractures develop, the affected muscles will never function normally.

IV Activities of Daily Living

16 Movement and Mobility

chapter outline

I. PHYSICAL ACTIVITY

A. Physical activity improves:
1. strength
2. ability to fight off disease and infection
3. breathing
4. circulation
5. kidney and bowel function
6. digestion
7. independence
8. positive attitude

B. Lack of physical activity may cause:
1. pressure sores
2. contractures and **muscle atrophy**
3. constipation and **fecal impaction**
4. edema
5. blood clots
6. urinary tract infections and kidney stones
7. pneumonia
8. mental and emotional problems

Muscle atrophy—decrease of muscle tissue
Fecal impaction—large amount of hard, dry stool in rectum

II. AMBULATION

Ambulation—walking or moving about

A. Ambulation helps:
1. strength
2. endurance
3. all body functions
4. improve independence
5. self-esteem

B. The resident who is unable to ambulate may become:
1. frustrated
2. angry
3. withdrawn
4. depressed

C. Causes of reduced ability to ambulate include:
1. head or back injuries
2. broken leg or hip
3. stroke
4. arthritis
5. confusion
6. fear of falling

D. Using a gait belt to assist the resident to ambulate:

1. Use the gait belt according to facility policy.
2. Use a gait belt if instructed by the nurse.
3. Apply the gait belt according to the manufacturer's instructions.
4. To use a gait belt:
   a. Assist the resident to sit at the edge of the bed.
   b. Allow the resident to gain his or her balance.
   c. Help the resident put on shoes.
   d. Fasten the gait belt around the resident's waist snugly.
   e. Place your fingers under the belt to check for fit.
   f. Stand in front of the resident.
   g. Put your knees against the resident's knees and block the resident's feet with your feet.
   h. Hold the gait belt from beneath and toward the back with both hands.
   i. Keep your knees bent and your back straight.
   j. Count to three, straighten your knees, stand, and assist the resident to stand.
   k. Allow the resident to gain balance.
   l. Change position of your hands, holding the belt in back and on one side.
   m. Stand at the resident's side and slightly behind him or her, holding the gait belt with both hands.
   n. Encourage the resident to stand and walk as normally as possible.
   o. Have the resident take the first step with the weak leg.
   p. Observe the resident for signs of tiring, including:
      • changes in normal breathing
      • sweating
      • dizziness
      • rapid heart rate
   q. If the resident becomes tired, have him or her sit in the closest chair and rest.
   r. Remove the gait belt when the resident finishes ambulating.
   s. Report to the nurse the distance the resident walked and how the resident tolerated the procedure.

E. If the resident begins to fall while ambulating:

1. Pull the resident close to your body.
2. Slowly slide the resident down your leg to the floor.
3. Bend your knees and straighten your back as you lower the resident to the floor.
4. Do not try to hold the resident up, which could hurt both of you.

Gait belt—a belt made of washable material with a safety buckle that is put around the resident's waist and used to assist the resident to walk or transfer

Why?
The strong leg will bear the weight.

Why?
— Lowering the resident to the floor helps you control the direction of the fall and prevent head injuries.
— Attempting to hold the resident up can cause injury to both the resident and you.

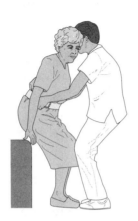
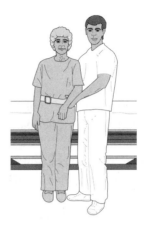
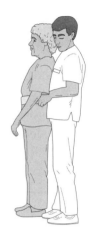

A Holding the falt belt with both hands, bring the resident to a standing position.

B Change the position of your hands so that one hand is holding the belt on the side and the other is holding the belt in the back.

C Stand at the resident's side and slightly behind her, holding onto the belt with both hands.

Figure 16–1 Using a gait/transfer belt to assist the resident in ambulation. (Source: From *The Long-Term Care Nursing Assistant* [2nd ed., p. 240], by P. Grubbs and B. Blasband, 2000, Upper Saddle River, NJ: Prentice Hall. Reprinted by permission.)

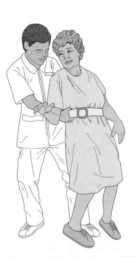
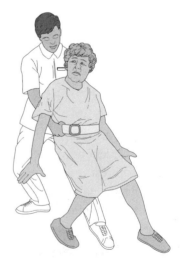

A If the resident begins to fall, pull her close to your body with the gait/transfer belt.

B Ease her to the floor by letting her slide down your leg.

Figure 16–2 Protecting a falling resident. (Source: From *The Long-Term Care Nursing Assistant* [2nd ed., p. 241], by P. Grubbs and B. Blasband, 2000, Upper Saddle River, NJ: Prentice Hall. Reprinted by permission.)

F. Assistive devices (ambulation devices):

1. increase independence
2. must be recommended by occupational or physical therapists
3. include:
   a. *brace*—limits movement of a body part
   b. *cane*—improves balance if the resident has weakness on one side of the body
   c. *crutches*—used to decrease weight bearing by one or both feet and legs
   d. *walker*—provides stability and support for residents with poor balance or general weakness
   e. *wheelchair*—provides mobility for residents who cannot ambulate
4. For safety, check that ambulation devices:
   a. have tips that are intact
   b. are in good repair
   c. are clean
   d. belong to that resident

III. BODY ALIGNMENT

A. Correct the resident's body alignment.

1. normal body alignment:
   a. when lying down:
      - shoulders and hips in a straight line
      - arms and legs in a position that is comfortable for the resident and supported if necessary
   b. when sitting in a chair:
      - back straight and against the back of the chair
      - feet flat on floor or stool
   c. when in a wheelchair:
      - hips back in the chair
      - shoulders and hips in a straight line
      - feet on footrests or flat on floor
      - arms on armrests or on a pillow if placed across the lap; pillows at sides to prevent sliding, if necessary
2. Equipment used to maintain proper body alignment:
   a. *foot supports*—keep feet and ankles aligned and prevent **footdrop**
   b. *bed cradle*—keeps top linen from pressing on toes
   c. *hand splints*—prevent contractures of hand and wrist
   d. *pillows*—placed to maintain proper body alignment

Footdrop—abnormal condition that occurs when foot is not in flexed position. Toes point downward and calf muscles tighten; may become permanent if ignored

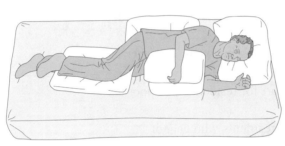
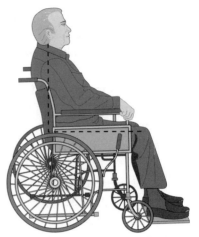

A The trunk of the body should be in a straight line.

B The resident should sit straight, with his back against the back of the chair.

Figure 16–3 Correct body alignment promotes comfort and helps to prevent complications. (Source: From *The Long-Term Care Nursing Assistant* [2nd ed., p. 218], by P. Grubbs and B. Blasband, 2000, Upper Saddle River, NJ: Prentice Hall. Reprinted by permission.)

Why?
Placing a pillow under the resident's knees prevents the resident from sliding down and reduces **shearing.**

Shearing—when the skin moves in one direction and the tissues below move in the opposite direction

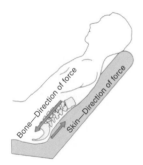

Figure 16–4 Shearing forces. (Source: From *The Nursing Assistant* [3rd ed., p. 166], by J. Pulliam, 2002, Upper Saddle River, NJ: Prentice Hall. Reprinted by permission.)

B. Positioning a dependent resident:

1. Change the resident's position at least every two hours to:
   a. prevent skin breakdown and contractures
   b. improve circulation
   c. prevent lung infections
   d. prevent discomfort and pain
   e. prevent edema
2. Body positions include:
   a. Fowler's position:
      • Raise the head of the bed to a 45°–90° angle.
      • Support the resident's head with a pillow; place a pillow under his or her knees; put pillows under the lower arms.
   b. semi-Fowler's position:
      • Raise the head of the bed to a 30°–45° angle.
      • Support the body as in Fowler's position.
   c. supine position:
      • Have resident lie flat on his or her back with arms and legs straight.
      • Support the head with pillows; use a footboard, if necessary, to prevent footdrop.
   d. lateral position:
      • Place the resident on the left or right side.
      • Put pillows under the head, against the back, between knees and ankles, and under the upper arm.

3. Other body positions:
   a. Sims' position (used when giving enemas):
      - Put the resident on the left side with the left leg extended, the left arm behind the resident, and the right leg and arm flexed.
      - Support the head and shoulder with a pillow; place pillows under the right leg and arm.
   b. Trendelenburg position (used to prevent shock):
      - Put the resident in a supine position with the mattress tilted so the head is below the feet.
   c. reverse Trendelenburg position:
      - Put the resident in a supine position with the mattress tilted so the feet are below the level of the head.
   d. prone position:

      CAUTION:

      —Do not put the resident into the prone position unless instructed by the nurse.

      —Never use the prone position if the resident has difficulty breathing, is debilitated, is obese, or has large breasts.

      —Check the resident frequently because many residents quickly become uncomfortable in the prone position or develop a feeling of suffocation and become apprehensive.

      —Never put both arms up next to the head, which may cause a painful strain on the shoulders and upper back.

      - Put the resident flat on the abdomen, legs straight, face turned to one side, and one arm bent upward.
      - Put a pillow under the head and under the lower legs to reduce pressure on the toes.

C. Moving the resident up in bed:

1. Move the resident to the head of the bed with the resident's assistance. See Procedure 16-1 in Appendix A.
   a. Raise the side rails and raise the bed to working height.
   b. Lower the head of the bed.
   c. Lean a pillow against the headboard.
   d. Lower the side rail on the side nearest you.
   e. Face the head of the bed, one foot in front of the other, 12 inches apart.
   f. Keep your knees and back straight.
   g. Place one arm under the resident's shoulder blades and the other arm under the resident's thighs.
   h. Ask the resident to bend the knees, put feet flat on the mattress, bend the arms, and brace on the bed.
   i. Tell the resident that, on the count of three, he or she should push with the feet and arms as you lift and shift your weight from your back foot to the front foot.

Why?
— Supporting arms and legs with pillows reduces stress on the joints and improves comfort.
— Pillows keep body in position and alignment, reduce stress on joints, and reduce pressure on bony areas.

Why?
A pillow against the headboard prevents injury if the resident moves too fast or too far and bumps his or her head into headboard.

    j. Place a pillow under the resident's head.

    k. Raise the side rail.

    l. Lower the height of the bed and position the side rails as appropriate for the individual resident.

2. Move a resident to the head of the bed with a lift sheet and an assistant. See Procedure 16-2 in Appendix A.

    a. Raise the side rails and raise the bed to working height.

    b. Lower the head of the bed.

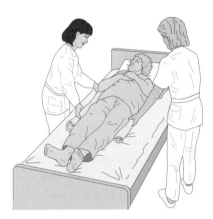

Figure 16–5 Roll the lift sheet close to the sides of the resident's body when moving her up in bed. (Source: From *The Long-Term Care Nursing Assistant* [2nd ed., p. 222], by P. Grubbs and B. Blasband, 2000, Upper Saddle River, NJ: Prentice Hall. Reprinted by permission.)

    c. Lean a pillow against the headboard.

    d. You and the assistant lower the side rails on both sides of the bed.

    e. Face the head of the bed, one foot in front of the other, 12 inches apart.

    f. Keep your knees and back straight.

    g. Be sure the lift sheet is under the resident's shoulders and hips.

    h. Roll the lift sheet as close as possible to the resident's body.

    i. Grasp the lift sheet with one hand at the resident's shoulder and the other at the hip.

    j. On the count of three, both you and the assistant move the resident to the head of the bed by shifting your weight from the back foot to the front foot.

    k. Put a pillow under the resident's head.

    l. Unroll, straighten, and tuck the lift sheet under the mattress.

m. Lower the height of the bed and position the side rails as appropriate for the individual resident.

D. Turning a resident in bed:

1. Move the resident to the side of the bed before turning or transferring. See Procedure 16-3 in Appendix A.
   a. Raise the side rails and raise the bed to working height.
   b. Lower the head of the bed.

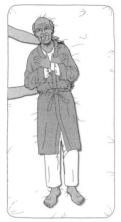 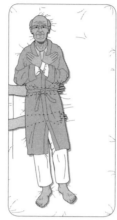 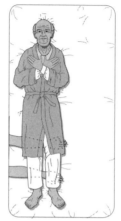

A Place your arms under the resident's neck and shoulders to move the upper part of the body toward you.

B Place your arms under the resident's waist and thighs as you move the middle of the body.

C Place your arms under the legs to move the lower part of the body.

Figure 16–6 Moving the resident to the side of the bed.
(Source: From *The Long-Term Care Nursing Assistant* [2nd ed., p. 223], by P. Grubbs and B. Blasband, 2000, Upper Saddle River, NJ: Prentice Hall. Reprinted by permission.)

   c. Lower the side rail; keep your feet apart, one in front of the other, knees bent, back straight.
   d. Place the resident's arms over the chest.
   e. Place your arms under the resident's shoulders and upper back and move the upper section of the body toward you.
   f. Place your arms under the resident's waist and thighs and move the middle of the body toward you.
   g. Place your arms under the resident's thighs and lower legs and move the lower part of the body toward you.
   h. Turn the resident away from you or raise the side rail, lower the height of the bed, lower the side rails, and begin the transfer.
2. Turning the resident away from you (see Procedure 16-4 in Appendix A):
   a. Place the resident in a supine position.
   b. Raise the side rails and raise the bed to working height.

     c. Lower the head of the bed.

     d. Lower the side rail on the side nearest you.

     e. Move the resident to the side of the bed nearest you.

     f. Bend the resident's farthest arm next to the head and place the other arm across the chest.

Why?
— If the resident has a problem with the hip, crossing the leg may be painful. By slightly bending the knee, the leg will turn in the appropriate direction when the resident is turned and will not put stress on the hip joint.
— Do not move a resident by grasping a joint because you may pull the joint out of alignment, causing pain and possible injury.

     g. Cross the resident's near leg over the far leg or bend the knee slightly.

     h. Place one hand under the resident's shoulder blade and the other hand under the buttocks.

     i. On the count of three, roll the resident away from you onto the side.

     j. Raise the side rail.

     k. Lower the height of the bed and position side rails as appropriate for the individual resident.

3. Turning the resident toward you (see Procedure 16-5 in Appendix A):

    SAFETY AND INFECTION CONTROL CAUTION: *Turn the resident away from you whenever possible. If you must turn the resident toward you, do not lean against the resident during the turn because he or she may be injured and will be contaminated by your uniform.*

     a. Place the resident in a supine position.

     b. Raise the side rails and raise the bed to a working height.

     c. Lower the head of the bed.

     d. Lower the side rail, move the resident to the side of the bed nearest you, and raise the side rail.

     e. Go to the other side of the bed.

     f. Leave the side rail up if possible.

Why?
For the resident's safety, leave the side rail up when turning the resident toward you to prevent him or her from accidentally rolling off the bed.

     g. Bend the resident's near arm next to the head and place the other arm across the chest.

     h. Cross the resident's far leg over the near leg or bend the knee slightly.

     i. Reach across the resident without leaning on him or her; place one hand under the resident's shoulder blade and the other hand under the buttocks.

     j. On the count of three, roll the resident toward you onto the side.

     k. Lower the height of the bed and leave the side rail up.

Why?
Never leave the resident rolled to the side of the bed if the side rail is down.

4. Logrolling a resident:

     a. a method of turning used for residents who must be moved without disturbing body alignment

     b. Get assistance.

     c. Raise the side rail on the side of the bed toward which the resident is to be turned and pad the rail with a pillow.

     d. Place a flat pillow lengthwise between the resident's knees.

     e. Cross the resident's arms over the chest.

     f. Have one person stand at the shoulders and the other at the hips.

     g. Lower the side rail, reach over the resident, and roll the turning sheet as close to the resident as possible.

    h. On the count of three, turn the resident toward you with the turn-ing sheet, treating the resident's body as a whole unit without bending the joints, hips, or spine.

    i. Use pillows to maintain the position.

E. Moving a resident out of bed:

1. Assist the resident to sit on the edge of the bed. See Procedure 16-6 in Appendix A.

    a. Place the bed at its lowest height and lock the wheels.

    b. Move the resident to the side of the bed closest to you.

    c. Raise the head of the bed and allow the resident to sit up for several minutes.

    d. Place one arm under the resident's shoulders and the other arm under the knees.

    e. On the count of three, turn the resident toward you so his or her legs dangle over the side of the bed.

    f. Tell the resident to provide support by pushing his or her fists into the mattress.

    g. Stand, blocking the resident's knees, and check for dizziness.

    h. Be certain the resident's shoes are on and feet are flat on the floor.

2. **Pivot transfer** the resident to the wheelchair (see Procedure 16-7 in Appendix A):

    a. Put the bed at its lowest height and lock the wheels.

    b. Place a wheelchair on the resident's strong side, braced firmly against the side of the bed.

    c. Lock the wheels and move the footrests out of the way.

    d. Assist the resident to sit on the edge of the bed.

    e. Stand in front of the resident and block his or her feet with your feet.

    f. Bend your knees and put your knees against the resident's knees.

    g. Place your hands under the resident's arms and under the shoulder blades.

    h. Ask the resident to push on the mattress with his or her hands or place the hands on your upper arms.

    i. On the count of three, help the resident into a standing position by straightening your knees.

    j. Allow the resident to gain balance and ask if he or she feels dizzy.

    k. Taking small steps, pivot the resident toward a chair.

    l. Help the resident back up until the backs of the legs touch the seat of the wheelchair.

    m. If he or she is able, have the resident hold the arms of the chair.

    n. Lower the resident into the wheelchair by bending your knees and leaning forward.

    o. Align the resident's body and position the footrests.

Why? Allowing the resident to sit up for a few minutes before moving to the edge of the bed may prevent dizziness from sudden change of posture.

Why? Holding the resident under the shoulders and knees allows you to move the body in good alignment. Never pull the resident's legs off the bed or pull up by the arms, which can cause severe injury.

Pivot transfer—method of transfer used for residents who can bear weight and as-sist with the move

Why? Lifting a resident by grasping under the arms can cause serious injury, including dis-located shoulder, skin tearing and bruising.

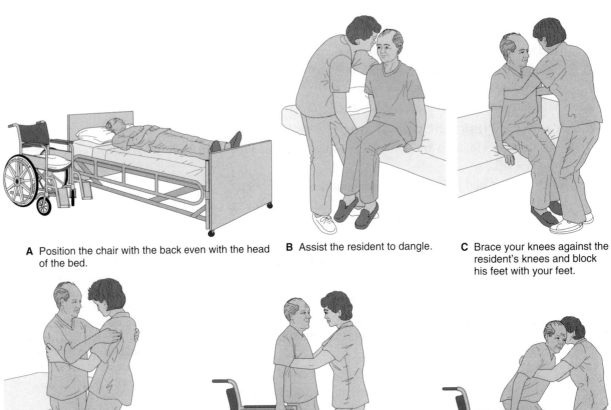

A Position the chair with the back even with the head of the bed.

B Assist the resident to dangle.

C Brace your knees against the resident's knees and block his feet with your feet.

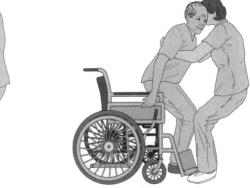

D Bring the resident to a standing position.

E Ask the resident to grasp the chair as you support him.

F Bend your knees as you lower the resident to the chair.

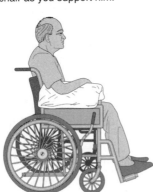

G Use pillows as necessary to position the resident in correct body alignment.

Figure 16–7 Assisting the resident to transfer from the bed to a chair. (Source: From *The Long-Term Care Nursing Assistant* [2nd ed., p. 229], by P. Grubbs and B. Blasband, 2000, Upper Saddle River, NJ: Prentice Hall. Reprinted by permission.)

3. Using a wheelchair:
   a. used for residents who cannot walk
   b. may be manual or motorized
   c. for safety:
      • Check that the chair is in good repair.
      • Lock the brakes when the resident is getting in or out.
      • Back the chair down ramps.
      • Back the chair into elevators.
      • Back the chair through closed doors.
      • Clean the chair regularly and immediately if it becomes soiled.
      • Use pillows to keep the resident in good body alignment.
4. Transferring with a mechanical lift:
   a. a procedure used for residents who are very heavy or unable to move
   b. requires at least two people to perform the procedure safely
   c. protects residents and staff
   d. Always operate a lift according to the manufacturer's guidelines.
   e. Explain the procedure and reassure the resident frequently.
   f. Stabilize the resident and the frame to prevent the sling from swinging back and forth.
   g. Never transport the resident down a hallway in a lift.
   h. Never leave the resident suspended in a lift unattended.
   i. Leave a sling under the resident when he or she is in the chair.
   j. Pad the edges of the sling to protect the resident's skin.

Why?
Backing a wheelchair down a ramp gives you control and prevents the resident from tipping forward and falling out of the chair.

IV. RANGE OF MOTION (ROM)

A. Range-of-motion exercises move each joint in all the ways it normally moves.
1. prevents loss of movement
2. helps to restore movement after illness
3. prevents contractures
4. The number of times each movement is repeated varies according to the resident's condition and tolerance.
5. Use slow, steady motions.
6. Stop if you feel resistance or if the resident complains of pain.
7. Watch the resident's face and body language for signs of pain or discomfort.
8. Report increase or decrease in range of motion to the nurse.

Range of motion—the distance a joint will move comfortably

B. Range-of-motion exercises may be:
1. *active*—done by the resident without assistance
2. *assistive*—done by the resident with assistance from you
3. *passive*—done by you for the resident

C. To perform range-of-motion exercises (see Procedure 16-8 in Appendix A):

1. Give support above and below the joint being exercised.
2. Move the joint in all ways it normally does move.
3. Start the exercise at the neck and work toward the toes:
   a. neck (if instructed by nurse)
   b. shoulders
   c. elbows
   d. wrists
   e. fingers
   f. hips
   g. knees
   h. ankles
   i. toes
4. Body movements and directions include:
   a. *extension*—straightening
   b. *flexion*—bending
   c. *abduction*—moving away from the midline of the body
   d. *adduction*—moving toward the midline of the body
   e. *external rotation*—rolling away from the body
   f. *pronation*—turning down
   g. *supination*—turning up
   h. *hyperextension*—extending beyond a straight line
   i. *internal rotation*—rolling in toward the body
   j. *radial deviation*—moving the hand toward the thumb
   k. *ulnar deviation*—moving the hand toward the little finger
   l. *plantar flexion*—bending the foot downward
   m. *dorsal flexion*—bending the foot upward

Why?
For some residents, moving the neck can be painful or frightening.

V. RESTRAINTS (PROTECTIVE DEVICES)

A. Federal and state laws limit the use of restraints. Unnecessarily restraining a resident is:

1. a violation of the resident's rights
2. abuse
3. false imprisonment

B. Using a restraint requires a doctor's order. The doctor decides:

1. the type of restraint
2. the length of time a resident can be restrained
3. in what circumstance a restraint may be used

C. Using restraints may cause:

1. pressure sores
2. changes in bowel and bladder function
3. weakness
4. loss of ability to move independently
5. illnesses, including pneumonia and blood clots
6. increased anxiety and confusion
7. loss of dignity and self-respect
8. withdrawal

D. Substitutes for restraints:

1. Address behaviors before they become out of control.
2. Reduce loud, disruptive situations.
3. Provide a calm environment.
4. Play calming music.
5. Encourage residents to participate in enjoyable activities.
6. Observe confused residents for signs of frustration.
7. Provide safe areas for residents to walk.
8. Be certain that bed, door, or arm band alarms are functioning.

E. Types of restraints include:

1. *soft belt restraint*—used to prevent the resident from falling out of a wheelchair or bed
2. *safety vest*—used for the same purpose as the soft belt restraint but providing more support than a belt
3. *wrist restraint*—used to prevent the resident from removing dressings or pulling out tubes that are part of treatment
4. *mitt restraint*—used for the same purpose as the wrist restraint, restricting finger movement without preventing movement of the hand or arm
5. *side rail on bed*—considered a form of restraint if it is left up when the bed is in its lowest position after care is complete
6. *sheet tucked under the mattress along the sides of the bed*—restricts the resident and considered a form of restraint

F. Safety guidelines for restraints include:

1. Apply a restraint only if instructed by the nurse.
2. Apply a restraint only according to the manufacturer's guidelines.
3. Visually check the resident every 30 minutes (check wrist restraints every 15 minutes).
4. Remove the restraint every 2 hours and provide exercise, skin care, repositioning, toileting, and fluids.
5. Observe for complications such as skin irritation, injury, restricted circulation, or increased anxiety.

Why?
Using a restraint incorrectly can cause injury or death.

6. Be certain the resident is in proper body alignment.
7. Have the call signal within reach.
8. Communicate with the resident frequently.
9. Accurately document the type of restraint and times of application and removal.

DIRECTIONS
A brief description of a resident is given followed by 10 questions related to the resident. Each question has four possible answers. Read each question and all answer choices carefully. Choose the one best answer.

Mrs. Irene Watkins is 58 years old. She has suffered a closed head injury during an automobile accident. Her left side is paralyzed.

1. Mrs. Watkins has paralysis on one side of her body. This is called:
   A. quadriplegia
   B. poliomyelitis
   C. multiple sclerosis
   D. hemiplegia

2. When preparing Mrs. Watkins to sit on the edge of the bed, you move her to one side of the bed by:
   A. moving her body in sections beginning with the head and shoulders
   B. asking her to slide over to the side of the bed as much as possible
   C. moving her hips, then her shoulders and arms
   D. moving her head first then moving her shoulders

3. Before sitting Mrs. Watkins on the edge of the bed, you should:
   A. unlock the wheels on the bed
   B. put the height of the bed in the lowest position
   C. set the chair on her weak side
   D. raise the bed to a working height

4. When transferring Mrs. Watkins, you position yourself so that her:
   A. paralyzed leg is between your knees
   B. arms can be around your neck
   C. strong leg is between your knees
   D. both legs are between your knees

5. Mrs. Watkins starts to fall. You should:
   A. call for help and try to hold her up until the nurse arrives
   B. step away and let her fall since you can hurt yourself if you try to stop her
   C. try to get a chair behind her so she can sit down
   D. hold her around the waist, pull her close, and slide her down your leg as you sit down

6. Mrs. Watkins is dependent. To prevent the development of contractures, you:
   A. reposition her at least every four hours
   B. move her as little as possible to prevent pain
   C. assist her with range-of-motion exercises
   D. support her body with pillows

7. A contracture is a permanent:
   A. loss of muscle tissue
   B. lesion
   C. spasm
   D. tightening of a muscle

8. To help Mrs. Watkins regain mobility, you encourage her to:
   A. try to transfer herself
   B. assist as much as possible during activities of daily living
   C. see the physical therapist
   D. try harder to walk

9. When Mrs. Watkins's strength and movement of joints improve:
   A. range-of-motion exercises need to be increased
   B. self-care activities will provide range of motion
   C. she should be encouraged to go home
   D. she will be in pain

10. Someone has tucked the top sheet under Mrs. Watkins's mattress along both sides of the bed. Mrs. Watkins is struggling to move. This is a form of:
    A. exercise
    B. mobility
    C. restraint
    D. physical therapy

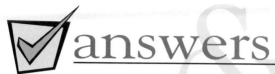

answers & rationales

1.

D. Hemiplegia is paralysis of one side of the body. Quadriplegia is paralysis from the neck down. Paraplegia is paralysis of the lower part of the body. Multiple sclerosis is a chronic disease of the central nervous system that results in many defects including loss of muscle coordination.

2.

A. Before sitting a resident on the edge of the bed, move the resident to the side of the bed where she will be sitting. Move the resident's body in sections from cleanest to dirtiest starting with the head and shoulders, then the waist and thighs, then the legs and feet. This position allows the resident to sit up directly on the edge of the bed instead of dangling from the middle of the bed and having to move forward for her feet to be flat on the floor.

3.

B. Before sitting the resident on the edge of the bed, the height of the bed should be in the lowest position for the resident's safety.

4.

A. When transferring a resident who has hemiplegia, have her paralyzed leg between your knees to stabilize the leg.

5.

D. If a resident begins to fall, grasp the resident around the waist, hold her close to you, and slide her down your leg as you sit down onto the floor. You control the fall and minimize injuries.

6.

C. Range-of-motion exercises help strengthen muscles and prevent contractures. Muscles move joints. Without movement, muscles can shorten and joints can no longer move. Loss of movement results in loss of independence.

7.

D. A contracture is a permanent shortening of a muscle. Muscle atrophy is the loss of muscle tissue. A lesion is an abnormality of the skin, such as a wound, sore, or rash. A spasm is a sudden, involuntary muscle contraction.

8.

B. To help a resident regain mobility, encourage her to do as much as possible with activities of daily living. Self-care helps mobility by moving joints and exercising muscles.

9.

B. As strength and movement in joints increase, self-care activities will provide good range-of-motion exercise for the joints and muscles. Encourage residents to participate in their own care by brushing hair and teeth, dressing, and eating independently.

10.

C. A top sheet tucked under the sides of the mattress to prevent the resident from getting out of bed is a form of restraint. Restraining the resident's movements causes loss of mobility, independence, and self-esteem. Restricting mobility will eventually negatively affect the resident's breathing, circulation, and skin condition.

Personal Care

chapter outline

I. HYGIENE AND GROOMING

A. Hygiene and grooming promote health and well-being by:
1. reducing odors
2. improving circulation
3. promoting comfort

B. While assisting with personal care:
1. Always provide for privacy.
2. Encourage residents to do as much as possible.
3. Offer choices.
4. Observe the condition of skin, scalp, mouth, hair, and nails and report changes to the nurse.
5. Respect cultural differences.

II. BATHING

A. Resident must be fully bathed at least twice per week. Benefits for the resident are that bathing:
1. increases movement
   a. stimulates circulation
   b. reduces chance of skin problems
   c. exercises joints and muscles
2. removes odor and pathogens
3. makes the resident feel clean and comfortable
4. helps the resident relax

B. Types of baths include:
1. complete bed bath
2. partial bed bath
3. tub bath
4. shower

C. Drape and undrape the resident when bathing (see Procedure 17-1 in Appendix A):
1. Raise the side rail, raise the bed to working height, lower the side rail on the side where you are working.
2. Place the drape over top linen and unfold it.
3. Ask the resident to hold the drape or tuck the drape under the resident's shoulders.
4. Roll top linen from head to foot of the bed.
5. Perform the procedure.
6. Cover the resident with top linen.
7. Ask the resident to hold the top linen or tuck it under the resident's shoulders.

Why?
Draping prevents top linen from being soiled, keeps resident warm, and provides privacy.

8. Roll drape from under the top linen to the foot of the bed and remove it.
9. Raise the side rail.
10. Lower the height of the bed and position side rails as appropriate for the resident.

D. Give a complete bed bath. (See Procedure 17-2 in Appendix A.)

1. Gather supplies, including:
   a. bed linen
   b. drape
   c. towels
   d. washcloths
   e. clean gown
   f. waterproof pad
   g. bath basin
   h. soap
2. Offer the resident a urinal or bedpan.
3. Raise the side rails before raising the bed to working height and lower the side rail on the side of the bed where care is being given.
4. Drape the resident and remove the gown from beneath the drape.
5. Fill a bath basin with warm water and ask the resident to check the water temperature.
6. If the resident has open lesions or wounds, put on gloves.
7. Fold and wet a washcloth.

Why?
Water stimulates the urge to urinate.

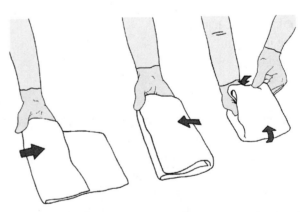

Figure 17–1   (Source: From *The Nursing Assistant* [3rd ed., p. 211], by J. Pulliam, 2002, Upper Saddle River, NJ: Prentice Hall. Reprinted by permission.)

Why?
Using soap will irritate the eye. Washing the eye from the inner corner out reduces pressure and pulling on the eyelid. Using a different part of the cloth for the other eye reduces the chance of spreading infection.

8. Gently wash one eye from the inner corner out. Wash the other eye using a different part of the cloth.
9. Wet the washcloth and apply soap, if requested.

10. Wash, rinse, and pat dry face, neck, ears, and behind ears.
11. Place a towel under the far arm.
12. Wash, rinse, and pat dry hand, arm, shoulder, and underarm.
13. Repeat steps 11 and 12 with the other arm.
14. Place a towel over the chest and abdomen and lower the bath blanket to waist.
15. Lift the towel and wash, rinse, and pat dry chest and abdomen.
16. Pull the drape up over the towel and remove the towel.
17. Place the towel under the far leg.
18. Wash, rinse, and pat the leg dry from hip to foot.
19. Repeat steps 17 and 18 with the other leg.
20. Change the water in the basin.
21. Turn the resident away from you onto his or her side.
22. Wash, rinse, and pat dry from neck to buttocks and turn the resident onto his or her back.
23. Change the bath water, put on clean gloves, and use a clean washcloth and towel.
24. Provide perineal care.
25. Remove your gloves.
26. Wash your hands.
27. Help the resident put on a clean gown.
28. Change the bed linen.
29. Raise the side rail, lower the height of bed and position the side rails as appropriate for the individual resident.

E. Provide perineal care (see Procedure 17-3 in Appendix A).

1. Offer the resident a urinal or bedpan.
2. Assist the resident to a supine position.
3. Gather supplies:
   a. waterproof pad
   b. bath basin
   c. towels
   d. washcloths
   e. drape
   f. soap
4. Drape the resident.
5. Place a waterproof pad under the resident's hips.
6. Fill a bath basin with warm water and ask the resident to check the water temperature.
7. Put on gloves.
8. Assist the resident to spread his or her legs and lift knees, if possible.

Why?
The perineum is delicate and hot water may be drying and irritating.

9. Wet and soap a folded washcloth.
10. If the resident has a catheter:
    a. Check for leakage, secretions, and irritation.
    b. Gently wipe the catheter from meatus out for 4 inches.
11. For females:
    a. Separate the labia.
    b. Wash from front to back with one stroke down the center of urethral area, then one stroke down each side using a different part of the washcloth for each stroke.
    c. With a clean washcloth, rinse in the same direction as when washing and thoroughly pat dry.
12. For males:
    a. Pull back the foreskin if the resident is uncircumcised.
    b. Wash and rinse the head of the penis, beginning at the urethra and washing outward.
    c. Using a clean washcloth, rinse and dry thoroughly.
    d. Put the foreskin of an uncircumcised resident back to its normal position.
13. Continue washing down the penis to the scrotum and inner thighs.
14. Use a clean washcloth to rinse the area and thoroughly pat dry.
15. Assist the resident to turn onto the side away from you.
16. Remove any feces with toilet tissue.
17. Wet and soap a washcloth.
18. Wash from vagina or scrotum to the anal area, using a different area of cloth for each stroke.
19. Rinse and thoroughly pat dry.
20. Remove the waterproof pad and undrape the resident.
21. Raise the side rail, lower the height of the bed, and position side rails as appropriate for the resident.
22. Remove gloves and wash your hands.

F. Assist with tub bath or shower (see Procedure 17-4 in Appendix A):
1. Gather supplies:
    a. towels
    b. washcloths
    c. soap
    d. shampoo
    e. shower chair if needed
    f. shower cap if needed
    g. rubber bath mat

Why?
A rubber bath mat may prevent slips and falls.

      h. personal toilet articles

      i. clean clothing

2. Assist the resident to the bathing area and close the door.

3. Clean the shower area and shower chair or tub.

4. Stay with the resident during the entire procedure.

5. Help the resident to remove clothing and drape him or her with a bath blanket.

6. Turn on the water and ask the resident to check the water temperature.

7. For a shower:

      a. Assist the resident into the shower chair.

      b. Remove the drape.

      c. Push the chair into the shower and lock the wheels.

8. For a tub bath:

      a. Place the bath mat on the floor beside the tub.

      b. Assist the resident into the tub.

9. Let the resident wash as much as possible, starting with the face, and assist him or her as necessary.

10. If directed by the nurse, help the resident to shampoo and rinse his or her hair.

11. For a shower:

      a. Turn off the water.

      b. Give the resident a towel and assist him or her to pat dry.

12. For a tub bath:

      a. Drain the tub.

      b. Help the resident out of the tub into a chair.

      c. Give the resident a towel and assist to pat dry.

13. Help the resident dress, comb his or her hair, and return to the room.

Why?
— Closing the door signals the need for privacy, but keep the door unlocked in case help is needed.
— The resident may become weak when bathing.

Why?
If the resident has hair done by a beautician, hair may not need to be washed or resident may become upset if hairstyle is ruined.

G. Assist in washing the resident's hair:

1. Hair must be shampooed at least once per week.

2. Ask the nurse before shampooing hair because some residents prefer their hair to be done by a barber or beautician.

3. Hair may be shampooed in the shower or bath.

4. Protect the resident's ears and eyes.

5. Massage the scalp while washing hair.

6. Thoroughly rinse shampoo out.

7. Dry hair and style hair according to the resident's preferences.

H. Partial baths are given on days the resident is not completely bathed. Partial baths include:

1. washing hands, face, back, and armpits

2. providing perineal care

I. Give a back rub (see Procedure 17-5 in Appendix A):

1. Gather supplies:
   a. towel
   b. lotion
   c. gloves, if the resident has open areas or rash on skin
2. Raise the side rails before raising the bed to working height and lower the side rail on the side of the bed where care is being given.
3. Turn the resident away from you onto the side and expose only his or her back and shoulders.
4. Rub lotion between your hands to warm it.
5. Apply lotion to the entire back with the palms of your hands.
6. Make long, firm strokes upward along the spine from buttocks to shoulders to relax muscles.
7. Make circular strokes on shoulders, upper arms, and down sides of the back to buttocks to increase circulation.
8. Observe skin, report abnormalities to the nurse, and do not rub reddened areas.
9. Repeat for 3–5 minutes.
10. Gently pat off excess lotion with a towel.
11. Cover the resident.
12. Lower the height of the bed and position the side rails as appropriate for the resident.

Why?
Reddened areas are a sign of decreased circulation and rubbing them may damage skin and underlying structures.

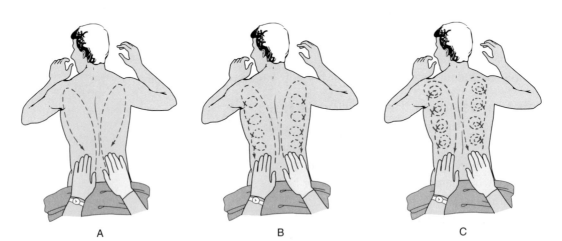

A   B   C

Figure 17–2 (Source: From *The Nursing Assistant* [3rd ed., p. 222], by J. Pulliam, 2002, Upper Saddle River, NJ: Prentice Hall. Reprinted by permission.)

III. ORAL HYGIENE

Why?
Frequent oral care keeps lips and oral tissues moist.

A. Oral care should be given:

1. before breakfast
2. after meals

3. at bedtime
4. more frequently, as often as every two hours, if resident:
    a. has a **nasogastric** tube
    b. is receiving oxygen
    c. is unconscious
    d. is taking certain medications

Nasogastric tube—tube that is inserted through nose into stomach

B. Observe the teeth, gums, tongue, and lips and report to the nurse:

1. unusual bad breath
2. cracked, blistered, or swollen lips
3. bleeding
4. loose, chipped, or broken teeth
5. damaged dentures
6. sores or white patches
7. coated tongue
8. complaints of pain or discomfort

C. When assisting a resident with oral care (see Procedure 17-6 in Appendix A):

1. Gather supplies, including:
    a. emesis basin
    b. towel
    c. toothbrush
    d. toothpaste
    e. mouthwash
    f. glass of water with straw if needed
    g. gloves
2. Place supplies on the overbed table or other clean surface.
3. Raise the head of the bed so the resident is sitting up.
4. Wash your hands and put on gloves.
5. Put a towel under the resident's chin.
6. Ask the resident to rinse the mouth with water and spit into an emesis basin.
7. Wet the brush and put on a small amount of toothpaste.
8. Brush all surfaces of the upper teeth and then the lower teeth.
9. Hold the emesis basin under the resident's chin.
10. Have the resident rinse the mouth with water and spit into the emesis basin.
11. If requested, give the resident mouthwash half diluted with water.
12. Check the teeth, mouth, tongue, and lips for:
    a. odor
    b. cracking
    c. sores
    d. bleeding

Why?
— If resident is lying flat or slightly elevated, fluids may drain down back of throat and cause gagging and breathing problems.
— Moistening the mouth before beginning the procedure prevents cracking and other damage to inside of mouth.
— Brush upper teeth before lower teeth because salivary glands near lower teeth may be stimulated by brushing, will produce too much saliva, and will be uncomfortable for the resident.

e. discoloration

f. loose teeth

13. Remove the towel and wipe the resident's mouth.

D. When giving oral care to the comatose resident (see Procedure 17-7 in Appendix A):

1. Gather equipment:

   a. towel

   b. emesis basin

   c. swabs

   d. cleaning solution

   e. glass of water

   f. padded tongue blade

   g. lubricating jelly

   h. gloves

2. Place supplies on the overbed table or other clean surface.

3. Drape a towel over the pillow and explain what you are doing to the resident.

4. Raise the side rails before raising the bed to working height.

5. Put the bed in its flattest position and turn the resident onto the side.

6. Put on gloves.

7. Place an emesis basin under the resident's chin.

8. Hold the mouth open with a padded tongue blade.

9. Dip a swab in cleaning solution and wipe:

   a. teeth

   b. gums

   c. tongue

   d. all inside surfaces of the mouth

10. Change the swab and repeat as needed.

11. Rinse with a clean swab dipped in water.

12. Check teeth, mouth, tongue, and lips for:

    a. odor

    b. cracking

    c. sores

    d. bleeding

    e. discoloration

    f. loose teeth

13. Cover lips with a thin layer of lubricating jelly.

14. Remove the towel.

15. Place the resident in a comfortable position and in good body alignment.

16. Remove your gloves.

17. Lower the height of the bed and position the side rails as appropriate for the resident.

Why?

Even if unconscious, the resident may be able to hear and understand what you say.

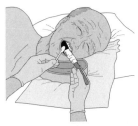

Figure 17–3 A padded tongue blade may be used to hold the mouth open during oral hygiene of the comotose resident. (Source: From *The Long-Term Care Nursing Assistant* [2nd ed., p. 265], by P. Grubbs and B. Blasband, 2000, Upper Saddle River, NJ: Prentice Hall. Reprinted by permission.)

E. When assisting with dentures (see Procedure 17-8 in Appendix A):

1. Gather equipment:
   a. towels
   b. denture cup
   c. emesis basin
   d. denture brush or toothbrush
   e. denture cleaner
   f. mouthwash
   g. swabs
2. Raise the head of the bed so the resident is sitting up.
3. Put on gloves.
4. Drape a towel under the resident's chin.
5. Remove the upper denture by gently moving it up and down with your thumb and forefinger to release suction. Turn the lower dentures slightly to lift them out of the mouth. Never put your finger between the denture and the resident's gums.
6. Put the dentures in the emesis basin and take it to the sink.
7. Line the sink with a towel and fill it halfway with water.
8. Never put dentures in the sink to soak.
9. Apply denture cleaner to a brush, hold the denture over the sink, and brush all surfaces.
10. Rinse the denture in cool water and place it in a denture cup filled with cool water.
11. Clean the resident's mouth with a swab if necessary.
12. Help the resident rinse the mouth with water or mouthwash half diluted with water if requested.
13. Check teeth, mouth, tongue, and lips for:
    a. odor
    b. cracking
    c. sores
    d. bleeding
    e. discoloration
    f. loose teeth
14. Help the resident place dentures in his or her mouth if requested.
15. Remove your gloves.

Why?

— You can scratch and damage the gum with your fingernail, which is very painful and takes a long time to heal.

— The sink is considered dirty and contains pathogens not normally found in the mouth. If you put the denture into the water in the sink, it is grossly contaminated.

— Hot water may cause dentures to change shape and if dentures become dry, they can warp.

IV. HAIR AND NAIL CARE

A. Combing and brushing hair:

1. Encourage residents to comb and brush their hair themselves as much as possible.
2. Never cut a resident's hair.

3. Place a towel over the pillow or around the resident's shoulders.
4. Remove glasses and hair clips.
5. Part the hair in sections and comb from roots to ends.
6. If hair is tangled, work from ends to scalp.
7. Style hair according to the resident's wishes.

B. Nail care:
1. Never perform nail care unless instructed by the nurse.
2. Never trim fingernails or toenails if the resident is diabetic.
3. Before beginning nail care check:
   a. for redness around nails
   b. for bluish color in nail bed
   c. if skin feels too hot or cold
4. If abnormalities are present, report to the nurse before continuing with the procedure.
5. Put on gloves.
6. Fill a bath basin with warm water and ask the resident to check the water temperature.
7. Soak the resident's hands in the bath basin for approximately 10 minutes or as tolerated.
8. Clean under the nails with an orange stick.
9. Dry hands thoroughly.
10. Trim nails straight across with clippers.
11. Gently file edges of nails with an emery board, shaping the nails into a curve.
12. Apply lotion and massage the resident's hands.
13. Remove your gloves.

C. Shaving a resident with safety razor (see Procedure 17-9 in Appendix A):
1. Gather supplies:
   a. towel
   b. washcloth
   c. bath basin
   d. shaving cream
   e. razor
   f. aftershave lotion
2. Raise the head of the bed so the resident is sitting up.
3. Fill a bath basin halfway with warm water and ask the resident to check the water temperature.
4. Drape a towel under the resident's chin.
5. Put on gloves.
6. Help the resident put his dentures in his mouth if necessary.
7. Moisten the beard with a washcloth and put shaving cream over the area.

Why?
Keeping the dentures in the resident's mouth maintains the normal contour of his face and makes shaving easier.

8. Hold the skin taut and shave the beard in the direction of hair growth (downward strokes on the face and upward strokes on the neck).

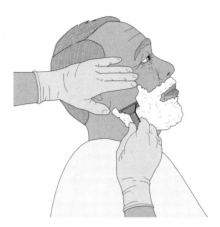

Figure 17–4   Hold the skin taut and shave in the direction that the hair grows. (Source: From *The Long-Term Care Nursing Assistant* [2nd ed., p. 276], by P. Grubbs and B. Blasband, 2000, Upper Saddle River, NJ: Prentice Hall. Reprinted by permission.)

9. Always shave away from your fingers.
10. Rinse the razor after each stroke.
11. Rinse the resident's face and neck and thoroughly pat dry.
12. Apply aftershave lotion if requested and remove the towel.
13. Remove your gloves.

Why?
Shave away from your fingers for safety. Shaving toward your fingers with a razor can cause cuts from a blade contaminated with body fluids.

D. Shaving with an electric razor:
1. *Caution:* Do not use a plug-in razor near a water source or oxygen.
2. If you use a foil head shaver, shave with a back and forth motion.
3. If you use a three-head shaver, shave in a circular motion.
4. Encourage the resident to do as much as possible for himself.

V. CLOTHING

A. Assist the resident to select clothing.
B. When assisting the resident to dress:

Why?
Clothing is a personal choice and affects self-esteem.

1. Remove clothing from unaffected limbs first and dress affected limbs first.
2. Gather sleeves and pant legs before inserting arms or legs.
3. Encourage residents to dress themselves as much as possible.
4. Assist if the resident is becoming frustrated.

5. Encourage the use of restorative personal care and dressing devices.
6. After the resident is dressed, assist with glasses and hearing aids.

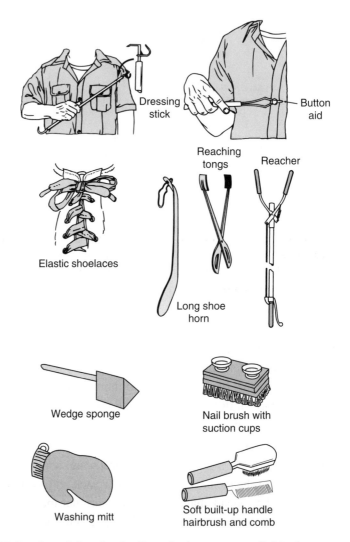

Figure 17–5 A variety of adaptive devices are available for personal care and dressing. (Source: From *The Long-Term Care Nursing Assistant* [2nd ed., p. 278], by P. Grubbs and B. Blasband, 2000, Upper Saddle River, NJ: Prentice Hall. Reprinted by permission.)

VI. DAILY CARE ROUTINES

A. Early morning care is performed before breakfast and includes:

1. oral hygiene
2. washing face and hands

3. toileting
4. straightening unit and linens

B. AM care is performed after breakfast and includes:
1. toileting
2. bathing
3. perineal care
4. oral hygiene
5. care of hair and nails
6. shaving
7. back rubs
8. dressing

C. HS care is performed at bedtime and includes:
1. toileting and perineal care if necessary
2. brushing teeth
3. washing face and hands
4. straightening linens
5. putting on night clothes
6. back rub for relaxation

HS—hour of sleep; bedtime

D. Residents may have their own preferences for care and routines.

DIRECTIONS A brief description of a resident is given followed by 10 questions related to the resident. Each question has four possible answers. Read each question and all answer choices carefully. Choose the one best answer.

Mr. Michael Holland is 73 years old. He has had a stroke and his left arm is paralyzed. He is occasionally incontinent. He has a feeding tube. You help him prepare for bed.

1. Mr. Holland has been incontinent. When doing perineal care, you use a small amount of soap because:
   A. too much soap may be irritating to his skin
   B. he has only been incontinent of urine
   C. you need to do the procedure quickly
   D. you will prevent odor by using talcum powder

2. Mr. Holland is uncircumcised. When doing perineal care, you should:
   A. wash the outer surface of the foreskin only
   B. have the nurse do the procedure
   C. ask Mr. Holland how he wants to be cleaned
   D. retract the foreskin and clean thoroughly

3. Mr. Holland is wearing a shirt that is fastened in the back with Velcro. The shirt is made especially for people who:
   A. are independent and mobile
   B. are confused and pace
   C. spend time in a wheelchair or in bed
   D. do not choose to dress themselves

4. Because Mr. Holland has a feeding tube, when undressing or dressing him you should:
   A. complete the procedure as quickly as possible
   B. be careful with the tube

   C. disconnect the tubes, undress him, then reconnect the tubes
   D. have the nurse do the procedure

5. You help Mr. Holland put on his pullover T-shirt. You should:
   A. put the shirt over his head, then put his arms in the sleeves
   B. put one arm into a sleeve, put the shirt over his head, then place the other arm into a sleeve
   C. put both his arms into the sleeves, grasp the neck opening, and slide the shirt over his head
   D. cut the shirt open in the back, put it on him like a hospital gown, and pin it closed

6. When assisting Mr. Holland, you use a restorative approach with personal care and dressing, which means:
   A. encouraging him to do as much as possible for himself
   B. doing all tasks for him
   C. discouraging the use of adaptive equipment
   D. working as fast as possible

7. You clean Mr. Holland's dentures. If you fail to use precautions and you break his dentures, you may:
   A. have to pay for new dentures
   B. be negligent

C. go to jail

D. be guilty of abuse

8. When performing oral hygiene for Mr. Holland, you observe his mouth for:

    A. bleeding, sores, and coated tongue

    B. skin rash, cracks, and stiffness

    C. swelling of joints

    D. jaundice, cyanosis, and coated tongue

9. When helping Mr. Holland prepare for bed, it is important to:

    A. bath

    B. brush teeth

C. shave

D. care for hair and nails

10. Mr. Holland is ready for bed. He gives you his hearing aid. You should:

    A. place it in a basin of antiseptic solution

    B. soak it in warm water

    C. place it in a container marked with his name

    D. take it to the nurse's station

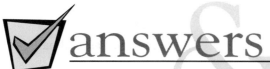

answers & rationales

1.

A. When performing perineal care for the male resident, use a small amount of soap because too much soap could be difficult to rinse off and may dry and irritate his skin.

2.

D. When providing perineal care for an uncircumcised male, retract the foreskin and clean the tip of the penis and the folds of the foreskin thoroughly.

3.

C. Clothing made with Velcro fasteners are used by residents who spend much of the time in bed or in a wheelchair.

4.

B. When dressing a resident who has a feeding tube, be very careful with the tube so it does not become dislodged or displaced. Do not pull on or put pressure on the tube.

5.

C. When assisting a resident with a pullover shirt, help the resident put both hands into the sleeves. Pull the shirt up the resident's arms, then grasp the neck opening and slide it over the resident's head.

6.

A. A restorative approach should be used when assisting a resident with personal care. Always encourage the resident to do as much as possible for himself. Assist as needed and praise even small accomplishments.

7.

B. You may be found negligent if you fail to use precautions such as lining the sink with a towel and filling it half full with water to reduce the chance of breaking dentures if dropped. Dentures are expensive to replace, and replacement may be extremely difficult or impossible for some elderly residents.

8.

A. When helping residents perform oral hygiene, observe the entire mouth including the lips, tongue, gums, and teeth. Check for mouth odor, bleeding of the gums, chapped lips, loose or chipped teeth, sores, or coated tongue. Report any unusual findings to the nurse. Painful problems with the mouth may cause the resident to avoid eating which can result in a poor nutritional status and increased possibility of infection and disease.

9.

B. Before bed, assist the resident with toileting needs. Help the resident wash his face and hands. Give the resident bedtime nourishment if ordered. Provide oral hygiene. Help the resident dress for bed and give the resident a back rub.

10.

C. When hearing aids are not in use, they should be stored in a container marked with the resident's name. Put the container in the resident's bedside stand or at the nurse's station according to facility policy.

CHAPTER

18 Nutrition and Hydration

chapter outline

I. NUTRITION

A. Factors affecting the resident's food choices include:

1. resident's likes and dislikes
2. resident's income
3. medical restrictions
4. culture
5. religious beliefs

B. Nutrition is the intake and use of food by the body.

Nutrient—chemical substance contained in food

1. A well-balanced diet provides all **nutrients** necessary for health.
2. Unmet nutritional needs may cause:
   a. irritability
   b. fatigue
   c. lack of energy
   d. fear and anxiety
3. Nutrients include:
   a. *carbohydrates*—provide energy (found in bread, cereal, pasta, wheat, oats and rice, fruits and vegetables)
   b. *proteins*—aid in growth and repair of tissue (found in meat, poultry, fish, eggs, cheese, milk, peanut butter, dry beans, and whole-grain cereals)
   c. *fats*—provide energy (found in meat, mayonnaise, butter, margarine, oil, and nuts)
   d. *vitamins and minerals*—build body tissue and regulate body fluids
      - *vitamin A*—needed for healthy skin, vision, and mucous membranes; helps fight infection (found in yellow fruits and vegetables, milk, cheese, liver, green leafy vegetables)
      - *B-complex vitamins (B_1, B_2, B_6, B_{12}, and niacin)*—used for digestion, muscle tone, growth, healthy nervous system; help form red blood cells (found in meat, fish, milk, eggs, cereals, bread, green leafy vegetables)
      - *vitamin C*—aids tissue formation, mineral absorption, healthy skin and mucous membranes, fighting infection (found in citrus fruits, tomatoes, strawberries, other fruits and vegetables)
      - *vitamin D*—builds healthy bones and teeth (found in milk, butter, eggs, liver, and bread)
      - *vitamin E*—helps in formation of red blood cells, healthy muscles (found in green leafy vegetables, liver, eggs, vegetable oils)
      - *vitamin K*—helps blood clotting (found in liver, eggs, green leafy vegetables)
      - *calcium*—helps build bones and teeth, muscles, and nerves (found in milk, cheese, sardines, green leafy vegetables)

- *sodium*—regulates body fluids (high amounts found in commercially prepared foods)
- *potassium*—regulates body fluids (found in bananas, oranges, prunes, cranberries, and the juice of these fruits)
- *iron*—necessary for hemoglobin in blood (found in meat, eggs, dry beans, whole-grain cereals, green leafy vegetables)

C. Types of diets include:

1. *regular diet*—balanced diet with no restrictions
2. *mechanical diet*—chopped, pureed, or blended foods if the resident has difficulty chewing or swallowing
3. *therapeutic diet*—special diets ordered by the doctor that eliminate or restrict certain foods

Diet	Description	Foods
Diabetic	Used to treat diabetes mellitus. Carbohydrates, fat, protein, and calories are controlled.	A variety is allowed as long as the calorie and nutrient count is maintained. Candy and desserts should be avoided.
Clear Liquid	Liquids that have no residue. Used after surgery, for nausea and vomiting, and for acute illness.	Water, broth, apple juice, tea, coffee, carbonated beverage, and Jell-O.
Full Liquid	All liquid foods and solids that will melt at room temperature. May be used for residents who have problems swallowing. Next diet after clear liquids.	Clear liquid, plus milk, custard, pudding, cream soup, and ice cream.
Low-Sodium	Used for residents who have heart problems, hypertension, or kidney disease. Restricts all salty foods and those with a high sodium content. Usually, no salt is added to food. Doctor orders amount of salt allowed.	Restricted: salt, ham, bacon, luncheon meat, hot dogs, pickles, mustard, canned soup, and vegetables that are not low-sodium.
Low-Cholesterol	Used for residents with heart disease, gallbladder problems, or a high cholesterol count.	Restricted: eggs, cheese, whole milk, butter, beef, and pork.
High-Residue/Fiber	Used for constipation and other bowel problems. Increase peristalsis and adds bulk.	Whole-grain bread and cereals, cheese, fruits and vegetables— especially green leafy vegetables.

Figure 18–1 Therapeutic diets. (Source: From *The Long-Term Care Nursing Assistant* [2nd ed., p. 307], by P. Grubbs and B. Blasband, 2000, Upper Saddle River, NJ: Prentice Hall. Reprinted by permission.)

D. Residents have the right to:

1. be served food according to their ethnic, cultural, and/or religious beliefs
2. be served food according to their personal preferences

3. be served attractive, tasty food at the correct temperature, in a pleasant environment, in a pleasant manner
4. participate in traditional holiday meals
5. be offered substitutions and snacks

II. ASSISTING THE RESIDENT TO EAT

A. Before serving food, help the resident:
1. with toileting
2. wash hands and perform oral care if needed
3. with grooming
4. with glasses, hearing aid, and dentures if needed
5. to the dining room whenever possible

Why?
The dining room provides an opportunity for the resident to meet social needs.

B. When serving trays:
1. Wash your hands.
2. Check the meal card for the resident's name, correct diet, likes and dislikes.
3. Check the tray for correct food and beverages, condiments, and utensils.
4. Be certain the name on the menu card matches the resident's ID.
5. Offer something else if the resident does not like the food.
6. Unwrap silverware and napkin.
7. Encourage the use of special equipment if suggested by the occupational therapist.
8. Open cartons and remove covers.
9. Offer salt, pepper, and other condiments as allowed.
10. Assist by buttering bread or cutting meat if needed.

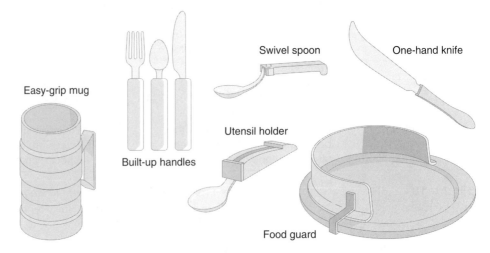

Figure 18–2 Assistive dining equipment. (Source: From *The Long-Term Care Nursing Assistant* [2nd ed., p. 311], by P. Grubbs and B. Blasband, 2000, Upper Saddle River, NJ: Prentice Hall. Reprinted by permission.)

C. Feed the resident (see Procedure 18-1 in Appendix A):

1. Assist the resident with elimination if necessary.
2. Assist the resident to wash his or her hands.
3. Place the resident in a comfortable sitting position.
4. Get the meal tray from the kitchen cart and check the meal card for:
   a. name
   b. diet
   c. likes and dislikes
5. Check the tray for:
   a. correct food and beverages
   b. condiments
   c. utensils
6. Serve the tray with the main course closest to the resident.
7. Sit at the resident's eye level.
8. Describe the food.
9. Place a napkin or clothing protector under the resident's chin and across the chest, if the resident wishes.
10. Ask the resident what food is wanted.
11. Fill the tip of the spoon half full with food.
12. Gently place food into the unaffected side of the mouth.
13. Allow the resident time to chew and swallow.
14. Tell the resident what food is being offered and whether it is hot or cold.
15. Offer fluids frequently.
16. Use a different straw for each liquid.
17. Wipe the resident's mouth as needed.
18. Encourage the resident to help.
19. Remove the napkin or clothing protector and tray.
20. Measure and record intake if directed by the nurse.

Why?
— If you stand over the resident, he or she may have to tilt the head back and bring the chin up to eat; the airway is open; and the resident may inhale and choke on food.
— Always use a spoon to feed because, if you use a fork, you may accidentally poke the resident, causing injury and pain.
— Fluids moisten the mouth and throat and help with swallowing.

D. Report symptoms of swallowing problems to the nurse immediately.

1. Symptoms of swallowing problems include:
   a. difficulty chewing food
   b. repeated coughing or clearing throat
   c. drooling
   d. holding food in the cheeks
   e. weakness of lips or tongue
   f. swallowing several times with each bite
   g. excessively slow eating
2. Use thickening products, if ordered.
3. If the resident has swallowing problems:
   a. Have the resident sit up as straight as possible.
   b. Be patient and give the resident extra time to chew.

Why?
Thickening products are used to increase the resident's ability to control fluid.

c. Check that food is swallowed before offering the next bite.

d. Gently stroke the throat to encourage swallowing.

e. Have the resident sit up for at least 30 minutes after eating.

E. Residents who do not eat well are given supplements.

Supplements—additional feedings or snacks throughout the day according to doctor's orders

F. For restorative dining programs, you should:

1. Have a quiet environment, free from distraction.

2. Use adaptive equipment as needed.

3. Give residents one dish at a time.

4. Use the clock method to identify food for vision-impaired residents.

5. Give one simple direction at a time and repeat them as necessary.

6. Guide the resident's hand with your hand if needed.

7. Allow time for the resident to chew and swallow.

8. Praise the resident.

G. Tube feedings may be ordered if the resident cannot swallow.

1. nasogastric (NG) tube placed through the nose into the stomach

2. gastrostomy (G) tube placed through a surgical opening directly into the stomach

3. Never give food or fluids to a resident with a feeding tube unless directed by the nurse.

III. HYDRATION

A. Fluids:

1. carry oxygen and food to the cells and waste products away from the cells

2. keep body tissues moist

3. help control body temperature

4. help regulate body chemistry and fluid balance

B. Fluid imbalance in the body may cause:

1. **edema**

   a. symptoms:
   - swelling
   - weight gain
   - increased blood pressure
   - wet noisy respirations

   b. treatment:
   - Elevate swollen extremity.
   - Restrict sodium and fluid intake.
   - **Diuretics** may be ordered.

Edema—swelling of the body, usually hands and feet, caused by poor circulation, fluid retention, or medication

Diuretics—medications that increase urination

2. **dehydration**

   a. symptoms:

   - thirst
   - very dry skin
   - pale or ashen skin color
   - sunken eyes
   - dry mouth and tongue
   - dry mucous membranes
   - weight loss
   - decreased urinary output
   - concentrated urine
   - constipation
   - rapid heart and respiratory rate
   - fever
   - irritability, confusion, and/or depression
   - weakness, twitching, or convulsions

   b. Fluid is lost through:

   - urine
   - respiration
   - perspiration
   - feces
   - vomiting
   - diarrhea
   - bleeding

   c. To help prevent dehydration:

   - Offer fluids frequently.
   - Offer residents the fluids they prefer.
   - Place fluids within reach on the resident's unaffected side.

3. Measure fluid intake if ordered.

   a. Fluids include:

   - water
   - all liquid foods
   - tube feedings
   - IV solutions
   - juice
   - milk
   - soup
   - coffee
   - tea
   - all solid foods that melt at room temperature
   - ice chips
   - popsicles

Dehydration—having too little fluid in the body

- ice cream
- sherbet
- pudding
- custard

b. Accurately record fluid intake.

c. Understand equivalent measurements for the metric system.

d. Measure fluid output if directed by the nurse so **fluid balance** may be determined.

Fluid balance—equal amounts of fluid are taken into the body and eliminated by the body

EQUIVALENT MEASUREMENTS

1 cc = 1 ml

30 cc = 1 oz

240 cc = 8 oz or 1 cup

1,000 cc = 1 liter

Figure 18–3 It is helpful to know equivalent measurements for the metric system. (Source: From *The Long-Term Care Nursing Assistant* [2nd ed., p. 325], by P. Grubbs and B. Blasband, 2000, Upper Saddle River, NJ: Prentice Hall. Reprinted by permission.)

DIRECTIONS A brief description of a resident is given followed by 10 questions related to the resident. Each question has four possible answers. Read each question and all answer choices carefully. Choose the one best answer.

Mrs. Ellen Walters has had a stroke and is paralyzed on her left side. You feed her at mealtime.

1. You feed Mrs. Walters lunch in her room. Before bringing in her tray, you should:
   A. clean the room
   B. bathe Mrs. Walters
   C. ask other residents to join her in her room
   D. remove any unsightly or odor-producing articles

2. You place the tray in front of Mrs. Walters and position yourself:
   A. sitting at her eye level
   B. standing over her
   C. directly in front of her
   D. close to the door

3. Before you feed Mrs. Walters, you describe what is on the tray. If she cannot see the tray clearly, you should:
   A. hold the plate up to her face
   B. name each mouthful of food before you give it to her
   C. get another lamp for her room so she can see better
   D. let her smell the food before you put it into her mouth

4. Mrs. Walters is paralyzed on the left side. When feeding her, you place the food:
   A. on her affected side
   B. on her unaffected side
   C. toward the back of her throat
   D. on the tip of her tongue

5. Mrs. Walters tells you that she wants her chocolate cake first. You should:
   A. tell her that you are giving her the cake but put a bite of meat into her mouth
   B. feed her the chocolate cake
   C. argue with her until she does what you want
   D. tell her that she can have one bite of chocolate cake but then must eat the main course

6. You feed Mrs. Walters her meal using:
   A. a spoon for liquids and a fork for solid foods
   B. a spoon that you fill half full
   C. assistive devices
   D. gastric tubes

7. Because Mrs. Walters has difficulty chewing and swallowing, she has a higher risk for choking. This condition is called:
   A. dyspnea
   B. apnea
   C. dysphagia
   D. aphagia

8. Symptoms that may indicate that Mrs. Walters has difficulty swallowing include:
   A. coughing, trying to clear the throat, drooling, and swallowing many times with each bite
   B. hoarding food and chewing quickly

C. tongue thrusts, spitting out food, and refusing to eat

D. gulping food quickly, playing with food, wheezing and sneezing

9. To help Mrs. Walters with chewing and swallowing, her meal may consist of:

A. solid foods that are cooked well-done and very cold liquids

B. liquids that have been thickened and solid foods that are softened or pureed

C. liquid and solid foods that are mixed together

D. solid foods that are cut into small pieces and very warm liquids

10. To minimize the chance that Mrs. Walters may aspirate food or choke after completing her meal, she should:

A. be put in lateral position immediately after finishing the meal

B. be encouraged to get up and walk as much as possible

C. lie flat on her back until her mouth is completely empty

D. sit up for at least 30 minutes after eating

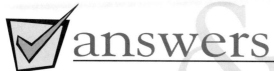

answers & rationales

1.

D. Before feeding a resident, remove any unpleasant or odor-producing items from the area. Unpleasant or odor-producing items may affect the resident's appetite and ability to enjoy mealtime.

2.

A. When feeding a resident, sit at the resident's eye level. If you stand higher than the resident when feeding, the resident may need to tilt her head back and bring up the chin to take the food. This position opens the airway and may cause the resident to choke and aspirate food. If the airway is open, food may enter the airway instead of the esophagus.

3.

B. When feeding a resident who cannot see the tray or recognize the different foods, name each mouthful of food before you give it to the resident.

4.

B. When feeding a resident who has an affected side of the mouth, place the spoon of food on the unaffected side so the resident can control chewing and swallowing better. If the left side of the mouth is paralyzed, place the food on the right side of the mouth.

5.

B. Residents have the right to choose what foods they prefer to eat. If a resident wants to eat dessert first, feed the resident the dessert.

6.

B. Use a spoon when feeding a resident. Fill the spoon half full to prevent giving the resident too much food that can cause choking. The tines of a fork may poke the resident and injure the mouth.

7.

C. Dysphagia means difficulty chewing and swallowing. Dyspnea means difficulty breathing. Apnea means periods of not breathing. Aphagia means the loss of the ability to express oneself usually caused by brain damage.

8.

A. Symptoms that may indicate that a resident is having difficulty swallowing include coughing, trying to clear the throat, drooling, and swallowing many times with each bite.

9.

B. If a resident has difficulty chewing and swallowing, meals may include liquids that have been thickened and solid foods that are softened or pureed to make eating easier.

10.

D. After eating, the resident with problems swallowing should be encouraged to sit up for at least 30 minutes to help food remain in the stomach and move into the intestines.

CHAPTER

Elimination

19

chapter outline

I. ASSISTING WITH TOILETING

A. The body eliminates waste through the:

1. *urinary system*—produces **urine**
2. *digestive system*—produces **feces**
3. *lungs*—eliminate gases (carbon dioxide) during breathing
4. *skin*—eliminates waste through perspiration

Urine—liquid waste product secreted by kidneys through urination

Feces—semisolid waste product eliminated from rectum by defecation

B. Equipment used for toileting includes:

1. bathroom toilet
   a. may have safety bars
   b. emergency signal within reach of toilet
   c. may have raised seat
2. **bedside commode**—used for residents who are weak or have poor balance
3. bedpans—used for residents who cannot get out of bed
   a. *fracture pan*—place flat end under resident; it is more comfortable and has less effect on body alignment
   b. *regular bedpan*—has seat resembling standard toilet seat
4. **urinal**—used by men when urinating

Why?
Raised seat makes use easier and promotes independence.

Bedside commode—portable chair with toilet seat that fits over a container and is used for elimination at the bedside

Urinal—portable container used by male while urinating

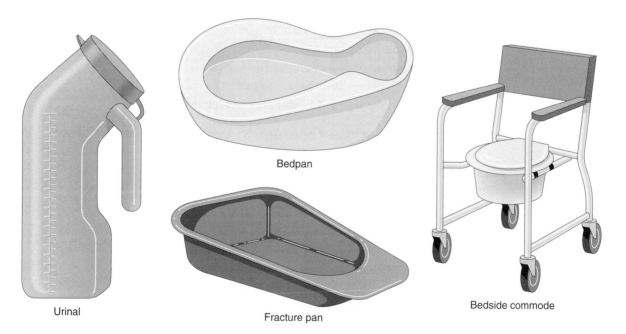

Urinal Bedpan Fracture pan Bedside commode

Figure 19–1 Devices used for elimination. (Source: From *The Nursing Assistant* [3rd ed., p. 252], by J. Pulliam, 2002, Upper Saddle River, NJ: Prentice Hall. Reprinted by permission.)

C. To assist the resident to the bathroom:

1. Walk with the resident into the bathroom.
2. Adjust the resident's clothing and help him or her sit on the toilet.
3. Place emergency signal and toilet tissue within reach.
4. Wash your hands and leave the room.
5. At the resident's signal, return to the bathroom, wash your hands, and put on gloves.
6. Help the resident clean the genital and anal areas.
7. Wipe from front to back.
8. Dispose of gloves, wash your hands, and assist the resident to stand, adjust clothing, and wash his or her hands.
9. Help the resident out of the bathroom and position him or her for comfort.

D. To assist the resident to use a bedside commode:

1. Place the commode next to the bed, open the cover, and be certain that the container is in place.
2. Help the resident onto the commode.
3. Put a blanket on the resident's lap.
4. Put call signal and toilet tissue within reach.
5. Wash your hands and leave the room.
6. At the resident's signal, return to the bedside, wash your hands, and put on gloves.
7. Help the resident clean the genital and anal areas.
8. Wipe from front to back.
9. Dispose of gloves and wash your hands.
10. Help the resident back into bed.
11. Help the resident wash his or her hands.

Why?
The blanket will keep the resident warm and provides privacy.

E. To assist the resident to use a bedpan/fracture pan (see Procedure 19-1 in Appendix A):

1. Lower the head of the bed.
2. Put on gloves.
3. Turn the resident away from you.
4. Place bedpan or fracture pan correctly.
5. Gently roll the resident back onto the pan and check for correct placement.
6. Raise the head of the bed to sitting position.
7. Give the resident call signal and toilet tissue.
8. Leave the resident and return when called.
9. Lower the head of the bed.
10. Press bedpan flat on the bed and turn the resident.
11. Wipe the resident from front to back.

Why?
Press the bedpan flat on the bed before turning resident to stabilize the bedpan so it does not spill as the resident rolls off it.

12. Check urine and/or feces for:
    a. color
    b. odor
    c. amount
    d. character (feces) or clarity (urine)
13. Cover the bedpan and take it into the bathroom.
14. If urine and/or feces is abnormal, save it and report to the supervising nurse immediately.
15. Dispose of urine and/or feces, sanitize the pan, and return pan according to facility policy.
16. Remove gloves and wash your hands.
17. Help the resident to wash his or her hands.

F. To assist a male resident with a urinal:
1. Put on gloves.
2. Give urinal to the resident or place urinal between the resident's legs so the penis is inside the urinal.
3. Put call signal and toilet tissue within reach.
4. Take off your gloves, wash your hands, and leave the room.
5. At the resident's signal, return to the room, wash your hands, and put on gloves.
6. Remove and cover the urinal.
7. Cover the resident.
8. Take urinal into the bathroom.
9. Check urine for:
    a. color
    b. odor
    c. amount
    d. clarity
10. Empty the urine into the toilet.
11. Clean the urinal according to facility policy.
12. Remove gloves and wash your hands.
13. Help the resident wash his hands.

G. Incontinence is the inability to control bladder or bowel function.
1. It may be caused by:
    a. disease
    b. confusion
    c. medications
    d. failure to toilet frequently
    e. nerve damage
    f. poor muscle tone

2. It may cause:
   a. skin breakdown
   b. infection
   c. embarrassment
   d. anger and frustration
   e. depression
   f. withdrawal
   g. fear of "having an accident"
3. Observe for signs that the resident may need to urinate:
   a. restlessness
   b. fidgeting
   c. pulling at clothes or undressing
   d. holding or pointing to the genitals
   e. crying
4. Observe for signs that the resident may need to defecate:
   a. perspiration
   b. goose pimples
   c. holding the abdomen
   d. frowning and straining movements
   e. crying
   f. complaining of fullness or abdominal cramps

II. URINARY ELIMINATION

A. Urine is normally pale yellow with a mild distinctive smell. Observe and report:
1. *color*—ranging from pale yellow to dark amber
2. *odor*—normal to very strong unusual smell
3. *clarity*—clearness of urine; note if urine contains blood, particles, mucus, stones, gravel, or sediment
4. *amount*—measure amount of urine if the resident is on intake and output
5. complaints of pain, burning, or itching in the perineal area

Why?
Complaints of pain, burning, or itching in the perineal area could indicate urinary tract infection.

B. Common urinary problems include:
1. *urinary frequency*—the urge to urinate often while passing only a small amount of urine at a time
2. *urinary urgency*—sudden, strong urge to urinate
3. difficulty starting to urinate
4. *nocturia*—urge to urinate frequently during the night

C. Urinary catheters include:
1. internal catheter
   a. tube inserted through the urethra to the bladder and kept in place by a balloon inflated inside the bladder

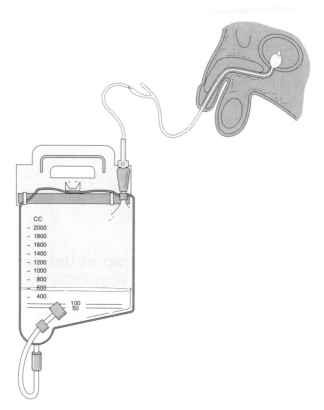

Figure 19–2 A ballon is inflated to hold the urinary catheter in place.
(Source: From *The Long-Term Care Nursing Assistant* [2nd ed., p. 338], by
P. Grubbs and B. Blasband, 2000, Upper Saddle River, NJ: Prentice Hall. Reprinted
by permission.)

b. When caring for a resident with an internal urinary catheter:
  • Keep the drainage tube below the level of the bladder.
  • Keep the catheter and drainage tubing free of kinks and
    pressure.
  • Do not pull on the catheter when moving the resident.
  • Keep the urinary drainage system closed and connected to pre-
    vent infection.
  • Report leaks to the nurse immediately.
  • Attach the drainage bag to the bed frame when the resident is in
    bed.
  • Do not allow the bag or tubing to touch the floor.
  • Use a drainage bag cover if available.
  • Clean catheter tubing during perineal care by washing the tubing
    3 to 4 inches beginning at the **urinary meatus** and working
    down the tube.

Why?
Urine drains from the bladder
by gravity.

Why?
— If urine can get out,
  pathogens can get in.
— Never attach the bag to
  the side rail or any other
  moving part of the bed.
— Allowing the bag to touch
  the floor would cause
  contamination.

Urinary meatus—external
opening of the urethra into
which a catheter may be
inserted

Why?
— Tape that is put completely
around the penis may cause
restricted blood flow, pain,
and injury.
— An external catheter left
on the penis for an excessive amount of time may
cause skin irritation and
infection.
Graduate—container used to
measure fluids

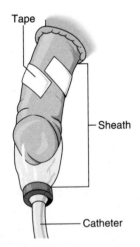

Tape

Sheath

Catheter

Figure 19–3 The ex-
ternal urinary catheter
must be applied and
taped correctly.
(Source: From *The Long-
Term Care Nursing
Assistant* [2nd ed., p.
341], by P. Grubbs and
B. Blasband, 2000,
Upper Saddle River,
NJ: Prentice Hall.
Reprinted by permission.)

2. external catheter—used by male if incontinent
   a. soft latex sheath applied over the penis with a tube leading
      to a urinary drainage bag
   b. When caring for a resident with an external catheter:
      • Wear gloves.
      • Provide perineal care.
      • Roll the sheath onto the penis leaving 1 inch of space at the
        end.
      • Apply tape spirally and do not completely encircle the penis
        with tape.
      • Attach the catheter to drainage tubing and bag.
      • Change it at least daily.

**D. Empty the urinary drainage bag at the end of each
shift. See Procedure 19-2 in Appendix A.**
   1. Collect equipment:
      a. **graduate**
      b. paper towel
      c. gloves
   2. Put on gloves.
   3. Place a paper towel on the floor below the bag and place the graduate
      on the paper towel.
   4. Detach the spout and point it into the center of the graduate without
      letting the tube touch the sides.
   5. Unclamp the spout and drain urine into the graduate.
   6. Clamp the spout and replace the spout in the holder.
   7. Take the graduate to the bathroom and check urine for:
      a. color
      b. odor
      c. clarity
      d. amount—by placing the graduate on a flat surface at eye level and
         noting amount of urine
   8. If urine is abnormal, save it and report to the supervising nurse
      immediately.
   9. Dispose of urine, sanitize the graduate, and return the graduate
      according to facility policy.
   10. Remove gloves.
   11. Wash your hands.

**E. Collect a routine urine specimen. See Procedure
19-3 in Appendix A.**
   1. Gather equipment:
      a. urine specimen container and lid
      b. label

    c. plastic bag for specimen

    d. laboratory requisition slip

    e. gloves

    f. clean bedpan or urinal

    g. plastic bag or wastebasket for disposal of toilet paper

    h. graduate

    i. intake and output sheet, if the resident has an order for intake and output

2. Print the resident's name on a label and put the label on the specimen container.

3. Put on gloves.

4. Ask the resident to urinate into a clean bedpan or urinal.

5. Tell the resident to put used toilet paper in the plastic bag or wastebasket.

6. Cover the bedpan or urinal and take it to the bathroom.

7. If the resident is on intake and output, measure and record the amount of urine.

8. Pour urine into the specimen container, filling the container about three-quarters full.

9. Put a lid on the specimen container and check label for accuracy.

10. Place the container in a plastic bag for transporting.

11. Dispose of urine, sanitize equipment, and return equipment according to facility policy.

12. Remove gloves.

13. Wash your hands.

14. Assist the resident to wash his or her hands.

15. Take the labeled specimen container with the requisition slip to the designated area.

III. BOWEL ELIMINATION

A. Normal feces are soft-formed and brown-colored. Observe for:

1. *color*—ranging from pale brown to black

2. *odor*—normal to very strong unusual smell

3. *consistency*—liquid to very hard; note blood or mucus

4. amount

5. complaints of pain when defecating

B. Common bowel problems include:

1. **constipation**

    a. caused by:

      • lack of fluid and exercise

      • not enough fiber from foods

Constipation—passage of hard, dry stool

Impaction—a large amount
of hard, dry stool

Diarrhea—loose, watery
stool because peristalsis
pushes food too rapidly
through intestines

Why?
A resident who has diarrhea
will need to defecate frequently and urgently.

Why?
Emptying bedpans immedi-
ately reduces odor and prevents spread of infection.

Enema—the introduction of
fluid into rectum and colon

- not taking time to defecate
- medication
- disease

b. must strain to defecate, which may cause pain and bleeding

c. To prevent constipation:
  - Increase fluid and exercise.
  - Offer high-fiber foods to stimulate peristalsis.
  - Answer call signals promptly and assist the resident as needed.
  - Remind the resident to toilet as needed.

2. **impaction**
  a. caused by prolonged constipation
  b. symptoms:
    - pain and nausea
    - swollen, hard abdomen
    - smears of stool on clothing and linen
    - dark liquid feces leaking from the anus
  c. may be treated with enemas or may have to be removed manually by the nurse

3. **diarrhea**
  a. caused by:
    - food
    - medication
    - infection
    - diseases
  b. may result in dehydration
  c. If the resident has diarrhea:
    - Answer call signal quickly.
    - Clean rectal and perineal area to prevent skin breakdown and infection.
    - Empty bedpans immediately.
    - Wear gloves.
    - Record time, amount, and frequency of diarrhea.

C. Enemas, which can only be given with a doctor's order, remove feces and cleanse the lower bowel. See Procedure 19-4 in Appendix A.

CAUTION:

Do Not perform this procedure unless properly trained and authorized. Some states do not permit certified nursing assistants to perform invasive procedures.

1. Gather equipment:
  a. commercially prepared enema or enema bag/bucket with tubing, clamp, and solution ordered by doctor

  b. gloves

  c. lubricating jelly

  d. bed protector

  e. toilet tissue

  f. bedpan

2. If administering a cleansing or oil retention enema:

  a. Prepare solution according to facility policy.

  b. Close clamp on tubing and fill bag/bucket with accurate amount of solution.

  c. Test temperature of solution to ensure that it is neither too hot nor too cold.

  d. Open clamp and allow solution to fill the tubing to remove air and then close the clamp.

3. Position the resident in Sims' position.

4. Protect the bed with disposable pads.

5. Have a bedpan within reach.

6. Keep the resident covered and expose only the buttocks.

7. Put on gloves.

8. Lubricate the tip (2 to 4 inches) of the enema tubing or the tip of a prepared enema with lubricating jelly.

9. Lift the upper buttock to expose the anal area.

10. Slowly insert the tip of tubing 2 to 4 inches using a gentle rotating movement. Stop if there is resistance.

Why?
Never push against resistance because you may injure the resident. Stop the procedure and call the supervising nurse.

11. If administering a cleansing or oil retention enema:

  a. Open the clamp and raise the enema bucket about 12 to 15 inches above the anus.

  b. Allow the solution to flow slowly into the anus.

  c. If the resident complains of discomfort, clamp the tubing and wait a minute or so before continuing the flow of solution.

  d. When the solution is almost gone, clamp the tube and slowly withdraw the tubing.

  e. Place the tubing into the enema bucket and do not allow the tip to come into contact with the bed or floor.

12. If administering a commercially prepared enema:

  a. Squeeze and roll the bottle from the bottom until all the solution is used.

  b. Place the squeeze bottle, tip first, into the original container and discard.

13. Assist the resident onto the bedpan.

14. Encourage the resident to retain the solution as long as possible.

15. Monitor the resident every few minutes.

16. When the resident is through:

a. Wearing gloves, remove the bedpan.

b. Assist the resident to clean the perineal area.

c. Remove the bed protector.

17. Empty the bedpan and observe feces for:

a. color

b. odor

c. amount

d. consistency

18. Remove supplies and clean equipment according to facility policy.

19. Remove gloves.

20. Wash your hands.

21. Assist the resident to wash his or her hands.

Colostomy—a surgical opening into the colon, which allows elimination of feces and flatus through the stoma on the abdomen.

Why?
Each resident may require a different type of care based on specific needs and doctor's orders.

D. Colostomy:

1. is necessary when disease or injury prevents normal elimination

2. To care for a colostomy:

   CAUTION:
   Do Not perform this care unless properly trained and authorized.

   a. Provide care every time the resident has a bowel movement to prevent skin irritation.

   b. Be sensitive to the resident's emotional needs.

   c. Wear gloves.

   d. Carefully and gently remove appliances that are applied to the skin.

   e. Clean around the stoma with soap and water or other solution.

   f. Empty and clean reusable bag with soap and water after each bowel movement.

   g. Observe skin around the stoma for redness and irritation.

   h. Use lubricant, skin protector, or skin cream around the stoma as ordered.

   i. Attach appliances securely to prevent leaking.

   j. Fasten clamp securely when finished.

   k. Observe feces for color, odor, consistency, and amount.

   l. Record and report to the nurse.

E. Collect a stool specimen. See Procedure 19-5 in Appendix A.

1. Gather equipment:

   a. stool specimen container and lid

   b. label

   c. plastic bag for specimen

   d. laboratory requisition slip

   e. gloves

f. clean bedpan

g. plastic bag or wastebasket for disposal of toilet tissue

h. tongue blades

2. Print the resident's name on a label and put the label on the specimen container.

3. Raise side rails before raising the bed to working height, and lower the side rail on the side of the bed where you are giving care.

4. Wash your hands and put on gloves.

5. Have the resident defecate into a clean bedpan.

6. Provide a plastic bag or wastebasket for disposal of toilet tissue.

7. Cover the bedpan and take it to the bathroom.

8. Use a wooden tongue blade to remove about 1 to 2 tablespoons of feces from the bedpan.

9. Take material from different areas of the stool.

   CAUTION: To avoid contamination, DO NOT touch the inside of the specimen container or lid.

10. Put a lid on the specimen container and check the label for accuracy.

11. Place the container in a plastic bag for transporting.

12. Dispose of urine, sanitize equipment, and return equipment according to facility policy.

13. Remove gloves and wash your hands.

14. Assist the resident to wash his or her hands.

15. Take the labeled specimen container with the requisition slip to the designated area.

IV. RETRAINING PROGRAMS

A. Restorative bladder retraining

1. program used to help minimize incontinence and establish a routine of urination at regular intervals

2. requires cooperation of staff and the resident

3. four-step program:

   a. determining normal voiding habits by observing and recording how often the resident voids

   b. establishing a routine based on the resident's voiding habits

   c. evaluating the results

   d. Adjust the routine if incontinence continues to occur prior to scheduled toileting.

Restorative bladder retraining—a program that is used to prevent incontinence and restore urinary elimination to as near normal as possible

B. Restorative bowel retraining

1. Determine a regular pattern of elimination.

2. Establish a schedule.

Restorative bowel retraining—a program used to prevent fecal incontinence, constipation, and other bowel problems

3. Take the resident to the bathroom and assist him or her to sit upright if possible to assist in complete emptying of the rectum.
4. A bowel retraining program includes:
   a. evaluating bowel function
   b. normalizing stool consistency
      • Encourage the resident to eat foods that create bulk.
      • Provide prune juice, orange juice, coffee, and tea.
      • Encourage ambulation and activity.
5. Stimulate the bowel to empty on schedule by using a combination of:
   a. stool softeners
   b. laxatives
   c. suppositories
   d. enemas
6. Retraining may take several weeks to accomplish.

DIRECTIONS
A brief description of a resident is given followed by 10 questions related to the resident. Each question has four possible answers. Read each question and all answer choices carefully. Choose the one best answer.

Mrs. Lonna Craig is 87 years old. She has arthritis. Her call signal is on. When you enter her room she tells you that she needs the bedpan.

1. When you help Mrs. Craig, with elimination, you communicate how you feel about helping her:
   A. with angry actions
   B. by discussing her unpleasant habits with other staff
   C. by telling her how disgusting it is to clean up after someone
   D. with body language and facial expressions

2. You check Mrs. Craig's urine. You notice what might be blood in her urine. You should:
   A. discard it immediately because all blood is infectious
   B. check if Mrs. Craig has an injury near the urethra
   C. save the urine and get the nurse
   D. ask Mrs. Craig if she recently drank any red juice

3. The doctor orders a urinalysis for Mrs. Craig. To collect the urine specimen, you have her urinate into:
   A. the collection bottle
   B. a clean bedpan
   C. a urinal
   D. an external catheter

4. The doctor diagnoses Mrs. Craig with a urinary tract infection. Women are much more likely to develop urinary tract infections because:
   A. bacteria commonly found in the vagina can infect the urethra
   B. women have shorter urethras making it easier for bacteria to get up into the bladder
   C. women have smaller bladders that allow bacteria to grow
   D. women urinate less frequently than men and bacteria stays in the bladder longer

5. The doctor orders an indwelling catheter for Mrs. Craig. She is upset and tells you that she is afraid. You understand that elderly residents:
   A. fear the loss of mobility and independence that may result from having catheter
   B. are afraid of most changes and procedures
   C. pretend to be afraid so you will pay attention to them
   D. should all have catheters to prevent incontinence

6. To help Mrs. Craig with her concerns about being catheterized, you should:
   A. listen to her and explain the procedure in terms she can understand
   B. get the social worker to talk with her
   C. have her family come and be with her during the procedure
   D. ask the doctor to reconsider the order because Mrs. Craig is too upset

7. You assist the nurse who is catheterizing Mrs. Craig. Once the closed system is in place, you make certain that the:
   A. drainage collection bag is emptied every hour
   B. catheter tubing is placed under her leg when she is in bed
   C. drainage collection bag is above the level of her bladder
   D. drainage collection bag and drainage tubing never touch the floor

8. Mrs. Craig has complained of constipation. The nurse tells you to give a commercial oil-retention enema. Mrs. Craig is currently having lunch in the dining room. You should:
   A. administer the enema as soon as she returns from the dining room
   B. go to the dining room and get Mrs. Craig so you can perform the procedure quickly
   C. announce over the intercom that Mrs. Craig needs to return to the unit for an enema

   D. wait one hour after she has eaten before giving the enema

9. You position Mrs. Craig in a side-lying Sims' position for the enema. You never give an enema to a resident who is seated on the toilet or commode because:
   A. you may cause skin breakdown from having her sitting too long
   B. the sitting position does not allow the solution to flow up into the colon
   C. she may stand up and make a mess
   D. you cannot control her as well as when she is lying down in bed

10. Before toileting, it is important that Mrs. Craig retain the oil for:
    A. 3 to 5 minutes
    B. 10 to 20 minutes
    C. 30 to 40 minutes
    D. at least 60 minutes

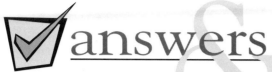

answers & rationales

1.

D. When assisting residents with elimination, you communicate how you feel about helping not only with words but also with body language and facial expressions. Treat residents with dignity, provide privacy, and control your reactions.

2.

C. If you notice any abnormality in the resident's urine, save the urine, and get the nurse immediately. A change in urine may indicate illness.

3.

B. When collecting a routine urine specimen, have the resident urinate into a clean bedpan or urinal. Pour the urine from the bedpan into a specimen bottle marked with the resident's name.

4.

B. Females develop bladder infections more frequently than males because the urethra is much shorter. Bacteria have less distance to travel to reach the bladder and cause infection.

5.

A. Residents who are elderly may fear the loss of independence and mobility that may result from having a catheter.

6.

A. Encourage the resident to talk about fears and reassure the resident. Explain the procedure to the resident in words she can understand.

7.

D. The drainage collection bag and drainage tubing should never touch the floor. The floor is always considered contaminated. Allowing the bag or tubing to touch the floor could cause infection. Empty the bag at the end of each shift or sooner if necessary. Place catheter tubing over the leg when the resident is in bed to prevent skin irritation and pressure on the back of the leg from the tubing. Always keep the drainage bag lower that the level of the bladder. If the bag is above the level of the bladder, urine could flow back up into the bladder and cause infection.

8.

D. Enemas should be administered at least 1 hour after the resident has eaten to avoid upsetting the stomach and prevent vomiting.

9.

B. Residents should not be given enemas while seated on a toilet or commode because sitting up does not allow the solution to flow up into the colon. The solution will remain in the rectum and be released quickly with little or no effect.

10.

B. When given a commercial oil-retention enema, the resident should retain the oil for 10 to 20 minutes before defecating.

Vital Signs and Measurements

chapter outline

I. VITAL SIGNS

A. Vital signs:

1. *temperature*—measurement of the amount of heat in the body
2. *pulse*—measurement of the number of heartbeats per minute
3. *respiration*—measurement of the number of breaths per minute
4. *blood pressure*—measurement of the force of the blood as it pushes against the walls of the arteries

B. Measure vital signs accurately because measurements:

1. are used by doctors when diagnosing
2. are used by nurses to assess a resident's physical condition
3. are used to determine the administration of some medications
4. may be the first indication of infection and illness

C. Report vital signs to the nurse immediately if:

1. you are not sure of a measurement
2. the measurement is very different from the previous one

II. MEASURING TEMPERATURE

A. Body temperature:

1. increases due to:
   a. infection
   b. exercise
   c. warmer external temperature
   d. **dehydration**
2. decreases due to:
   a. **shock**
   b. colder external temperature
   c. age
   d. drugs such as aspirin and acetaminophen

B. Temperature is measured in degrees:

1. **Fahrenheit**, abbreviated F
2. centigrade or Celsius, abbreviated C
3. Average adult temperatures are:
   a. oral: 98.6°F (37°C)
   b. rectal: 99.6°F (37.5°C)
   c. axillary: 97.6°F (36.5°C)
   d. aural (tympanic): 98.6°F (37°C)
4. Report immediately to the nurse if:
   a. oral temperature is at least 100°F or 37.6°C
   b. rectal temperature is at least 101°F or 38°C
   c. axillary temperature is at least 99°F or 37.2°C

Vital signs—measurements used to evaluate a resident's physical condition

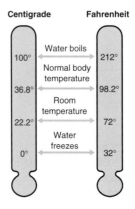

Figure 20–1   A comparision of the Fahrenheit and centigrade temperature scales. (Source: From *The Nursing Assistant* [3rd ed., p. 149] by J. Pulliam, 2002, Upper Saddle River, NJ: Prentice Hall. Reprinted by permission.)

Dehydration—lack of enough fluid in the body

Shock—decreased circulation

Why?
Older people tend to have a lower "normal" body temperature.

Fahrenheit—scale generally used in the United States for measuring temperature

C. Methods of measuring body temperature include:

1. *oral*—most common; thermometer is inserted under tongue. Do not take oral temperature if resident:
   a. is receiving oxygen
   b. is unconscious
   c. has seizures
   d. is vomiting
   e. is confused
   f. breaths through mouth
   g. has cough
   h. has difficulty breathing

2. *rectal*—most invasive; thermometer is inserted into rectum. Do not take rectal temperature if resident has:
   a. diarrhea
   b. a fecal impaction
   c. a rectal disorder or injury
   d. had recent rectal surgery

3. axillary or groin—least accurate; thermometer is placed under armpit (axilla) or in fold of groin. Take axillary temperature if unable to take oral or rectal temperature:

4. aural (tympanic)—accurate; probe is inserted into ear canal. Avoid taking aural temperature if resident complains of earache

D. Types of thermometers include:

1. glass thermometer
   a. NOT frequently used because of risk of mercury contamination
   b. used to take oral, rectal, and axillary temperatures
   c. disinfected according to facility policy and reused

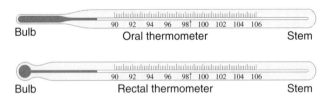

Figure 20–2 Glass oral and rectal thermometers with Fahrenheit scales. (Source: From *The Long-Term Care Nursing Assistant* [2nd ed., p. 285], by P. Grubbs and B. Blasband, 2000, Upper Saddle River, NJ: Prentice Hall. Reprinted by permission.)

2. electronic thermometer
   a. used to take oral, rectal, or axillary temperatures
   b. displays temperature on screen in less than a minute
   c. Probe is covered by disposable plastic cover that is discarded after every use.

Why?
CAUTION:
DO NOT perform rectal temperature unless properly trained and authorized. Some states do not permit certified nursing assistants to perform invasive procedures.

3. aural (tympanic)
   a. inserted into ear
   b. measures body temperature at eardrum
   c. Probe is covered by disposable plastic cover that is discarded after every use.

E. To take a temperature with a glass thermometer (see Procedure 20-1 in Appendix A):

1. Gather equipment:
   a. mercury-free or glass thermometer
   b. tissue
   c. thermometer sheath
   d. watch
2. If the resident has had hot or cold drinks or has been smoking, wait 20 minutes before taking oral temperature.
3. Position the resident comfortably.
4. Rinse the thermometer in cool water and dry with a clean tissue if necessary.
5. Hold the thermometer at the stem end and shake down to below the lowest number.
6. Put on a disposable sheath, if available.
   a. For oral temperature:
      • Place bulb end of thermometer under the resident's tongue and ask the resident to close his or her lips.
      • Leave in place for at least 3–5 minutes or longer.
   b. For rectal temperature:
      • Place the resident in Sims' position.
      • Wear gloves.
      • Lubricate the thermometer.
      • Lift the upper buttock and gently insert the bulb end of thermometer 1 to $1\frac{1}{2}$ inches into the rectum.
      • Hold thermometer in place for at least 3 minutes.
   c. For axillary temperature:
      • Remove the resident's arm from the sleeve of his or her gown and wipe axillary area with a towel.
      • Place the bulb end of thermometer in center of the armpit and fold the resident's arm over the chest.
      • Hold in place for at least 10 minutes.
7. Remove the thermometer, wipe with tissue from stem to bulb end, or remove sheath and dispose of tissue and sheath.
8. Hold thermometer by the stem end at eye level and slowly rotate it until a line appears. Accurately read and note the temperature.
9. Shake down the thermometer. Clean and store the thermometer according to facility policy.

Why?
Hot or cold drinks and smoking change the surface temperature inside the mouth and will give an inaccurate reading.

Why?
If you hold the stem end of the thermometer, your body heat can alter the temperature.

10. Remove gloves and wash your hands.

11. Report an unusual reading to the supervising nurse immediately.

12. Document the procedure according to facility policy.

F. To take a temperature with an electronic thermometer (see Procedure 20-2 in Appendix A):

1. Assemble equipment:
   a. battery-operated electronic thermometer
   b. attachment (blue for oral, red for rectal)
   c. disposable probe covers
   d. gloves, if necessary

2. If the resident has had hot or cold drinks or has been smoking, wait 20 minutes before taking an oral temperature.

3. Position the resident comfortably.

4. Remove the appropriate probe from its stored position and insert it into the thermometer.

5. Place the probe cover on the probe.
   a. For oral temperature:
      • Place probe under the resident's tongue and ask him or her to close lips.
      • Leave in place until the electronic thermometer beeps or flashes.
   b. For rectal temperature:
      • Place the resident in Sims' position.
      • Wear gloves.
      • Lubricate the thermometer.
      • Lift the upper buttock and gently insert probe $\frac{1}{2}$ inch into rectum.
      • Lower upper buttock and hold the thermometer in place until the electronic thermometer beeps or flashes.
   c. For axillary temperature:
      • Remove the resident's arm from the sleeve of his or her gown and wipe axillary area with a towel.
      • Place the probe of the thermometer in the center of the armpit and fold the resident's arm over the chest.
      • Leave in place until the electronic thermometer beeps or flashes.

6. Read the temperature on the digital display.

7. Eject probe cover into a wastebasket without touching it and replace the probe in the holder.

8. Remove your gloves and wash your hands.

9. Return the probe to its stored position. Return the thermometer unit to its storage location.

10. Report any unusual reading to the supervising nurse immediately.

11. Document the procedure according to facility policy, labeling R for rectal temperature and A or Ax for axillary temperature.

G. To take a temperature with a tympanic thermometer (see Procedure 20-3 in Appendix A):

1. Gather equipment:
   a. battery-operated tympanic thermometer
   b. disposable probe cover
   c. watch
2. Check that the probe is connected to the unit.
3. Insert the cone-shaped end of the thermometer into a probe cover.
4. Position yourself so the resident's ear is directly in front of you.
5. Gently pull ear up and back and insert the probe into the ear canal as far as possible to seal the ear canal.
6. Leave in place until the electronic thermometer beeps or flashes.
7. Remove the probe from the resident's ear.
8. Accurately note temperature on the digital display.
9. Eject the probe cover into the wastebasket without touching it and re-place the probe in the holder.
10. Return the tympanic thermometer to the battery charger or base unit.
11. Report an unusual reading to the supervising nurse immediately.
12. Document the procedure according to facility policy.

III. MEASURING PULSE AND RESPIRATIONS

A. Pulse:

1. Affected by:
   a. illness
   b. mobility
   c. medications
   d. position of body
   e. stress
2. Note:
   a. *rate*—number of beats per minute
   b. *rhythm*—if the beats are regular or irregular
   c. *force*—the strength of the beat:
      • weak
      • hard to feel
      • strong
      • very full (bounding)
3. Normal range of pulse:
   a. *children*—80 to 115 beats per minute
   b. *adults*—72 to 80 beats per minute
   c. *elderly*—60 to 70 beats per minute
4. Report abnormal pulse including:
   a. rate of under 60 or over 90 beats per minute

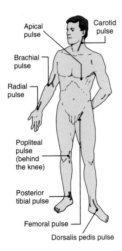

Figure 20–3 Pulse points. (Source: From *The Nursing Assistant* [3rd ed., p. 155] by J. Pulliam, 2002, Upper Saddle River, NJ: Prentice Hall. Reprinted by permission.)

b. changes from previous readings

c. an irregular, weak, or bounding pulse

5. Sites for pulses include:

   a. radial pulse at wrist

   b. apical pulse over apex of heart

   c. brachial pulse at bend of elbow

B. Respirations:

1. Affected by:

   a. stress

   b. mobility

   c. hot and cold

   d. medications

   e. illness

2. Note:

   a. *rate*—how many respirations per minute

   b. *rhythm*—if breaths are regular or irregular

   c. *character*—if respirations are:

   - shallow

   - deep

   - labored (difficult)

3. Normal range of respiration rate—12 to 20 breaths per minute

4. Report abnormal respirations to the nurse immediately:

   a. uneven breathing

   b. rapid breathing

   c. complaints of shortness of breath or pain upon respiration

   d. abnormal noises (snoring, gurgling) when breathing

   e. gasping

   f. blue color to skin, especially around lips, nose, or fingernails

C. Always count pulse and respirations for a full 60 seconds if the resident has:

1. irregular heartbeat

2. difficulty breathing

3. diagnosed heart diseases or abnormalities

4. diagnosed respiratory diseases or abnormalities

5. chronic illnesses

6. limited mobility

7. diabetes

8. stroke

9. previous circulatory problems

D. To take the resident's radial pulse and respiration rate (see Procedure 20-4 in Appendix A):

1. Use a watch with a second hand.

2. Place the resident's hand on a comfortable surface.

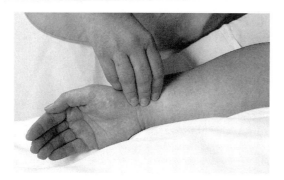

Figure 20–4 (Source: From *The Nursing Assistant* [3rd ed., p. 156], by J. Pulliam, 2002, Upper Saddle River, NJ: Prentice Hall. Reprinted by permission.)

3. Feel for a pulse on the thumb side of the wrist with the tips of your first three fingers.
4. Count beats for 60 seconds and note:
   a. *rate*—number of beats
   b. *rhythm*—regularity of beats
   c. *force*—strength of beats
5. Continue holding the wrist as if feeling for a pulse.
6. Count each rise and fall of the chest as one respiration.
7. Count respirations for 60 seconds, noting:
   a. *rate*—number of breaths
   b. *regularity*—pattern of breathing
   c. *sound*—shallowness or depth of breathing
8. Accurately note pulse and respiration rates.
9. Report an unusual reading to the supervising nurse immediately.
10. Document the procedure according to facility policy.

Why?
Never use your thumb to take a pulse. It has its own pulse that might be confused with the resident's and result in an inaccurate reading.

Why?
If the resident knows that you are counting respirations, the breathing pattern and rate may change voluntarily or involuntarily.

E. To take the resident's apical pulse:
1. Clean earpieces and diaphragm of a stethoscope.
2. Turn earpieces slightly forward to fit snugly into your ears.
3. Put diaphragm of the stethoscope flat against the skin on the left side of the chest under the left breast, just below the left nipple.
4. Count heartbeats for one full minute.
5. Record pulse rate and label Ap next to the rate to indicate apical pulse.
6. Clean earpieces and diaphragm of the stethoscope with antiseptic wipes.

IV. MEASURING BLOOD PRESSURE

A. Blood pressure:
1. Affected by:
   a. age
   b. body size

    c. emotions

    d. pain and illness

    e. heredity

    f. exercise

    g. diet

    h. medications

    i. condition of the blood vessels

    j. volume of blood in the system

2. Note:

    a. *systolic pressure*—highest pressure, which measures the pressure of the blood during the heart's contraction

    b. *diastolic pressure*—lowest pressure, which measures the blood flowing during the heart's relaxation

3. Normal range of blood pressure:

    a. systolic: 100–140

    b. diastolic: 60–90

4. Problems with blood pressure:

    a. *hypertension*—abnormally high blood pressure

    b. *hypotension*—abnormally low blood pressure

B. Equipment for measuring blood pressure includes:

1. sphygmomanometer (blood pressure cuff), made up of:

    a. cuff

    b. tubes

    c. bulb to inflate cuff

    d. manometer or gauge

2. stethoscope—magnifies the sounds of the pulse at the inner elbow (brachial artery)

C. To take a blood pressure reading (see Procedure 20-5 in Appendix A):

1. Gather equipment:

    a. antiseptic wipe

    b. stethoscope

    c. sphygmomanometer

2. Have the resident rest for approximately 15 minutes before taking blood pressure.

3. Clean earpieces and diaphragm of the stethoscope with an antiseptic wipe.

4. Uncover the resident's arm to the shoulder.

5. Rest the resident's arm, level with the heart, palm upward, on a comfortable surface.

6. Wrap the cuff around the upper unaffected arm approximately 1–2 inches above the elbow.

Why?

— Place the cuff on skin, not over clothing, for the most accurate reading.

— Avoid taking blood pressure on the affected arm (with a wound, cast, IV, paralyzed, or has skin problems) to prevent further injury and pain.

7. Put earpieces of the stethoscope snugly into your ears.
8. Locate the brachial pulse with your fingertips at the bend of the elbow.
9. Place diaphragm of the stethoscope over the brachial artery and hold it firmly in place, being sure that the stethoscope does not touch the cuff.
10. Close the valve on the bulb:
    a. If blood pressure is known, inflate the cuff to 30 mm/hg above the usual systolic reading.
    b. If blood pressure is unknown, inflate the cuff to 160 mm/hg.
11. Slowly open valve on the bulb.
12. Watch the gauge and listen for the sound of a pulse.
13. Note gauge reading at the first pulse sound.
14. Note gauge reading when the pulse sound disappears.
15. Completely deflate and remove the cuff.
16. Accurately note systolic and diastolic readings.
17. Clean earpieces and diaphragm of the stethoscope with an antiseptic wipe.
18. Report an unusual reading to the supervising nurse immediately.
19. Document procedure according to facility policy.

Why?
The pressure of the stethoscope on the inflating cuff can alter the reading.

Why?
NOTE:
If you are unable to hear sounds, completely deflate cuff, wait 1 minute for normal circulation to be reestablished, and begin again. **DO NOT** inflate cuff that has been partially deflated because reading will not be accurate, and the skin and underlying structures may be damaged, causing bruising.

V. MEASURING WEIGHT AND HEIGHT

A. Weight may be affected by:
1. medications
2. fluid balance
3. disease
4. diet

B. Weigh residents:
1. at the same time of the day
2. wearing the same type of clothing
3. using the same scale

C. Types of scales include:
1. standing scale
2. mechanical lift scale
3. wheelchair platform scale

D. When weighing the resident:
1. Balance the scale.
2. Depending on the scale used:
   a. Assist the resident to stand on the platform.
   b. Have the resident sit in the chair with feet on the footrest.
   c. Transport wheelchair onto the scale and lock the brakes.

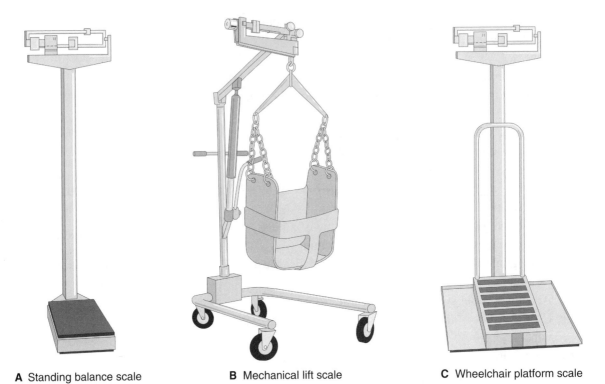

A Standing balance scale   **B** Mechanical lift scale   **C** Wheelchair platform scale

Figure 20–5 A. Standing balance scale. B. Mechanical liftscale. C. Wheelchair platform-scale. (Source: From *The Long Term Care Nursing Assistant* [2nd ed., p. 258], by P. Grubbs and B. Blasband, 2000, Upper Saddle River, NJ: Prentice Hall. Reprinted by permission.)

3. When using a standard scale:
   a. Move the lower weight to the pound mark that causes arm to drop; then move weight back one mark.
   b. Move the upper weight to pound mark that balances the pointer in the middle of the square.
   c. Add lower and upper numbers to determine accurate weight.
   d. Accurately note resident's weight.
4. When using a digital scale:
   a. Press the weigh button.
   b. Wait until numbers remain constant.
   c. Accurately note the resident's weight.
5. If weighing a resident in a wheelchair, subtract the weight of the wheelchair from the total weight.

E. The resident's height:
   1. usually only taken upon admission
   2. If the resident is able to stand:
      a. Take the resident to the standing scale.
      b. Raise height bar above the level of the resident's head.

    c. Have the resident stand with his or her back against the measuring bar.

    d. Lower bar until it touches the top of the resident's head.

    e. Record height.

    f. Assist the resident off the scale.

3. If the resident is not able to stand:

    a. Help the resident into supine position.

    b. Mark at top of head and at feet.

    c. Measure the distance between marks with a tape measure.

DIRECTIONS

A brief description of a resident is given followed by 10 questions related to the resident. Each question has four possible answers. Read each question and all answer choices carefully. Choose the one best answer.

Mr. Jeffrey Patrick is 85 years old. He is diagnosed with hypertension. He is being admitted to the facility.

1. The nurse tells you to take Mr. Patrick's vital signs. The correct abbreviation for vital signs is:
   A. RPT and BP
   B. PRT and BP
   C. TPR and BP
   D. T&P and BP

2. Mr. Patrick is drinking hot coffee. Before taking his oral temperature you:
   A. give him a glass of ice water, then take his temperature
   B. ask him to avoid hot or cold drinks and return in 15 minutes
   C. wait 3 to 5 minutes and then take his temperature
   D. take his temperature rectally

3. You take Mr. Patrick's temperature with an electronic thermometer. After removing the probe from his mouth, you should:
   A. discard the probe cover
   B. shake the thermometer several times
   C. ask Mr. Patrick if he can speak or cough
   D. provide oral care

4. You take Mr. Patrick's radial pulse, which is located:
   A. on the thumb side of the wrist
   B. on the left side of the chest
   C. at the bend of the elbow
   D. on the side of the neck

5. When taking Mr. Patrick's pulse, you note the pulse force, which is:
   A. the number of beats per minute
   B. the regularity of the pulse beats
   C. whether the beat is weak or bounding
   D. whether the beats are labored or shallow

6. You take Mr. Patrick's respiration rate. You count:
   A. every beat you hear
   B. the systolic sound
   C. the amount of heat in his body
   D. each rise and fall of the chest as one respiration

7. If Mr. Patrick knows that you are taking his respirations, he may not breathe naturally. You should:
   A. leave your fingers on his wrist after taking the pulse and count the respirations
   B. watch his respirations from the other side of the room
   C. ask him to close his eyes so he cannot see you
   D. leave the room and watch him breathe from the hallway

8. When you take Mr. Patrick's blood pressure, you wrap the cuff:
   A. around his wrist
   B. below his elbow
   C. at least 1 inch above his elbow
   D. over his elbow

9. You weigh Mr. Patrick. Knowing his weight helps the health care team:

A. monitor his nutritional status

B. calculate his vital signs

C. determine a prognosis

D. decide on an exercise program for him

10. You measure Mr. Patrick's height:

A. upon admission

B. upon admission and then monthly

C. upon admission and daily

D. weekly

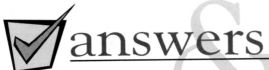

answers & rationales

1.

C. Vital signs include temperature, pulse, and respiration (TPR) and blood pressure (B/P).

2.

B. Ask the resident to avoid eating or drinking and return in 15 minutes to take his temperature. Eating and drinking can alter an oral temperature reading.

3.

A. After taking the resident's temperature with an electronic thermometer, discard the probe cover by ejecting it directly into a waste receptacle. The probe cover is contaminated and should not be touched or reused to prevent the spread of infection.

4.

A. The radial pulse is taken on the thumb side of the wrist. The apical pulse is taken on the left side of the chest under the breast. The brachial pulse is taken at the bend of the elbow. The carotid pulse is taken at the neck.

5.

C. When taking a resident's pulse, observe and report the force of the beat. The force or strength of the pulse will vary from weak to strong or bounding.

6.

D. Count one respiration each time the chest of the resident rises and falls. Count for a full 60 seconds.

7.

A. When counting a resident's respirations, leave your fingers on the wrist after taking the pulse. If the resident is unaware that you are counting his respirations, he will breathe naturally.

8.

C. When you take a resident's blood pressure, wrap the cuff of the sphygmomanometer around the arm at least 1 inch above the elbow. The cuff should not cover the elbow nor should the bladder of the stethoscope be put beneath the cuff. This will cause the reading to be inaccurate.

9.

A. The resident's weight is taken at admission, and at least monthly afterward, to help the health care team monitor the resident's nutritional status. Also, many medication doses are calculated according to weight.

10.

A. The nursing assistant may measure the resident's height during admission to provide a baseline for calculating nutritional needs and medication doses.

21 Restorative Care

I. PRINCIPLES OF RESTORATIVE CARE

A. Restorative care is routine care provided in a way that helps residents attain and maintain their highest level of function and independence.
1. Focus during care is on fostering independence and improving quality of life.
2. Principles of restorative care include:
   a. Treat the whole person.
   b. Meet physical, mental, emotional, social, sexual, and spiritual needs.
   c. Treat each resident as an individual.
3. Encourage activity to:
   a. strengthen mind and body
   b. improve bodily functions
   c. improve mental alertness
   d. prevent depression and withdrawal
   e. increase independence

B. Rehabilitation is a combination of methods determined by therapists to help residents attain maximum physical functioning.
1. needed by residents with impairments or disabilities
2. The rehabilitation process:
   a. encourages independence
   b. emphasizes abilities, not disabilities
   c. provides therapies to promote physical function and strength
3. The rehabilitation team:
   a. includes all members of the health care team
   b. *physical therapists*—help residents strengthen muscles and regain physical independence
      • evaluate muscle strength and mobility
      • develop approaches to help residents regain muscle strength and mobility
      • measure, fit, and help residents to use prosthesis
      • teach the use of canes, crutches, and walkers
   c. *occupational therapists*—help residents improve performance of activities of daily living.
      • evaluate abilities
      • help residents relearn skills or develop new skills
      • recommend equipment that helps residents function with a disability
   d. *speech therapists*—work with residents who have communication problems

- plan and direct treatment of residents with speech impairments
- work with residents with swallowing disorders
- work with residents who have hearing loss

4. The role of the nursing assistant in rehabilitation includes:
   a. Encourage independence when residents are performing activities of daily living.
   b. Prepare residents for and transport residents to occupational, physical, or speech therapy.
   c. Encourage rest between therapy sessions if needed.
   d. Do range-of motion exercises as instructed by the nurse.
   e. Observe and report resident's condition and progress to the nurse.
   f. Be supportive and praise residents' efforts.

II. RESTORATIVE PROGRAMS

A. Restorative programs:

1. are developed to meet the needs of residents who have difficulty performing activities of daily living
2. include:
   a. personal care and grooming programs
   b. restorative dining programs
   c. bowel and bladder programs
   d. range-of-motion exercise programs
   e. ambulation programs
   f. communication programs

B. Personal care and grooming programs:

1. help residents become more independent with grooming needs
2. Assistive devices include:
   a. electric toothbrushes
   b. suction toothbrushes
   c. long-handled combs, brushes, and sponges
   d. long-handled shoehorns
   e. buttonhooks
   f. sock pullers
   g. zipper pullers
3. When assisting:
   a. Encourage choice.
   b. Offer assistance if the resident becomes frustrated.
   c. Assist the resident to look in the mirror after finishing grooming tasks.

C. Restorative dining programs:

1. help residents learn to become more independent when eating
2. When assisting:
   a. Arrange equipment and food within the resident's reach.
   b. Encourage the resident to try.
   c. Offer finger foods.
   d. Don't point out mistakes.

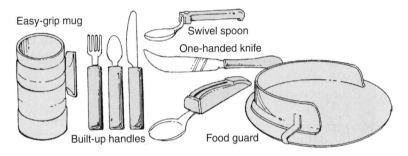

Figure 21–1 Assistive eating devices include mugs designed for easy gripping, silverware with built-up or curved handles, and plates with a food guard attached so patients can push food against it. (Source: From *The Nursing Assistant* [3rd ed., p. 284], by J. Pulliam, 2002, Upper Saddle River, NJ: Prentice Hall. Reprinted by permission.)

D. Bowel and bladder programs:

1. help to restore control of bowel and bladder functioning
2. Review bowel and bladder retraining in Chapter 19, *Elimination.*

E. Range-of-motion exercise programs:

1. help improve mobility
2. Review range-of-motion exercises in Chapter 16, Movement and Mobility.

F. Ambulation programs:

1. help residents increase or maintain the ability to walk
2. Supportive devices for walking include:
   a. walkers
   b. canes
   c. crutches
   d. braces
3. Review ambulation in Chapter 16, Movement and Mobility.
4. When assisting:
   a. Offer to assist the resident to walk frequently or as ordered.
   b. Be positive and encouraging.

c. Allow the resident to do as much as possible.
d. Understand the use of supportive devices for walking.

G. Communication programs:
1. are individually developed for residents who have sight, hearing, or speech impairments
2. When assisting:
    a. Follow the program as outlined in the care plan.
    b. Report to the nurse if you are unable to understand residents' requests.
    c. Be positive and supportive.
    d. Be empathetic.
    e. Speak slowly and clearly.

III. RESTORATIVE ENVIRONMENT

A. A restorative environment promotes independence because the room is arranged to foster self-care.
1. Position furniture and personal care items in safe, convenient places.
2. Have the call signal within reach at all times.
3. Position the bed at its lowest height.
4. Always provide for privacy.
5. Keep the room clean and free of clutter.
6. Encourage and help the resident to display personal possessions to make the room homelike and familiar.

B. A restorative environment fosters wellness by encouraging independence, reducing stress, and improving trust.
1. Know the signs and symptoms of disease and report to the nurse immediately if you note them in the resident.
2. Be certain the resident is clean and neat.
3. Keep the environment and resident safe.
4. Follow infection control policies and standard precautions to lessen the chance of infection.
5. Encourage the resident to eat and drink to maintain good nutrition and adequate fluids.
6. Prevent the resident from becoming overly tired, which may result in accidents and lower resistance to disease.
7. Provide continuity of care.

DIRECTIONS A brief description of a resident is given followed by 10 questions related to the resident. Each question has four possible answers. Read each question and all answer choices carefully. Choose the one best answer.

Mr. John Baldwin is 73 years old. He is recovering from injuries he received during an automobile accident. His left leg was amputated and he wears a prosthesis.

1. When caring for Mr. Baldwin, it is most important that you:
   A. tell him frequently how sorry you are that he lost his leg
   B. tell him that you do not believe that the accident was his fault
   C. perform all procedures for him so he can rest and recuperate
   D. encourage him to do as much as possible for himself

2. When you help Mr. Baldwin clean the prosthesis, you should:
   A. soak the prosthesis in hot water and disinfectant solution
   B. have the physical therapist teach you how to clean the leg
   C. ask Mr. Baldwin how to clean the leg and follow his instructions
   D. call housekeeping and they will clean the prosthesis

3. You notice that the foot of Mr. Baldwin's prosthesis is damaged. You should:
   A. report the damage to the nurse
   B. tell Mr. Baldwin that he should be careful because something is wrong with the artificial leg
   C. inform him that the prosthesis is very expensive and he needs to be more aware of how he is using it
   D. call maintenance and have them fix the prosthesis

4. You assist Mr. Baldwin to take a whirlpool bath. This type of bath is of most benefit for him because it will help:
   A. stimulate circulation to the stump
   B. help him relax
   C. remove dirt without having to use a washcloth
   D. prevent injury to the stump

5. When using a whirlpool tub, you should always:
   A. use a mechanical lift to get Mr. Baldwin into the tub
   B. have another CNA train you in the use of the tub
   C. put soothing medications into the water
   D. follow the manufacturer's guidelines for use of the tub

6. The whirlpool bath is used by several residents as a way to cleanse wounds. Special infection control procedures are necessary when sanitizing the tub to prevent:
   A. the spread of scabies
   B. the spread of infection
   C. upper respiratory infections
   D. skin cancer

7. You assist Mr. Baldwin with range-of-motion exercises. He can do most of the exercises himself. You help him only when necessary. This type of range-of-motion exercise is called:

A. active

B. passive

C. assistive

D. active assistive

8. When doing the exercise, you notice that Mr. Baldwin's knee is swollen and reddened. You would:

   A. stop the exercise and report to the nurse

   B. have Mr. Baldwin move the knee as much as possible to reduce the swelling

   C. do the exercise but stop when Mr. Baldwin complains of pain

   D. just push the joint to the point of resistance

9. Mr. Baldwin does most of his ADLs without assistance. When his family is visiting, his wife dresses him, his daughter feeds him, and his son lifts him. You should:

   A. tell them that they are harming him by making him dependent

   B. understand that, in his culture, the family is expected to provide care

   C. get the physical therapist to talk with the family about their actions

   D. tell Mr. Baldwin to stop acting so dependent and start doing things for himself

10. You answer Mr. Baldwin's call signal. He says that he has pain in the amputated leg. He says that the pain is severe and begins to cry. You should:

   A. listen with empathy

   B. ask Mr. Baldwin to tell you where it hurts

   C. have Mr. Baldwin exercise the stump to try to relieve the pain

   D. understand that the pain is phantom limb pain and get the nurse

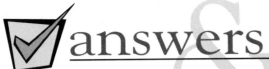

answers & rationales

1.

D. The nursing assistant's role in restorative care is to encourage residents to do as much as they can for themselves.

2.

C. To care for a resident's prosthesis, ask the resident for instructions whenever possible. The resident has been trained in the best way to take care of the prosthesis.

3.

A. Check the resident's prosthesis for wear and damage. Report any problems to the nurse immediately. A damaged prosthesis can cause an accident and injury.

4.

A. The whirlpool bath may be used to stimulate circulation to the stump of the amputated leg. Whirlpool baths are a form of therapy.

5.

D. Always follow the manufacturer's guidelines for use of the whirlpool tub. The resident may be injured if equipment is not used properly.

6.

B. Special infection control procedures must be followed to properly clean and sanitize the whirlpool between baths. Open wounds are treated with whirlpool therapy and there is a potential for the spread of infection.

7.

D. The nursing assistant helps, when necessary, with active assistive ROM exercises. The resident moves the limbs through as much range-of-motion as possible and the nursing assistant helps with the rest.

8.

A. If the resident's knee is swollen and reddened, do not exercise the joint. Report to the nurse immediately.

9.

B. As a nursing assistant, understand that in some cultures, the family is expected to provide care for family members. In those same cultures, independence may not be valued or considered important. Knowing this will help you to avoid becoming frustrated or annoyed by the actions of the family.

10.

D. Some amputees experience phantom limb pain in the amputated limb. Although the limb is gone, the resident actually feels pain in the absent part. The pain is real and can be quite severe. Report complaints of pain to the nurse immediately.

V Residents with Special Needs

22 Cognitively Impaired

chapter outline

I. COGNITIVE IMPAIRMENTS

A. Types of cognitive impairment include:

Cognitive impairment—a diminished ability to think and remember

1. periods of temporary confusion
   a. caused by acute disorders including:
   - dehydration
   - high fever
   - infection
   - pneumonia
   - drug reaction
   - stress
   b. Episodes usually stop once the condition is treated.
2. mild memory loss
   a. common with normal aging, may begin in middle age
   b. difficulty remembering names, dates, numbers
   c. Memory can be improved by:
   - concentration
   - association
   - repetition

Dementia—chronic, organic decline of mental ability

3. **dementia**
   a. Symptoms include:
   - memory loss
   - disorientation
   - inability to concentrate
   - inability to follow directions
   - poor judgment and reason
   - changes in mood and personality
   b. The person becomes progressively worse.
   c. Most common causes of dementia include:
   - **Alzheimer's disease**
   - Parkinson's disease
   - Lewy disease
   - Binswanger's disease
   - Huntington's disease
   - Pick's disease
   - stroke

Alzheimer's disease—a disease of the brain cells that, over time (2–25 years), destroys tissue and function

B. Alzheimer's disease (AD)

1. A definite diagnosis can only be made after examination of brain tissue during an **autopsy.**
2. A probable diagnosis is made by evaluation of:
   a. medical, social, and family history
   b. lab tests

Autopsy—the examination of a body after death to determine cause of death

    c. physical examination

    d. psychosocial assessment

3. It may begin as early as middle age.

4. No cure is known.

5. It passes through three stages:

    a. Early-stage symptoms include:

- short-term memory loss
- difficulty concentrating
- inability to remember or follow instructions
- getting lost and losing things
- loss of spontaneity or enthusiasm
- loss of initiative—unable to start things
- mood and personality changes
- poor judgment and decision making
- unable to organize, plan, follow through
- thoughts of persecution **(paranoid)**
- possible feelings of anger, frustration, withdrawing

    b. Middle-stage additional symptoms include:

- long- and short-term memory loss
- short attention span
- restlessness, especially in late afternoon and at night **(sundowning)**
- making repetitive statements and/or movements
- trouble with language and communication, possible **aphasia**
- **disorientation**
- more difficulty performing ADLs
- **catastrophic reactions**
- weight fluctuation, usually gaining and then losing weight
- changes in sleep patterns, confusing days and nights
- seeing or hearing things that are not there and being convinced they are real **(hallucinations)**
- generally requiring full-time supervision

    c. Late-stage symptoms include:

- unable to recognize family or self in mirror
- severe memory loss
- may be unable to eat, significant weight loss
- loses the ability to communicate with words
- loses control of bowel and bladder functions
- loss of coordination and inability to provide any self-care
- more susceptible to infection
- may be unable to sleep
- coma
- requires constant care and supervision

Paranoid—overly suspicious

Sundowning—increase in confusion, restlessness, and wandering as day progresses

Aphasia—inability to speak or express oneself

Disorientation—being unable to remember person, place, and time

Catastrophic reactions—overreacting to situations with anger and violence

Hallucination—seeing or hearing things that don't exist

II. COMMUNICATION AND BEHAVIORS

A. Communication with residents with Alzheimer's disease or related disorders (ADRD):

1. They may be unable to communicate verbally.
2. They depend on nonverbal communication.
3. To communicate with ADRD residents:
   a. Be patient.
   b. Never argue, threaten, or frighten a resident.
   c. Give one short, simple direction at a time.
   d. Watch for nonverbal responses from the resident.
   e. Repeat the resident's name frequently.
   f. Tell the resident your name frequently.
   g. Do not offer a variety of choices.
   h. Give the resident adequate time to respond.
   i. Make eye contact.
   j. Be calm and positive.
   k. Use simple words and phrases.
   l. When giving directions, point to items and visually cue the resident.
   m. Touch the resident.
   n. Smile frequently.
   o. Try to understand what the resident is trying to communicate.
   p. Help the resident with glasses and hearing aids if necessary.
   q. Encourage and praise the resident.
   r. Watch the resident's facial expressions and body language.

B. Managing behaviors of residents with ADRD:

1. Behaviors may change as the disease progresses.
2. Record problem behavior.
3. Identify causes for behavior:
   a. having unmet needs
   b. being unable to communicate needs
   c. being overstimulated by or uncomfortable in the environment
   d. having physical discomfort or pain
   e. being fearful or anxious
4. Address behaviors:
   a. Look for the cause of the behavior.
   b. Remove the cause and distract the resident.
   c. Decrease noise levels.
   d. Remove the resident from crowded areas.
   e. Limit choices.
   f. Keep a standard routine.

Why?
Residents with dementia have short-term memory loss and can quickly forget information.

Why?
A record of the behavior, the circumstances at the time of the behavior, the measures used to resolve the behavior, and the results gives staff information about prevention of the behavior and approach to be used that may be incorporated in the resident's care plan.

g. Remain calm and protect the resident from injury.

h. Report increased anger or **agitation** to the nurse immediately.

5. Manage sexually aggressive behaviors:

a. Understand human sexuality and sexual needs of the elderly.

b. Note patterns of sexual behavior.

c. Determine if your behavior may have affected the resident.

d. Remain professional and calm and tell the resident to stop.

e. Tell the resident that the behavior is not acceptable.

f. Distract the resident.

g. Provide privacy if the resident is aroused.

h. Do not embarrass or criticize the resident.

i. Report the situation to the nurse.

6. Manage aggressive behaviors:

a. The behavior may be sudden.

b. Know the signs of anger.

c. Be certain the resident understands why you are there and what you are going to do.

d. Speak in a calm, quiet voice.

e. Explain everything you are going to do just before you do it.

f. Do not make sudden moves that could be frightening.

g. Try to distract the resident.

h. Keep the resident's schedule as constant as possible.

i. Stay at eye level with the resident.

j. Always treat the resident with respect and as an adult.

k. Be aware of your body language.

l. Build a trusting relationship.

m. Allow the resident to safely wander or pace.

n. Call for help quickly if the resident becomes physically aggressive.

o. Report aggressive behaviors to the nurse.

7. Helping a resident who is depressed:

a. Symptoms of depression include:

• withdrawal

• overwhelming sadness

• low self-worth and self-esteem

• negative feelings

• lack of interest in personal appearance

• change in sleep patterns, weight, appetite, mobility

b. Encourage socialization.

c. Listen to the resident and let him or her express feelings.

d. Do not be judgmental.

e. Let the resident cry.

Agitation—a state of restlessness and excitement with no apparent cause

Why?

— The resident has a shortened attention span. A slow, soothing voice can calm the resident, promote understanding, and prevent frustration.

— Once distracted, the resident may forget the outburst because of short-term memory loss.

f. Encourage the resident to participate in care.

g. Provide opportunities for the resident to feel useful and needed.

III. RESTORATIVE APPROACHES TO ADLS

A. Help the resident with ADRD to assist with personal care.

1. Treat each resident as an individual.
2. Keep a constant schedule.
3. Use short sentences.
4. Give simple directions.
5. Try to continue the resident's normal routine.
6. Never force or argue with the resident.
7. Distract a resident who is not cooperating.
8. Provide privacy.
9. For safety, have the resident sit or lie down when dressing.
10. Help the resident with hair care, makeup, and shaving.
11. Encourage the resident to help.
12. Give the resident a choice of two outfits.

B. Help the resident with ADRD with eating.

1. Observe for chewing and swallowing problems.
2. Assist the resident to feed himself or herself.
3. Offer foods the resident likes.
4. Give the resident one food at a time if necessary.
5. Have the resident hold finger foods.
6. Keep the environment calm and quiet during meals.
7. Encourage the use of assistive equipment.
8. Offer snacks if ordered.
9. If the resident is restless or upset, stop trying to feed and report to the nurse.

C. Help the resident with ADRD with toileting and elimination.

1. The resident may become incontinent.
2. Take the resident to the bathroom on a regular schedule.
3. Look for nonverbal cues that the resident needs to go to the bathroom.
4. Answer call signals quickly and take the resident to the bathroom each time it is requested.
5. Report incontinence to the nurse.

D. Help the resident with ADRD with sleeping.

1. The resident may confuse day and night.
2. Provide activities to prevent frequent naps during the day.
3. Increase exercise in the afternoon.
4. Allow the resident to pace in a safe environment.

5. Avoid caffeine products in the evening.

6. Offer a backrub to help the resident relax.

7. Keep the environment quiet at night.

IV. MEETING THE RESIDENT'S PSYCHOSOCIAL NEEDS

A. Residents with ADRD have the same emotional, social, and spiritual needs as other residents.

1. Needs become more difficult to meet because of problems with:
   a. communication
   b. comprehension
   c. attention
   d. behavior

2. Provide opportunities for activities that are:
   a. structured
   b. repetitive
   c. visual
   d. predictable
   e. enjoyable
   f. of short duration
   g. based on previous favorites of the resident
   h. offered at intervals that allow time for rest
   i. Give the resident the opportunity to succeed.

3. Use **reality orientation** methods to help the resident focus.

4. Encourage the resident to **reminisce** to improve attention and self-esteem.

Reality orientation— program that helps the resident to maintain awareness of person, place, and time

Reminiscing—talking about past experiences, especially pleasant ones

B. Help the resident with ADRD cope with stress.

1. Stress may increase:
   a. confusion
   b. agitation
   c. aggressive behaviors
   d. combative behaviors

2. Avoid activities that:
   a. are competitive
   b. are conducted in large, noisy, crowded spaces
   c. involve TV or movies with violence

V. MEETING THE FAMILY'S NEEDS

A. The resident's family is experiencing the gradual death of their loved one.

1. Family members may:
   a. complain about quality of care

        b. become angry

        c. be hostile

        d. cry

    2. Family members' reactions reflect their feelings of:

        a. loss of care

        b. sense of failure

        c. frustration at their inability to make things better

        d. inadequacy

        e. grief

B. Provide emotional support for the family.

1. Encourage the family to talk about their feelings.
2. Ask family members for input into how to care for the resident.
3. Let family member assist with care.
4. Remind the resident of family members' names before visits.
5. Encourage family members to participate in facility programs.
6. Be empathetic.
7. Develop a trusting relationship with families.
8. Treat the family with respect.
9. Keep family information confidential.

C. Refer the family to the nurse or social worker if you are unable to answer their questions.

VI. ENVIRONMENT

A. The environment affects the behavior of residents with ADRD. The environment should be:

1. homelike
2. calm
3. predictable
4. stimulating
5. safe
6. free of clutter

B. The environment should be comfortable enough so the resident may:

1. safely wander
2. be encouraged to socialize
3. be allowed choices

DIRECTIONS
A brief description of a resident is given followed by 10 questions related to the resident. Each question has four possible answers. Read each question and all answer choices carefully. Choose the one best answer.

Mrs. Jessica Farmer is 81 years old. She has Alzheimer's disease and moderate dementia.

1. Mrs. Farmer is unaware of the day and date. She cannot identify where she is living. She is:
   A. in denial
   B. disoriented
   C. dehydrated
   D. depressed

2. You call Mrs. Farmer by name. You remind her of where she is living. You tell her the date and year. Reminding her of person, place, and time is:
   A. validation therapy
   B. depression therapy
   C. reality orientation
   D. remediation

3. When you communicate with Mrs. Farmer, she does not use words appropriately. You can improve communication by:
   A. speaking clearly and using smaller words
   B. watching her facial expressions and body language
   C. asking her questions so you can assess her level of awareness
   D. telling her whenever she uses a wrong word

4. You are behind with your work and your day is not going well. When caring for Mrs. Farmer, you speak softly to her but you are tense and impatient. She may:
   A. withdraw from you and become very quiet
   B. report you for not doing your job well
   C. sense your tension and impatience
   D. request another CNA

5. Because of her difficulty with communication, you observe Mrs. Farmer's physical condition more closely. Mrs. Farmer is:
   A. more likely to become ill
   B. less able to express discomfort
   C. less able to feel discomfort
   D. more susceptible to infection

6. Mrs. Farmer is agitated and says to you, "I have to go home and take care of my baby. She is very sick." This is an example of:
   A. pillaging
   B. anxiety
   C. sundowning
   D. hallucinations and delusion

7. After Mrs. Farmer tells you about her sick baby, you should:
   A. tell her that you will take care of the baby
   B. ask her if her daughter could take care of the baby
   C. call the nurse immediately
   D. calmly speak about the present

8. If you try to make Mrs. Farmer understand that she has no baby, you will:
   A. improve her sense of reality
   B. increase her agitation
   C. help her become less confused
   D. cause her to hallucinate

9. Because Mrs. Farmer has Alzheimer's disease, she tends to tire easily. You should:
   A. have her exercise more to improve her tolerance
   B. let her sleep longer in the morning
   C. provide opportunities for naps or rest periods
   D. be certain she goes to bed early

10. Mrs. Farmer's family must watch their mother's personality and memory deteriorate. They are coping with:
    A. negative feelings toward their mother
    B. the loss of the person they knew
    C. their own confusion and disorientation
    D. anger and hostility toward you

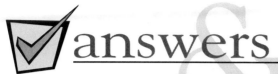
answers & rationales

1.

B. Disorientation means confusion about person, place, and time. Denial is a refusal to believe what is happening. Dehydrated means not having enough fluid in the body. Depression is a state of sadness, grief, or low spirits.

2.

C. Reality orientation (RO) helps the resident to maintain awareness of person, place, and time. It assists the confused resident to stay in touch with reality.

3.

B. When you communicate with a resident who is confused, observe facial expressions and body language for clues to how the resident feels and what the resident wants.

4.

C. If the nursing assistant is tense and impatient, the resident may sense that tension and impatience and become upset. To make communication easier with confused residents, slow down, relax, use appropriate body language, and keep eye contact.

5.

B. Residents with confusion have difficulty with communication. Observe residents physical condition closely because they may be unable to express discomfort.

6.

D. Hallucinations and delusions are common behaviors of people with dementia. The resident sees, hears, or feels things that are not real (hallucinations) or insists on a false belief (a delusion). Pillaging is collecting items. Anxiety is a state of apprehension. Sundowning is increased confusion, restlessness, and wandering as the day progresses.

7.

D. The nursing assistant should not reinforce a confused resident's fantasies. Be calm and speak to the resident about what is currently happening.

8.

B. Trying to convince a confused resident that hallucinations or delusions are not real will increase agitation and frustration. Do not reinforce the resident's fantasies; merely redirect the conversation toward what is currently happening around the resident. Remind the resident of the date and location. Speak of the weather, current events, scheduled activities, or impending family visits.

9.

C. Residents with dementia tire easily and they are less able to function. To keep confused residents from becoming overly tired, help them prepare for scheduled naps or rest periods.

10.

B. The family of a resident with Alzheimer's disease may be grieving over the loss of the person their loved one once was. The person is gone but the body is intact. Treat the family with empathy and kindness.

Visually Impaired

chapter outline

I. VISUAL IMPAIRMENTS

A. Visual impairments:
1. affect approximately 80% of residents
2. affect the resident's ability to meet:
   a. physical needs
   b. social needs
   c. emotional needs
   d. safety needs
   e. the need for independence

Visually impaired—having diminished vision or being blind

B. Some vision problems include:
1. *myopia*—nearsightedness
2. *hyperopia*—farsightedness
3. *astigmatism*—blurred vision
4. *glaucoma*—increased pressure in the eye that eventually leads to blindness
5. *cataract*—disorder in which the lens becomes cloudy so light cannot enter the eye, blurring and dimming vision

C. Visual changes with aging cause:
1. the eyes to take longer to adjust to changes in:
   a. light
   b. distance
   c. direction
2. increased difficulty reading small print
3. the need for brighter light in order to see

II. COMMUNICATION NEEDS

A. When communicating with the vision-impaired resident:
1. Announce your presence.
2. Be sure the resident knows that you are approaching.
3. State your name each time you begin a conversation.
4. Allow the resident to touch and handle unfamiliar objects.
5. Provide good lighting and avoid glare.
6. Face the person to whom you are speaking.
7. Explain everything that you are going to do.
8. Be sure the resident's glasses are clean.
9. Describe the resident's environment.
10. Describe events that are occurring.

B. When caring for a resident who wears eyeglasses:

1. Remind the resident to wear the glasses.
2. Hold glasses by the frame, not the lens.
3. Polish lenses with a soft cloth.
4. Clean lenses with soap and water and dry with a soft cloth.
5. Store eyeglasses in a container on the bedside table within the resident's reach.

III. PREVENTING WITHDRAWAL AND DEPENDENCY

A. Assist the resident with grooming:

1. Describe the location of personal items.
2. Assist with makeup.
3. Provide a predictable schedule so the resident has a sense of security and control.
4. Be sure that the resident's appearance is neat, clean, and appropriate.

B. Keep the resident's environment safe:

1. Describe the surroundings.
2. Describe the location of furniture.
3. Do not move furniture or belongings.
4. Increase independence by putting frequently used items in the same place.
5. Help the visually impaired resident learn to use the call signal.
6. Identify and report safety hazards.
7. Give special assistance to vision-impaired residents during emergencies.

C. Encourage the resident to be independent when dining:

1. Describe the location of food at mealtime by using the clock method.
2. Remove very hot items and serve them separately to avoid burns.
3. Use a plate with a lip-guard to help with self-feeding.
4. Ignore spills.
5. Praise success.
6. If you are feeding a visually impaired resident:
   a. Describe the food on the plate and describe each bite.
   b. Tell the resident the temperature of the food.
   c. Ask the resident what he or she wants next.
   d. Allow the resident to make as many choices as possible.
   e. Allow the resident to use his or her fingers to identify the food on the plate.

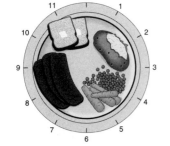

Figure 23–1 Describe the food on the plate in terms of a clock face. "Baked potato at 2 o'clock" for example also allow blind patients to identify the food on their plate with their fingers. (Source: From *The Nursing Assistant* [3rd ed., p. 241], by J. Pulliam, 2002, Upper Saddle River, NJ: Prentice Hall. Reprinted by permission.)

D. Assist the resident with ambulation:

1. Let the resident take your arm.
2. Describe where you are going.
3. Identify obstacles.
4. Show the resident how to locate raised numbers or symbols for rooms or bathrooms.
5. Explain the location of items inside and outside of the room.
6. Encourage the resident to walk.
7. Keep the resident's room free of clutter.

Why?
Your body movements communicate to the resident when and where to move.

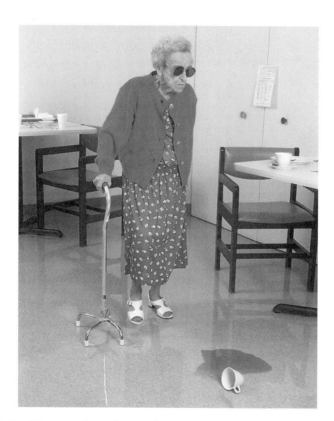

Figure 23–2   The confused or vision-impaired resident may not be aware of spills. (Source: From *The Long-Term Care Nursing Assistant* [2nd ed., p. 65], by P. Grubbs and B. Blasband, 2000, Upper Saddle River, NJ: Prentice Hall. Reprinted by permission.)

DIRECTIONS A brief description of a resident is given followed by 10 questions related to the resident. Each question has four possible answers. Read each question and all answer choices carefully. Choose the one best answer.

Mr. Edward Joseph is 73 years old. He is a new resident. He is diabetic, has heart disease, and is visually impaired.

1. Mr. Joseph is visually impaired. Visual complications are common for residents that:
   A. are diabetic
   B. are newly admitted to the facility
   C. have heart disease
   D. are over the age of 70

2. The nurse wrote in Mr. Joseph's admission notes that he has a "communication impairment." This means that:
   A. the nurse should have written "visual impairment"
   B. he has difficulty communicating
   C. he is aphasic
   D. you should not attempt to communicate with him

3. When admitting Mr. Joseph, you improve his ability to communicate by:
   A. checking on him every hour
   B. telling him to call if he needs you
   C. placing a sign on his door that says "Blind Resident"
   D. teaching him how to locate and use the call signal

4. Because Mr. Joseph has a vision impairment, you check that his room has:
   A. proper ventilation
   B. several very bright lights to help him see
   C. good lighting without glare
   D. hand rails

5. Mr. Joseph is very frustrated being in a long-term care facility. He is talking to you about his feelings. You should:
   A. continue doing other things while you listen
   B. listen to him and face him when you are talking
   C. speak loudly into his ear
   D. stand at the door and monitor other residents during the conversation

6. You know that you should provide a routine schedule for Mr. Joseph to help him:
   A. learn to take care of himself
   B. reduce his need to use the call signal
   C. feel a sense of security and control
   D. help him regain his vision

7. When caring for Mr. Joseph, it is most important that you:
   A. speak to him as little as possible
   B. explain everything that you are going to do
   C. ask him if he understands what you are telling him
   D. tell him to repeat directions to you

8. To help Mr. Joseph see as well as possible:
   A. encourage him to eat carrots
   B. keep his door open when you are giving care
   C. keep the lighting dim
   D. be certain that his glasses are kept clean

9. The furniture in Mr. Joseph's room is in your way. You want to move it for safety reasons. You should:

   A. call housekeeping and tell them to change the furniture

   B. move the furniture only if necessary and tell him where you are placing them

   C. contact the administrator and report Mr. Joseph's family for bringing in too much stuff

   D. remove everything but the bed and dresser from his room for his safety

10. All of the staff should explain to Mr. Joseph the location of items inside and outside of his room so he will be able to:

    A. avoid bumping into things

    B. be more dependent

    C. function more independently

    D. know when to call for help

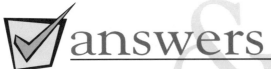

answers & rationales

1.

A. Common complications for the resident with diabetes include impaired vision and blindness.

2.

B. If a resident has a communication impairment, it means that the resident has difficulty communicating because of one or more impairments, diseases, or disabilities.

3.

D. If the resident is visually impaired, the nursing assistant improves his ability to communicate by teaching him to locate the call signal. The call signal gives the resident a sense of security and promotes trust, independence, and safety.

4.

C. Check the room of a resident with visual impairment for good lighting without glare to improve his ability to communicate. Not enough light or glare from lights that are too bright can distort vision.

5.

B. To communicate with a resident who is visually impaired, face him when you are communicating. A resident with a visual impairment depends on other senses to improve communication, especially hearing.

6.

C. Provide a predictable, routine schedule for a resident with visual impairment to improve his sense of security and control.

7.

B. When caring for a resident with a visual impairment, explain everything that you are going to do. The resident will not become startled or surprised and you will reduce anxiety.

8.

D. Keeping the resident's glasses clean increase the ability to see as much as possible, increasing independence and promoting safety.

9.

B. If a resident has a visual impairment, only move possessions or furniture if necessary and tell the resident where you are placing them. Because the resident has difficulty seeing, changing where things are placed can be a safety problem and cause accidents. The resident will be more dependent until comfortable with the new arrangement.

10.

C. When health care team members explain the location of items inside and outside of the room, most residents who are vision impaired develop a mental image of the surroundings and will be able to function more independently.

24 Hearing Impaired

chapter outline

Hearing impaired—having diminished hearing or being totally deaf

I. HEARING IMPAIRMENTS

A. Hearing loss can:

1. involve the inability to hear low-, medium-, or high-pitched sounds
2. affect one or both ears

B. A person with hearing loss may:

1. speak too loudly
2. ask to have things repeated
3. lean forward to hear
4. turn and cup the better ear toward the speaker
5. respond inappropriately to questions

C. Hearing loss may be caused by:

1. disease
2. noise
3. injury

D. Hearing loss can lead to:

1. withdrawal
2. suspicion
3. depression
4. isolation

II. COMMUNICATION NEEDS

A. Those with hearing impairments may communicate through:

1. use of hearing aids
2. reading lips
3. sign language
4. writing

B. Improved communication prevents:

1. isolation
2. withdrawal
3. deprivation

Why?

— Your expressions give visual cues that can help the hearing-impaired resident understand what you are communicating.

— The hearing-impaired resident may depend on lip reading to increase understanding.

— Chewing gum distorts the movements of your mouth and lips and decreases understanding.

C. When communicating with the hearing-impaired resident:

1. Approach the resident so he or she sees you.
2. Face the resident when speaking.
3. Look at the resident so your lips can be seen.
4. Never chew gum when communicating.
5. Speak into the resident's better ear if appropriate.
6. Use gestures and body movements to help increase understanding.
7. Use different words to say the same thing if the resident does not understand you.

8. Decrease background noise:
   a. Turn off the radio or TV.
   b. Close windows and doors.
9. Speak slowly and clearly.
10. Never exaggerate your lip movements.
11. Never shout.
12. Check that the resident is wearing a hearing aid if required.
13. Check the batteries in the hearing aid.
14. Slowly explain what you are going to do, one step at a time.
15. Stimulate the senses of vision, touch, and smell.
16. Use written messages when necessary.

Why?
Speaking loudly does not make the words understandable.

III. HEARING AIDS

A. Hearing aids may help some residents with certain types of hearing loss.

B. Basic parts include:

1. microphone
2. amplifier
3. speaker
4. battery

Hearing aid—a device used to make certain sounds louder

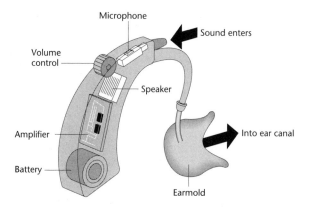

Figure 24–1 Basic parts of a hearing aid. (Source: From *The Long-Term Care Nursing Assistant* [2nd ed., p. 95], by P. Grubbs and B. Blasband, 2000, Upper Saddle River, NJ: Prentice Hall. Reprinted by permission.)

C. When assisting a resident with a hearing aid:

1. Place the hearing aid into the ear with the volume on low.
2. Slowly turn the volume up until it is comfortable for the resident.
3. If whistling occurs, turn the volume down until it stops and check for proper positioning of the earpiece in the ear.

4. To remove the hearing aid, turn it off with the volume set on low and pull it toward you by holding the earpiece.
5. Check the resident's ear for irritation or wax buildup.
6. Check the tubing of the hearing aid for ear wax.
7. Clean the earpiece by:
    a. wiping it with soap and water
    b. keeping water out of the tubing
    c. not placing the hearing aid in water
8. Check the battery regularly.

Why?
Sprays can clog the microphone opening of hearing aids.

9. Do not use hair spray or medical spray when the resident is wearing a hearing aid.
10. Keep the hearing aid away from heat.

D. Hearing aids may distort sound in noisy environments. The resident may:
1. avoid noisy situations
2. turn off the hearing aid in a noisy environment

DIRECTIONS

A brief description of a resident is given followed by 10 questions related to the resident. Each question has four possible answers. Read each question and all answer choices carefully. Choose the one best answer.

Mr. Michael Hammond is hearing impaired. He is 87 years old and occasionally confused.

1. You face Mr. Hammond when speaking because this:
   A. lets him know that you like how he looks
   B. provides visual cues and increases understanding
   C. allows him to see that you are neat, clean, and professional
   D. makes him feel that you care about him

2. When communicating with Mr. Hammond, who is hearing impaired, you:
   A. speak slowly and clearly
   B. shout so he can hear you better
   C. overarticulate to make lip reading easier
   D. look away from him frequently

3. Because Mr. Hammond is hearing impaired, the sounds he hears are distorted. If you shout when speaking to him:
   A. it is easier for him to understand you
   B. sounds will be more distorted
   C. other residents will complain about you
   D. you will breach his right to confidentiality

4. Mr. Hammond is deaf in his right ear and partially deaf in his left ear. When communicating with him, you should:
   A. speak into the left ear
   B. speak into his right ear
   C. stand directly behind him to speak
   D. cup your hands around his left ear when you speak

5. Mr. Hammond depends on you to do all you can to improve his ability to communicate. When communicating with him you should NEVER:
   A. touch him
   B. show emotion
   C. spend extra time with him
   D. chew gum

6. To help you communicate with Mr. Hammond when he is wearing his hearing aid, you should:
   A. turn off the radio or television
   B. take him into the hallway
   C. repeat everything you say twice
   D. approach him when he is having lunch

7. If whistling occurs when you help Mr. Hammond with his hearing aid, you should:
   A. turn the volume down until it stops
   B. turn the volume up until it stops
   C. turn the volume off and begin again
   D. replace the battery

8. When eating in the dining room, Mr. Hammond often turns off his hearing aid because large, noisy rooms:
   A. distort sounds for the residents who wear hearing aids
   B. enhance sounds so he doesn't need the hearing aid

C. are often a favorite location for resident's who are hearing impaired

D. help the resident who is hearing impaired to communicate better with other residents

9. Mr. Hammond is talking with another resident who is telling him about a baseball game. Later, Mr. Hammond tells you that he thinks the other resident has a problem because he kept talking about hitting and running. You know that Mr. Hammond:

A. is correct

B. can become suspicious of other people

C. does not like other residents and is very critical

D. is becoming confused

10. Because of his difficulty with hearing, Mr. Hammond begins avoiding other residents and refuses to attend activities. He is:

A. being realistic

B. isolating himself

C. withdrawing from reality

D. expressing his anger

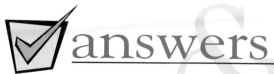

answers & rationales

1.

B. Face the resident who is hearing impaired when speaking. Facing the resident allows the resident to see your facial expressions and read your lips that provide visual cues and increases understanding.

2.

A. Speaking slowly and clearly to a hearing-impaired resident improves communication. Shouting makes the hearing impaired resident hear distorted sounds. Overarticulation prevents the resident from interpreting the sounds. Looking away prevents the resident from lip reading.

3.

B. When communicating with residents who are hearing impaired, do not shout. Shouting further distorts sounds, making it even more difficult for the resident to understand.

4.

A. When communicating with a resident who is partially deaf, speak into the resident's better ear to improve communication.

5.

D. Avoid chewing gum when communicating with a hearing-impaired resident. Chewing gum distorts the sounds the resident hears and limits the ability to read lips.

6.

A. Minimize background noise by turning off the radio or television when communicating with a resident who is hearing impaired. Reducing the background noise will improve the resident's ability to hear and communication.

7.

A. While assisting a hearing-impaired resident with a hearing aid, turn the volume down if whistling occurs. Recheck the position of the aid in the resident's ear and slowly increase the volume.

8.

A. Residents with hearing aids experience distortion of sound in noisy environments. They may turn off the hearing aid during those times or avoid such situations.

9.

B. Hearing loss may cause withdrawal, suspicion, depression, and isolation. Because the resident only hears part of the conversation, he may misunderstand what the other person actually says.

10.

B. A resident with hearing loss may avoid others because communication is difficult and confusing. The resident then becomes isolated, lonely, and depressed.

CHAPTER

25

The Developmentally Disabled

chapter outline

I. TYPES OF DEVELOPMENTAL DISABILITIES

A. Developmental disability is a severe, chronic disability that:

1. occurs before the person is 22 years old
2. will last a lifetime
3. results in significant limitations in important activities, including:
   a. activities of daily living
   b. **receptive and expressive language**
   c. **learning**
   d. **mobility**
   e. **self-direction**
   f. ability to live independently
   g. **economic self-sufficiency**
4. requires:
   a. services and treatment that last a long time or for life
   b. individual planning
   c. coordination of services

B. Developmental disabilities include:

1. **mental retardation**
   a. can occur before, during, or after birth
   b. causes include:
      • heredity
      • difficult birth
      • illness
      • accidents
      • physical abuse

2. **cerebral palsy**
   a. causes may:
      • occur during pregnancy or birth
      • be due to prematurity, lack of oxygen, or injury to head
   b. may or may not involve mental retardation

3. **epilepsy**
   a. causes may include:
      • brain injury before, during, or after birth
      • infection of the brain and surrounding membranes (encephalitis, meningitis)
      • high fever
      • pressure in the brain from tumor, blood clot, or bleeding
      • presence of toxic chemicals in the blood (poisons, drugs)
      • may have no known cause

Receptive and expressive language—understanding others and making self understood

Learning—ability to acquire new skills and new knowledge

Mobility—ability to move from place to place without assistance

Self-direction—ability to make decisions about one's own life

Economic self-sufficiency—ability to support oneself

Mental retardation—defined as having IQ of 70 or below and limitations in ability to learn, be independent, be socially responsible

Cerebral palsy—damage to the brain that results in person having difficulty controlling muscles of the body

Epilepsy—condition or disorder in the electrical functioning of the brain that results in various kinds of seizures

b. seizures:
  - are not disfiguring
  - are not painful
  - do not shorten life
  - do not cause insanity
  - do not cause mental retardation
  - do not affect intelligence
  - are not contagious

c. The risk of seizures can be lessened by avoiding:
  - illness
  - lack of physical activity
  - fatigue
  - constipation
  - emotional stress

d. types of seizures:
  - *Tonic-clonic seizure*—limbs become stiff and rigid with jaw clenched (tonic phase), followed by violent, rhythmic jerking of limbs (clonic phase) and loss of consciousness
  - *Absence seizure*—episodes of staring for a few seconds while being out of contact with surroundings
  - *Atonic seizure*—loss of muscle tone resulting in falling to the ground
  - *Tonic seizure*—body stiffens, may or may not be followed by loss of consciousness
  - *Complex partial seizure*—change in level of consciousness, being unable to respond, some uncontrolled movements

e. If the resident is having a seizure:
  - Call for help.
  - Move objects away from the resident.
  - Loosen clothing, especially around the resident's neck.
  - Put a pillow under the head to prevent injury.
  - After the seizure stops, turn the resident on side to keep the airway clear.
  - Reassure the resident as consciousness returns.
  - Observe and report length of the seizure, parts of body involved, if incontinence occurs, any injury.

CAUTIONS:
  - DO NOT put any implements into the mouth.
  - DO NOT attempt to give liquids during or just after a seizure.
  - DO NOT hold the person down or try to restrain movement.

4. autism
  a. cause not clearly understood

Why?
— The tongue cannot be swallowed but the resident can bite down on a tongue blade or other objects, and damage teeth and inside of mouth.
— During or just after a seizure, the resident may be unable to swallow and will choke if liquids are given.
— Attempting to restrain a person who is having a seizure could cause injury to the resident and to you.

b. Signs of autism include:
- occurring before the age of 3 years
- unresponsiveness to human contact
- overreaction or underreaction to environmental stimuli
- responding in unpredictable ways to things seen or heard
- rigid or flaccid muscle tone while being held
- little or no interest in human contact
- lack of attachment to parents or caretakers
- language impairment
- repetitive behavior patterns such as head banging, screaming, arm flapping
- self-destructive behavior
- delayed mental and social skills

Autism—defined as a disability related to lack of organization in the functioning of the brain

II. PHILOSOPHY OF CARE

A. Philosophy of care includes:

1. normalization
   a. Emphasize approved positive qualities of the individual.
   - Groom and dress residents based on their chronological age, not mental or developmental age.
   - Acknowledge the resident's culture.
   b. Ways to identify normalization include:
   - Treat residents with dignity and respect.
   - Take the role of an assistant, not a parent.
   - Encourage residents to do all they can for themselves.
   - Encourage residents to have age-appropriate personal belongings.
   - Residents' clothing is individualized and age appropriate, not uniform.
   - Respect residents' privacy and confidentiality.
   - Encourage residents to make choices when possible.
   - Encourage residents to become involved in their community.

Normalization—creating an atmosphere and environment that is as close as possible to what is perceived as normal for those who do not have developmental disability

2. developmental model
   a. based on philosophy that all human beings have potential
   b. Change and growth may seem very small but be enormous to the resident.
   c. Help each resident achieve as much growth as possible.
3. **least restrictive alternative**

B. Programming

1. IPP—individual program plan
   a. based on assessment of each resident's abilities
   b. interdisciplinary team headed by a **QMRP**

Least restrictive alternative—choice of treatment, activities, or living arrangement that least limits the freedom and independence of the individual

Programming—plan that describes in writing how the principles of normalization, least restrictive alternative, and developmental model will be made a reality

QMRP—qualified mental retardation professional

    c. A plan includes:
- functional life skills, including ADL skills
- fine motor skills—using fine muscles for tasks such as buttoning, writing, feeding
- gross motor activities—using larger muscles for walking, swimming, or dancing
- sensory-motor activities—to improve thinking by improving information coming into the brain through the senses

  2. least restrictive environment
    a. as close to normal as possible
    b. allows maximum use of living skills
    c. allows for most personal freedom

  3. active treatment
    a. Each client has:
- an interdisciplinary professional evaluation
- an individual written plan of care

    b. Facilities are surveyed yearly to:
- determine if the program is being followed
- assess if residents are reaching their goals

C. When communicating with residents with developmental disabilities:

1. Consider each resident as an individual.
2. Treat each resident with respect and dignity.
3. Remain calm and use touch if acceptable.
4. Offer praise and encouragement.
5. Treat each resident as an adult, regardless of behavior.
6. Use short, simple sentences.
7. Repeat actions and words to ensure understanding.

D. When caring for residents with developmental disabilities:

1. Follow each resident's plan of care.
2. Encourage independence and self-care.
3. Assist with ADLs.
4. Treat each resident with respect and dignity.
5. Be patient.
6. Know each resident's plan of behavior management.
7. Respond appropriately to each resident's behavior.

III. BEHAVIOR MANAGEMENT

A. Behavior modification:

1. Change behavior patterns by eliminating useless behaviors and reinforcing useful ones.

2. The ABC's of behavior modification are:
   a. *A*—antecedent to the behavior, what happened before the behavior occurred
   b. *B*—the behavior
   c. *C*—the consequence or result of the behavior

B. Increasing behaviors:
1. Follow the desired behavior with a reinforcer (reward).
2. Reinforcers can be:
   a. *primary*—foods
   b. *social*—praise, smiles
   c. *physical*—touch, hug, pat on the shoulder

C. Behavior shaping:
1. creating a new set of behaviors
2. Techniques include:
   a. *modeling*—showing the resident how to perform a task
   b. *graduated guidance*—gradually reducing the amount of assistance offered
   c. *shadowing*—staff member keeps his or her hands within 1 inch of the resident's hands as the task is performed
   d. *prompting*—staff member verbally reminds the resident what to do next

D. Undesirable behaviors:
1. Always respect the resident's rights.
2. Modify an undesirable behavior by reinforcing other behaviors.
3. If a behavior cannot be controlled and is harmful to the resident or others, physical restraint may be necessary.
4. Punishment is rarely used and only under very special, approved circumstances.

DIRECTIONS

A brief description of a resident is given followed by 10 questions related to the resident. Each question has four possible answers. Read each question and all answer choices carefully. Choose the one best answer.

Mr. Daniel Swanson is 17 years old. He has a developmental disability and epilepsy with uncontrolled seizures several times a day. The doctor has ordered side rails for his safety.

1. To ensure that he does not hurt himself when having a seizure, you should:
   A. raise the head of the bed
   B. tape a padded tongue blade on the headboard
   C. apply soft wrist restraints
   D. wrap the side rails with a soft cloth

2. Daniel had a seizure. To keep his airway clear following the seizure, you should:
   A. raise the head of the bed
   B. turn him on his side
   C. put him in the prone position
   D. hyperflex his neck

3. You observed the seizure. When you report your observations to the nurse, you include:
   A. the length of the seizure
   B. which residents were there
   C. what activity he did that day
   D. who visited him that day

4. Following the seizure, Daniel appears:
   A. more alert
   B. excited
   C. angry
   D. to have amnesia

5. When caring for Daniel and the other residents with developmental disabilities, your role is that of:

A. a health care professional
B. an associate or assistant
C. a parent
D. the best friend

6. You help Daniel dress for the day. He should wear:
   A. the standard uniform
   B. a hospital gown
   C. a T-shirt and bib
   D. clothing of his choice

7. Daniel's roommate, Tom, has moderate mental retardation. He is beginning a job today at the local grocery store and he is apprehensive. You:
   A. caution him about the way other people may treat him
   B. encourage him to become involved in the community
   C. tell him that you expect him to succeed
   D. ignore him so you do not make him more nervous

8. Tom has been successful with a behavior modification program that has:
   A. changed his personality and physical image
   B. improved his social skills and communication skills
   C. helped him learn to dress himself
   D. enhanced his ability to function in a normal environment

9. You were responsible for data collection during Tom's behavior modification program. You:
   A. counted and recorded behaviors to measure the results
   B. documented what Tom said when he was told to perform tasks a certain way
   C. reported to the nurse any of Tom's behaviors that you did not like
   D. had Tom write down all behaviors that were not acceptable

10. Because you believe in the philosophy of normalization for your residents, you treat Daniel, Tom, and all people under your supervision:
    A. as adults
    B. with respect and dignity
    C. exactly alike
    D. with stern authority

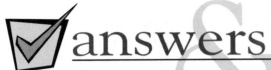

answers & rationales

1.
D. Side rails on a resident's bed may be wrapped with soft cloth to provide padding to prevent injury during a seizure.

2.
B. After a seizure, turn the resident to one side to keep the airway open, allow fluids to drain from the mouth, and prevent choking or aspiration.

3.
A. Report to the nurse everything you observed during the resident's seizure. Report how long the seizure lasted, what body parts were involved, and any injuries that occurred during the seizure.

4.
D. Residents may experience short-term amnesia after a seizure. Amnesia is memory loss. The nursing assistant's role is to help the resident regain awareness of person, place, and time.

5.
B. When assisting a resident with a developmental disability, your role is that of an associate or assistant. You encourage the resident to be independent. You treat the resident with dignity and respect.

6.
D. Residents with developmental disabilities should choose their own clothing with the assistance of the nursing assistant. Clothing should be age appropriate.

7.
B. The nursing assistant should encourage the resident with a developmental disability to be a part of the community. Working, shopping, and attending community functions help create a normalized environment for the resident.

8.
D. Behavior modification programs help residents with developmental disabilities learn skills that promote greater independence and enhance the ability to function in a normal environment.

9.
A. In a behavior modification program, data collection means counting and recording behaviors. The nursing assistant is the team member that spends the most time with the resident. It may be the nursing assistant's responsibility to collect data.

10.
B. The philosophy of normalization is based on the belief that all human beings are treated with dignity and respect.

26

The Abusive Resident

chapter outline

I. AGGRESSIVE BEHAVIORS

A. Factors that affect residents' behavior include:
1. unmet needs
2. life experiences
3. attitudes
4. prejudices
5. frustration
6. fears
7. culture

B. Residents may be:
1. physically aggressive
2. verbally aggressive
3. combative

C. Residents who display combative behavior may:
1. believe that someone is trying to harm them
2. mistake one person for someone else with whom they are angry
3. have hearing or vision loss and may not understand what is happening to them
4. be angry due to:
   a. loss of control over their life
   b. feeling dependent
   c. being rushed
   d. physical discomfort
   e. physical changes in the nervous system
   f. illness
   g. medications

D. Signs of aggressive behavior include:
1. muscle tension
2. clenched jaw
3. glaring eyes
4. clenched fists
5. rigid posture
6. pacing
7. rocking
8. kicking
9. loud, rapid speech

E. To manage the aggressive behavior:
1. Be certain the resident understands what you are going to do before you do it.
2. Offer choices and encourage decision making.
3. Pat or hold the resident's hands.

Why?
— The resident may forget what is being done or not understand what you are doing and react with anger.
— Choice gives the resident a sense of control, which can minimize anger.

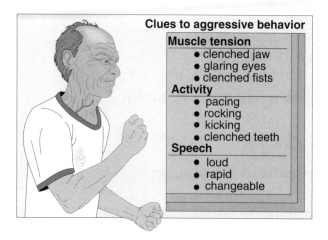

Figure 26–1 Learn to recognize signs of anger. (Source: From *The Long-Term Care Nursing Assistant* [2nd ed., p. 175], by P. Grubbs and B. Blasband, 2000, Upper Saddle River, NJ: Prentice Hall. Reprinted by permission.)

4. Maintain a routine.
5. Avoid standing over or talking down to the resident.
6. Speak in a soothing tone.
7. Keep your gestures calm and slow.
8. Be respectful.
9. Listen to the resident.
10. Never argue with the resident.
11. Use nonaggressive body language.
12. Establish **rapport** with the resident.
13. Offer the resident food.
14. Use restraints only as a last resort.
15. Avoid making the resident feel cornered.
16. Face the angry resident and don't turn your back.
17. Stay an arm's length away from the angry resident when possible.
18. Let the resident pace.
19. Report signs of anger and aggression to the nurse immediately.

Why?
A soothing voice is not threatening and can calm the resident.

Rapport—mutually trusting relationship
Why?
— Food can distract the resident and lessen anger.
— Restraints remove all control from the angry individual and usually worsens combativeness.
— Pacing is an outlet for emotional energy and may reduce anger.

II. DIFFICULT BEHAVIORS

A. Demanding residents:
1. never seem happy or satisfied and:
   a. ring the call signal frequently
   b. are critical of your efforts and their care

    2. Their behavior may be due to fear of being alone.

        a. Involve them in care.

        b. Let them make decisions.

        c. Visit them frequently, even when they do not light the call signal.

B. Coping with a crying resident:

    1. Allow the resident to cry.

    2. Let the resident know that crying is acceptable.

    3. Listen to the resident.

    4. Encourage the resident to participate in activities.

    5. Report to the nurse.

C. To better understand difficult behaviors:

    1. Recognize your own feelings.

    2. Put yourself in the resident's place as much as possible.

    3. Anticipate the resident's needs.

    4. Explain everything you are doing.

    5. Allow the resident to express thoughts and feelings.

    6. Do not take the resident's behavior personally.

    7. Be tolerant and patient.

    8. Do things the resident's way, not your way.

    9. Praise accomplishments.

    10. Treat residents the way you would like to be treated.

    11. Learn about the resident's culture.

III. SEXUAL BEHAVIORS

A. Residents may:

    1. touch inappropriately

    2. flirt

    3. make sexual comments

B. Causes of sexual aggression may include:

    1. illness

    2. medications

    3. confusion

    4. poor self-image

    5. cultural differences

C. Residents who become sexually aggressive may have:

    1. difficulty understanding the difference between care giving and affection

    2. an unmet need to be loved

    3. poor vision or confusion and mistake you for a sexual partner

    4. mental changes that cause inappropriate sexual behavior

D. Deal with sexual behavior professionally.

1. Understand sexuality in the elderly.
2. Accept your own sexuality and reactions.
3. Determine if your behavior may be affecting the resident's behavior.
4. Firmly and calmly tell the resident to stop the behavior.
5. Explain that the behavior makes you uncomfortable.
6. Never yell at, embarrass, shame, or criticize the resident.
7. Remain calm.
8. Provide privacy for a resident who is sexually aroused.
9. Check the care plan for approaches to be used.

IV. DEPRESSION

A. Elderly residents may be depressed because of:

1. loss of role in life
2. loss of freedom
3. loss of independence
4. loss of family and friends
5. loss of home and income
6. loss of dignity, privacy, independence, and personal routine
7. loss of health
8. loss of mobility and sensory stimulation

B. Symptoms of depression include:

1. deep sadness
2. feelings of hopelessness and uselessness
3. fear and confusion because of changes
4. low self-esteem
5. feelings of worthlessness
6. lack of interest in activities
7. social withdrawal
8. negative reactions
9. difficulty in decision making

C. Physical symptoms of depression include:

1. poor hygiene and grooming
2. slow movement
3. sleep problems
4. changes in appetite
5. changes in weight
6. constipation
7. fatigue

Depression—a state of sadness, grief, or low spirits that may or may not cause a change in activity

D. Severe depression can lead to:

1. confusion
2. chronic illness
3. death

E. Restorative care for the depressed resident includes:

1. encouraging the resident to talk about feelings
2. listening attentively
3. allowing the resident to cry
4. encouraging and praising the resident
5. helping the resident feel accepted and appreciated

DIRECTIONS

A brief description of a resident is given followed by 10 questions related to the resident. Each question has four possible answers. Read each question and all answer choices carefully. Choose the one best answer.

Mr. Kurt Simon is 73 years old. He has had a closed head injury. He can be both physically and verbally abusive.

1. Mr. Simon's difficult behavior may be his attempt to:
   A. control a situation in which he feels powerless
   B. let you know that he does not like you
   C. intentionally cause you and other residents pain
   D. get the attention that he wants

2. Mr. Simon is becoming aggressive. If you think that he may be a threat to himself or others, you should:
   A. put him in restraints
   B. lock him in his room
   C. call his family
   D. get assistance from the nurse

3. The best thing to do if Mr. Simon becomes physically aggressive, is to:
   A. hit him first
   B. hold him down
   C. yell at him
   D. back away

4. You may be able to tell when Mr. Simon is becoming combative by observing:
   A. how much he eats
   B. his body language
   C. his vital signs
   D. his level of activity

5. Fidgeting, picking at clothing, wringing hands, pacing, and wandering are signs of:

A. aggression
B. mental illness
C. anxiety
D. Alzheimer's disease

6. When you help Mr. Simon shower he begins yelling that you are trying to set him on fire with the water. You should:
   A. listen without argument or defense and check the water
   B. tell him to stop yelling because he is being inconsiderate
   C. leave him in the shower and get the nurse
   D. wash him quickly and take him back to his room

7. When Mr. Simon verbally abuses you, you should:
   A. answer him by raising your voice so he can hear you
   B. argue with him until he understands how wrong he is
   C. listen calmly and take care of his safety and comfort
   D. ask him why he is being so difficult

8. Working with Mr. Simon is very stressful and exhausting. If you lose control and threaten him, slam doors, or shove furniture, your behavior would be considered:
   A. appropriate
   B. abusive
   C. neglectful
   D. expected

9. If you feel yourself becoming frustrated with Mr. Simon, you should:

    A. threaten to restrain him

    B. lock yourself in the bathroom

    C. refuse to care for him again

    D. provide for his safety, leave the room, and calm down

10. Mr. Simon has been exceptionally aggressive. He has used vile language, called you names, scratched your arm, and tried to kick you. You are upset, afraid, and angry. You should discuss your feelings with:

    A. your supervisor

    B. the other residents

    C. Mr. Simon's family

    D. the other CNAs

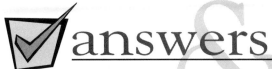

answers & rationales

1.

A. The resident may exhibit difficult and aggressive behavior in an attempt to control a situation that he perceives as threatening to him. When the resident feels powerless, he may become aggressive to gain control.

2.

D. If an aggressive resident appears to be a threat to himself or others, get the nurse immediately. The nurse will assess the resident and decide what should be done.

3.

D. If a resident becomes aggressive slowly back away. Do not turn your back on the resident or try to reason with him. Protect yourself, the resident, and other residents from possible injury.

4.

B. When caring for a resident who is disruptive, observe body positioning and nonverbal body language. You can sometimes predict a resident's combative behavior by carefully observing body language.

5.

C. When the resident's anxiety level is increasing, he may begin fidgeting, picking at clothing, wringing hands, pacing, and wandering. Report these observations to the nurse immediately.

6.

A. To cope with a resident's verbal aggression, listen carefully without argument or defense. The resident may be unable to communicate appropriately. Try to determine if what the resident is saying could actually be a valid problem. Correct the problem immediately.

7.

C. Do not raise your voice or argue when a resident verbally abuses you. Remain calm. Provide for his safety and comfort, and report to the nurse.

8.

B. Abusive behavior includes any act that intentionally harms a resident verbally or physically. If you lose control and do or say anything that threatens or frightens the resident or causes loss of self-esteem, you are guilty of abuse.

9.

D. If you feel yourself becoming frustrated with a difficult resident, be certain that the resident is safe, leave the room, and calm down. If you lose control and respond negatively to the resident you may be considered abusive.

10.

A. You discuss the resident's behavior with your supervisor. Your supervisor is the person to hear your concerns. Extreme behavior by the resident needs a united response from the health care team. The nurse needs the facts.

CHAPTER

27

The Young Resident

chapter outline

I. GROWTH AND DEVELOPMENT

A. Growth and development continues throughout life.

1. infant (first year of life):
   a. body weight triples by end of first year
   b. temporary teeth start appearing
   c. learns to roll over, sit up, crawl, and walk
   d. learns to recognize familiar faces and voices
   e. tends to cling to mother or primary caregiver
   f. developmental task is developing trust
2. toddler (age 1 to 3 years):
   a. has all the temporary teeth
   b. growth slows, muscle strength and energy increase
   c. learns to run, jump, and climb stairs
   d. moves quickly and has little concept of danger
   e. has no clear idea of right or wrong
   f. developmental task is to gain independence
3. play age (preschool age) (age 3 to 6 years)
   a. grows more in height than in weight
   b. muscular development increases
   c. language and social skills increase
   d. more concerned with playmates than home
   e. developmental task is developing initiative—trying new and different things
4. school age (6 to 12 years)
   a. arms and legs lengthen
   b. muscle tissue increases
   c. gains strength
   d. may enter **puberty**
   e. acceptance in peer group is more important
   f. major developmental task is to gain competency in basic intellectual skills (reading, writing, and arithmetic)

   > **Puberty**—period when sex characteristics appear and reproductive organs begin to function

5. teenage years:
   a. changes from child to adult
   b. body proportions change
   c. secondary sex characteristics appear
   d. psychosocial growth is as great as physical growth
   e. has poor emotional control
   f. major developmental task is separating from parents and developing independence
6. young adult:
   a. body systems are fully developed and functioning
   b. major developmental task is to establish intimacy in a close personal relationship
7. middle age:
   a. body starts showing signs of aging

b. women go through menopause

c. may experience midlife crisis (fear that time is running out, resulting in confusion about self)

d. interests move from meeting own needs to caring for society as a whole

e. major developmental task is to achieve productivity

8. old age

a. physical changes of aging become more obvious

Life review—remembering and discussing past events

b. experiences **life review:**
   - helps person let go of past and adjust to present
   - raises self-esteem and improves quality of life

c. major developmental task is to find meaning in life's experiences

ERIKSON'S LIFE STAGES AND DEVELOPMENTAL TASKS	
Stage	**Developmental Task**
1. Infancy	Develop trust
2. Early childhood	Develop independence and self-direction
3. Play age	Develop initiative
4. School age	Develop competence
5. Adolescence	Develop self-identity
6. Early adulthood	Develop intimacy and love
7. Middle adulthood	Develop concern for others and continue productivity
8. Old age	Develop integrity

Figure 27–1   The developmental tasks according to Erik Erikson. (Source: From *The Long-Term Care Nursing Assistant* [2nd ed., p. 119], by P. Grubbs and B. Blasband, 2000, Upper Saddle River, NJ: Prentice Hall. Reprinted by permission.)

II. AGE-SPECIFIC NEEDS

A. Consider age-specific considerations regarding communicating with and caring for residents.

B. Provide care to residents in an age-appropriate way:

Age-appropriate—appropriate to the chronological age of the person

1. Never treat adults like children.
2. Never speak to adults as if they were children.
3. Dress, grooming, and activities should be age appropriate.
4. Address adults by title and name.

C. When communicating with children:

1. Call children by first name or nickname.
2. Do not use commands.
3. Attempt to understand by listening to and assessing sounds and gestures.
4. Be empathic, smile, and be friendly.

DIRECTIONS A brief description of a resident is given followed by 10 questions related to the resident. Each question has four possible answers. Read each question and all answer choices carefully. Choose the one best answer.

Miss Tracy Christensen is 16 years old. She is recovering from extensive injuries received in an automobile accident.

1. Because she is an adolescent, when speaking with Tracy, you should:
   A. try to use current slang
   B. use adult vocabulary
   C. speak to her as a child
   D. try to be her best friend

2. Tracy becomes very upset when she is unable to take care of herself. It is important for her to:
   A. accept dependency
   B. realize that her life will never be normal again
   C. express her anger toward you and her family
   D. strive to be independent

3. Tracy is very worried about the scars on her legs and arms. You should:
   A. tell her that she is lucky the scars are not on her face
   B. suggest that she see a plastic surgeon
   C. understand that body image is very important to her
   D. tell her to put vitamin E cream on the scars

4. When caring for and communicating with Tracy, it is important that you treat her:
   A. with respect
   B. as an equal
   C. as an adult
   D. as a child

5. Tracy needs to use the bedpan. As an adolescent, she:
   A. is very modest and needs privacy
   B. doesn't care about privacy
   C. has no sense of modesty
   D. should accept the fact that privacy cannot exist

6. Tracy's friends come to visit. She ignores you and her family and talks with her friends. You should:
   A. tell her that she is rude
   B. ask her family if she is always this inconsiderate
   C. understand that this is normal for an adolescent
   D. ask her friends to leave

7. Because of her age, it is common for Tracy to experience:
   A. panic when her parents leave
   B. turmoil with rapidly changing moods
   C. anxiety when her friends ask her questions about the accident
   D. fear when a new caregiver is assigned

8. The doctor wants Tracy out of bed for meals and she refuses. You should:
   A. ask for help and get her out of bed
   B. refuse to give her food unless she does what you want
   C. respect her decision and leave her in bed
   D. tell her that she is acting like a child

9. Tracy is verbally abusive to you. You should:
   A. talk to her as if she is a small child
   B. understand that mood swings are common
   C. tell the nurse that Tracy needs medication
   D. tell Tracy that you will not care for her

10. Tracy's parents do not appear to care about her behavior or her language. They only come to see her twice a week and never ask how she is doing. You should:
   A. suggest that they visit more frequently
   B. avoid being judgmental about their attitudes or behavior
   C. report them to Child Protective Services
   D. visit them at home

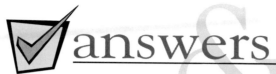
answers & rationales

1.

B. When speaking with an adolescent resident, use adult language. Do not speak to the resident as a child.

2.

D. It is important for the adolescent resident to try to be independent. Independence is a developmental task at this age. As a nursing assistant, your role is to patiently assist the resident with self care.

3.

C. As a nursing assistant, express interest in the resident's concerns. Body image is very important to the adolescent.

4.

A. When caring for an adolescent resident, it is important that you treat her with the same respect that you would any other resident.

5.

A. An adolescent resident is very modest and needs privacy. As a nursing assistant, you need to be sensitive to an adolescent's needs.

6.

C. An adolescent resident is more interested in peers than family. As a nursing assistant, show interest in the resident's peers and encourage them to visit.

7.

B. An adolescent resident experiences turmoil with rapidly changing moods and behavior due to hormonal changes at this developmental stage.

8.

C. Respect the resident's decision to disregard the doctor's order. The resident has the right to refuse and choose to remain in bed. Explain the importance of following doctor's orders and the value of getting out of bed and increasing mobility and independence but do not force the resident.

9.

B. An adolescent resident experiences turmoil with changing moods and behavior due to hormonal changes. Do not take the situation personally. Remain calm and patiently complete her care.

10.

B. As a nursing assistant, do not make judgments about the family members' attitudes or behavior, even if they seem strange to you. Each family has its own cultural beliefs and practices.

The Dying Resident

28

chapter outline

I. ATTITUDE TOWARD DEATH

A. Death and dying involve emotions including:
1. fear
2. anger
3. guilt
4. empathy
5. compassion

B. Attitude toward death is influenced by:
1. *culture*—learned very early in life
2. *religion*—defines beliefs about what happens after death
3. *personal experience*—grieving is learned through experience
4. *age*—very young and very old seem to fear death less

C. The resident may have:
1. a **DNR** order
2. an **advance directive**

DNR—do not resuscitate, which means that no extraordinary means should be used when death occurs

Advance directive— prewritten instructions regarding life-prolonging measures

D. Dying residents may fear:
1. abandonment
2. dying alone
3. pain
4. loss of control
5. the unknown
6. being a burden on their family

II. STAGES OF GRIEF

A. Stages of grief include:
1. *denial stage*—refusal to believe what is happening
   a. Denial delays shock until the grieving resident has more emotional control.
   b. Do not rush the resident through the denial stage.
   c. Listen with empathy and make neutral statements.
2. *anger stage*—grieving resident expresses hostility
   a. A target of anger may be the person with whom the grieving resident spends the most time (you).
   b. The anger is about dying, not about you.
   c. Listen and encourage the resident to express anger.
3. *bargaining stage*—attempt to gain more time by promising something in return
   a. Bargaining is often between the resident and a higher power.
   b. It may be expressed in the form of prayer.

Grief—intense emotional suffering caused by a loss

      c. Encourage hope and respect beliefs.

      d. Notify the nurse if the resident wants spiritual assistance.

   4. depression stage—deep sadness because of thoughts of loss of health, independence, and life

      a. The resident may be unable to communicate.

      b. The resident may experience withdrawal.

      c. Spend time with the resident.

   5. acceptance stage—calmness because the resident accepts dying

      a. The resident becomes peaceful.

      b. The resident understands the situation.

      c. Offer emotional support and caring.

B. The resident's family will be experiencing all the stages of grief.

C. Other residents in the facility may be affected by the death of another resident:

1. may become irritable and angry
2. may withdraw and become depressed
3. may develop anxiety and fear
4. Show concern and understanding.
5. Take time to listen.
6. Assure residents that these feelings are normal.

D. Staff can develop emotional conflicts:

1. feelings of frustration, anger, and guilt
2. physical and emotional stress
3. Staff should support one another.
4. Listen and encourage coworkers to discuss their feelings.

III. MEETING NEEDS

A. To meet the dying resident's physical needs:

1. Keep the resident comfortable.
2. Observe for signs of pain, including restlessness or facial expressions.
3. Give a backrub or help the resident to change position.
4. Observe for **dyspnea:**

    a. caused by disease, anxiety, and fear

    b. Encourage the resident to take slow, deep breaths.

    c. Do not leave the resident alone until the dyspnea is relieved.

5. Offer frequent small amounts of food.
6. Provide mouth care frequently.
7. Lubricate lips to prevent cracking.

Why?
Backrubs and repositioning improve comfort and help the resident relax.

Dyspnea—difficulty breathing

Why?
— Mouth care can help keep the mouth moist and improve the resident's comfort.
— Keeping the lips lubricated prevents cracking, which is very painful and will lessen the resident's desire to speak.

8. Keep skin clean and dry.
9. Massage the resident with lotion.
10. Change bed linen whenever necessary.

B. To meet the dying resident's psychosocial needs:

1. Be caring, gentle, and empathetic.
2. Listen carefully.
3. Allow the resident to make decisions.
4. Ensure privacy for spiritual visits.
5. Be courteous to the spiritual counselor.
6. Handle religious objects carefully and respectfully.

C. To meet the needs of the dying resident and the family:

1. Encourage the resident and family to share memories, discuss the future, make apologies, say goodbye.
2. Provide for comfortable, private visits.
3. Encourage the family to take an active role in caring for the dying resident.
4. Help the family by communicating and being courteous.
5. Never impose your own beliefs on the family.

D. To meet the resident's communication needs:

1. Talk to and with the dying resident.
2. Do not whisper.
3. Only say things you would want the resident to hear.
4. Continue to touch the resident.
5. Respect the need for spiritual support.
6. Offer assistance without taking control.
7. Let the resident and family express grief.
8. Focus on comfort.

E. Provide hospice care/palliative care:

1. includes:
   a. pain control
   b. comfort measures
   c. continuity of care
2. The goal is to improve the resident's quality of life.
3. It can be provided in:
   a. resident's home
   b. long-term care facility
   c. hospital
   d. freestanding hospice unit
4. It is offered when the person has 6 months or less to live.

Why?
When you give a massage, the touch of your hands may be comforting and relaxing for the resident.

Why?
The resident needs to talk, wants you to listen, but does not want or expect answers to questions.

Why?
Caring for the dying resident lets the family maintain some power and control and increases their self-esteem.

Hospice care—a special program designed to provide supportive care for terminally ill individuals and their families
Palliative care—care designed to comfort, instead of cure, the resident

The Dying Person's Bill of Rights

As we face death, what are our rights as human beings? This bill of rights was created at a workshop on "The Terminally Ill Patient and the Helping Person," sponsored by the Southwestern Michigan Insurance Education Council and conducted by Amelia J. Barbus.

- I have the right to be treated as a living human being until I die.
- I have the right to maintain a sense of hopefulness, however changing its focus may be.
- I have the right to be cared for by those who can maintain a sense of hopefulness, however changing this might be.
- I have the right to express my feelings and emotions about my approaching death in my own way.
- I have the right to participate in decisions concerning my care.
- I have the right to expect continuing medical and nursing attention even though "cure" goals must be changed to "comfort" goals.
- I have the right not to die alone.
- I have the right to be free from pain.
- I have the right to have my questions answered honestly.
- I have the right not to be deceived.
- I have the right to have help from and for my family in accepting my death.
- I have the right to die in peace and dignity.
- I have the right to retain my individuality and not be judged for my decisions which may be contrary to beliefs of others.
- I have the right to discuss and enlarge my religious and/or spiritual experiences, whatever these may mean to others.
- I have the right to expect that the sanctity of the human body will be respected after death.
- I have the right to be cared for by caring, sensitive, knowledgeable people who will attempt to understand my needs and will be able to gain some satisfaction in helping me face my death.

Figure 28–1 The dying person's bill of rights. (Source: From *Being A Long-Term Care Nursing Assistant* [2nd ed., p. 480], by C. Will-Black and J. Eighmy, 2000, Upper Saddle River, NJ: Prentice Hall. Reprinted by permission.)

IV. SIGNS THAT DEATH IS NEAR

A. Common signs of death:
1. circulatory system:
   a. cyanosis, a blue color of the lips, nails, and skin.
   b. pulse may be weak, rapid, and irregular
   c. blood pressure drops
   d. skin feels cold but temperature may rise

Why?
The dying person's breathing becomes shallow, taking in less oxygen. Cyanosis results from lack of oxygen.

2. respiratory system:
   a. dyspnea may be present with shallow, noisy respirations
   b. **Cheyne-Stokes respirations**
3. digestive system:
   a. loss of senses of hunger and thirst
   b. swallowing becomes difficult
   c. peristalsis slows
   d. abdomen becomes swollen
   e. nausea and vomiting may occur
   f. bowel incontinence may develop
4. urinary system:
   a. urinary incontinence
   b. urine output decreases
   c. urine can become darker and have a strong odor
5. muscular system:
   a. decrease in muscle tone
   b. jaw muscles relax and cause mouth to remain partly open
6. sensory system:
   a. ability to feel pain decreases
   b. pupils may be dilated
   c. hearing may be last sense to fail
7. confusion:
   a. doesn't know day, place, or people
   b. may hallucinate and see people whom no one else can see

Cheyne-Stokes respirations—repetitious pattern of breathing; shallow breathing followed by deeper breathing and then apnea (no breathing)

B. Death occurs when there is no:
1. pulse
2. respirations
3. blood pressure

C. After death, changes include:
1. permanently fixed and dilated pupils
2. gradual loss of body heat
3. release of urine, feces, and flatus
4. blood pools, causing purplish skin discoloration
5. **rigor mortis** usually occurs within 6 to 8 hours
6. unless body is embalmed or cooled within 24 hours, body tissue begins to break down

Rigor mortis—stiffening of a person's body and limbs that occurs after death

V. POSTMORTEM CARE

A. The purpose of postmortem care is to preserve the appearance of the body.

B. Postmortem care can include:
1. positioning the body
2. straightening the room
3. collecting the personal belongings

C. When providing postmortem care:
1. Wear gloves and follow standard precautions.
2. Treat the body with respect and privacy.
3. Remove tubes and catheters according to facility policy.
4. Bathe the body if needed.
5. Place protective pads under the body to absorb urine and feces.
6. Comb or brush the hair.
7. Place the body in a supine position with the bed flat.
8. Close the eyes.
9. Elevate the head on a pillow and place the arms at the sides.
10. Place the dentures in the mouth if possible.
11. Cover the body with a clean sheet, leaving the head and shoulders exposed.
12. Be certain the room is neat and clean.
13. Provide privacy if the family wishes to view the body.
14. Place identification on the body according to facility policy.
15. Wrap the body in a shroud or sheet according to facility policy.
16. Dispose of belongings as directed by the nurse.
17. Prepare the room for cleaning after the body has been removed.

DIRECTIONS
A brief description of a resident is given followed by 10 questions related to the resident. Each question has four possible answers. Read each question and all answer choices carefully. Choose the one best answer.

Mr. Jon Poole has a terminal illness. He is 82 years old and his two sons are with him.

1. Mr. Poole tells you that he hopes a cure for his illness will be found before he dies. You should:
   A. tell him that he is being unrealistic
   B. listen and encourage feelings of hope
   C. take his sons aside and tell them to speak with him about dying
   D. ask Mr. Poole why he is afraid of death

2. Mr. Poole tells you that his greatest need is to be with his family. They:
   A. share memories, make apologies, and say goodbye
   B. are taking over his care and should be restricted in their visits
   C. are not his caregiver and Mr. Poole should understand how much he needs you
   D. sometimes make him cry and need to be supervised

3. Mr. Poole and his sons are meeting with a spiritual advisor. You should:
   A. stay with them
   B. provide for their privacy
   C. tell the sons to leave the room
   D. ask them to leave until you finish care

4. Mr. Poole is receiving hospice care. The philosophy of the hospice program is that a comforting environment makes dying:
   A. quicker
   B. easier
   C. less lonely
   D. more relaxing

5. To be part of a hospice program, Mr. Poole must have:
   A. 6 weeks or less to live
   B. 3 months or less to live
   C. 6 months or less to live
   D. one year or less to live

6. Mr. Poole has an advance directive, which is his prewritten instructions regarding:
   A. who will inherit his possessions
   B. his funeral
   C. life-prolonging measures that can be used
   D. the medications he can take

7. Mr. Poole refuses all medications and refuses to eat. He tells you that he is ready to die. You should:
   A. tell him that he doesn't have a right to do this to himself
   B. recognize that this is his right and honor that right
   C. get a spiritual advisor to talk with him again
   D. tell him that he needs to fight harder to live

8. Mr. Poole is becoming less responsive. His sons are with him constantly. The nurse asks you to get coffee for Mr. Poole's sons. You:
   A. tell the nurse that you are not a waitress
   B. refuse because you are there to care for Mr. Poole

C. tell another nursing assistant to get the coffee

D. understand that anything you do for his family also helps Mr. Poole

9. Mr. Poole begins Cheyne-Stokes breathing. This is a sign that he is:

A. starting to recover

B. near death

C. uncomfortable

D. developing an upper respiratory infection

10. Another resident, is upset and pacing outside his room. She says, "I'm afraid that I may be next." You should:

A. tell her not to be so self-centered

B. reassure her that she is not sick

C. ask her if she wants to see her doctor

D. understand that her concern is appropriate

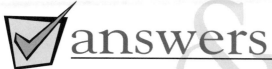

answers & rationales

1.

B. As a nursing assistant, you should encourage feelings of hope by being a supportive listener and allowing the resident to express feelings. Hope is a necessary belief for all humans.

2.

A. A great need of the dying resident is to be with family members to share memories, make apologies, and say goodbye.

3.

B. If a spiritual advisor is visiting the dying resident, the nursing assistant's role is to provide privacy for their visits.

4.

C. The philosophy of the hospice program is that a comforting environment makes dying less lonely and frightening for the dying resident.

5.

C. Hospice residents generally have 6 months or less to live.

6.

C. An advance directive is a resident's prewritten instructions regarding life-prolonging measures, such as resuscitation and the use of feeding tubes.

7.

B. Dying residents may refuse all medications and refuse to eat. As a nursing assistant, recognize that this is their right and honor that right.

8.

D. Anything that a nursing assistant does for the family also helps the resident. Assisting the family to meet their needs is as important as meeting the resident's needs. The family plays an important part in the resident's life and at the time of death. Be empathetic and help the family as much as possible.

9.

B. Cheyne-Stokes breathing is a kind of breathing that occurs when a resident is near death. The breathing is slow and shallow at first followed by faster and deeper breathing that reaches a peak, then stops completely. The pattern then repeats until breathing stops completely.

10.

D. When a resident is dying, other residents may be upset. Understand that the concern is appropriate and that anxiety and fear affect their feelings and reactions.

Procedures

A

5-1 Wash your hands

5-2 Hand hygiene using an alcohol-based hand rub

5-3 Use gloves

5-4 Apply and remove personal protective equipment

8-1 Respond to an adult resident who is choking

13-1 Make an unoccupied bed (open or closed)

13-2 Make an occupied bed

16-1 Assist resident to move to head of bed

16-2 Assist resident to move to head of bed using lift sheet and assistant

16-3 Move resident to one side of bed

16-4 Turn resident away from you

16-5 Turn resident toward you

16-6 Assist resident to sit on edge of bed

16-7 Pivot transfer resident to wheelchair

16-8 Perform range-of-motion exercises

17-1 Drape and undrape resident

17-2 Administer a bed bath

17-3 Perform perineal care

17-4 Assist resident with shower/tub bath

17-5 Rub resident's back

17-6 Assist resident with oral care

17-7 Perform oral care for unconscious resident

17-8 Assist resident with denture care

17-9 Shave resident with safety razor

18-1 Feed the resident

19-1 Assist resident to use a bedpan/fracture pan

19-2 Empty a urinary drainage bag

19-3 Collect a routine urine specimen

19-4 Administer an enema

19-5 Collect a stool specimen

20-1 Take a temperature with a glass thermometer

20-2 Take a temperature with an electronic thermometer

20-3 Take a temperature with tympanic thermometer

20-4 Take resident's radial pulse and respiration rate

20-5 Take resident's blood pressure

PROCEDURES

Before and after performing procedures, the student is expected to take steps to:

- guarantee that the resident is receiving proper care
- ensure that the resident's rights are respected
- provide for the resident's privacy, safety, and comfort
- prevent the spread of infection
- establish positive communication with the resident

Before beginning procedures:

1. Get a report from the supervising nurse.

   The nurse will share the most current information about the resident's needs, care, and abilities, enabling you to provide quality care and continuity of care for the resident.

2. Knock before entering the resident's room.

   By knocking, you respect the resident's right to privacy, give the resident control, and improve the resident's self-esteem.

3. Address the resident by name and title.

   Using a proper name shows respect and reinforces personal identity for the resident.

4. Introduce yourself by name and title.

   The resident has a right to know who you are and that you are qualified to provide care.

5. Identify the resident according to the procedure established by the employer (wrist band, picture, or alternative identification).

   To provide for safety and well-being, you must give the right care to the resident.

6. Explain to the resident what you will be doing.

   Communicating with the resident reduces anxiety, increases trust, and shows respect.

7. Encourage the resident to do as much as possible.

   The restorative approach to care improves the resident's independence and self-esteem.

8. Get all the supplies you need before beginning a procedure.

   Leaving a resident during a procedure to get necessary supplies creates a safety hazard, may be uncomfortable for the resident, and indicates that you are unorganized.

9. Check all the equipment that you will be using.

   Damaged, unsafe equipment can cause injury to the resident and you.

10. Close the bed curtain, window drapes, and door.

    Respect the resident's right to privacy.

11. Wash your hands.

    By controlling infection, you maintain good health and protect the resident and yourself.

12. Wear gloves if indicated by standard precautions.

    Gloves must be worn if you may come into contact with blood, body fluids, secretions, and excretions except sweat, nonintact skin, and mucous membranes, to prevent the spread of pathogens.

13. Use good body mechanics.

Using good body mechanics reduces strain on your spine, joints, and muscles, and decreases the chance of injuries to yourself and the resident.

14. Raise the side rails if you elevate the bed to a working height.

Side rails provide safety for the resident when the bed is elevated.

15. Keep the resident covered and expose only the smallest area necessary to perform the procedure.

Keeping the body covered preserves the resident's right to privacy and maintains dignity.

After completing procedures:

1. Check the resident for proper body alignment and comfort.

Proper alignment reduces stress on joints and muscles, decreases discomfort and pain, and lessens the risk of injury for residents.

2. Put the bed in the lowest position.

A resident can be severely injured if attempting to get into or out of an elevated bed.

3. Be certain that the side rails are positioned according to the resident's care plan and doctor's orders.

Side rails are a form of restraint and can only be used with a doctor's order.

4. Place the call light, water, and frequently used items within reach on the resident's unaffected side.

The call light is an important means of communication for the resident. Accidents can be prevented if residents can easily reach what they want.

5. Remove supplies and clean equipment.

Keeping the resident's environment clean reduces the chance of infection.

6. Remove gloves and wash your hands.

By controlling infection, you maintain good health and protect the resident and yourself.

7. Open the curtains, drapes, and door, if the resident desires.

Give the resident choices to preserve dignity and self-respect.

8. Check the room for safety hazards.

An unsafe environment increases the risk of accidents for staff, residents, and visitors.

9. Thank the resident and ask if anything else is needed.

Always treat the resident with respect.

10. Report any unusual circumstances to the nurse.

The nurse uses your observations to assess the resident's needs.

11. Document the care you provided for the resident according to the employer's policy.

Documentation is the legal method of proving that appropriate care was given. If care is not documented, care was legally not given.

PROCEDURE 5-1: WASH YOUR HANDS

Name _____ **Date** _____

Directions: Practice this procedure, following each step. When you are ready to have your performance evaluated, give this sheet to your instructor.

Procedure	Pass	Redo	Date Competency Met	Instructor Initials
1. Stand away from the sink. *The sink is contaminated. If your uniform touches the sink, you carry the pathogens throughout the facility.*	☐	☐	_____	_____
2. Turn on faucet with a clean paper towel and dispose of towel.	☐	☐	_____	_____
3. Adjust water to comfortable temperature. *Frequent exposure to hot water can damage skin and result in cracking and infection.*	☐	☐	_____	_____
4. Angle arms down, holding hands lower than elbows, and wet hands and wrists.	☐	☐	_____	_____
5. Put soap in hands.	☐	☐	_____	_____
6. Lather all areas of hands and wrists, rubbing vigorously and lacing fingers for at least 15–20 seconds. *Lather and friction loosen pathogens from the surface of the skin.*	☐	☐	_____	_____
7. Clean nails by rubbing them in palm of other hand.	☐	☐	_____	_____
8. Rinse thoroughly, running water down from wrists to fingertips. *Rinsing flushes the loosened pathogens from the skin.*	☐	☐	_____	_____
9. Thoroughly dry hands with paper towels.	☐	☐	_____	_____
10. Turn off faucet with a dry paper towel and discard towel immediately. *The faucet is contaminated. Hands become contaminated if dried with the paper towel after turning off faucet or if paper towel is transferred from hand to hand after turning off faucet.*	☐	☐	_____	_____

PROCEDURE 5-2: HAND HYGIENE USING AN ALCOHOL-BASED HAND RUB

Name _____ **Date** _____

Directions: Practice this procedure, following each step. When you are ready to have your perform-ance evaluated, give this sheet to your instructor.

Procedure	Pass	Redo	Date Competency Met	Instructor Initials
1. Put alcohol-based hand rub into hand.	☐	☐	_____	_____
2. Use the amount of product recommended by the manufacturer.	☐	☐	_____	_____
3. Rub product into hands, covering all surfaces of hands and fingers.	☐	☐	_____	_____
4. Continue rubbing hands until they are dry.	☐	☐	_____	_____

PROCEDURE 5-3: USE GLOVES

Name _____ **Date** _____

Directions: Practice this procedure, following each step. When you are ready to have your perform-ance evaluated, give this sheet to your instructor.

Procedure	Pass	Redo	Date Competency Met	Instructor Initials
1. Wash hands.	☐	☐	_____	_____
2. Put on gloves.	☐	☐	_____	_____
3. Check gloves for fit, tears, holes, cracks, or discoloration. *Improperly fitting gloves can result in contamination. Damaged gloves do not provide a barrier and protection.*	☐	☐	_____	_____
4. Perform procedure.	☐	☐	_____	_____
5. Remove one glove by grasping outer surface just below the cuff.	☐	☐	_____	_____
6. Pull glove off so that it is inside out.	☐	☐	_____	_____
7. Hold the removed glove in your gloved hand.	☐	☐	_____	_____
8. Place two fingers of ungloved hand under cuff of other glove and pull down so first glove is inside second glove. *When the gloves are inside out and one inside the other, pathogens are contained.*	☐	☐	_____	_____
9. Dispose of gloves without contaminating hands. *If your skin comes into contact with the outside surface of the contaminated gloves, you are contaminated.*	☐	☐	_____	_____
10. Wash hands.	☐	☐	_____	_____

PROCEDURE 5-4: APPLY AND REMOVE PERSONAL PROTECTIVE EQUIPMENT

Name _____ **Date** _____

Directions: Practice this procedure, following each step. When you are ready to have your performance evaluated, give this sheet to your instructor.

Procedure	Pass	Redo	Date Competency Met	Instructor Initials
1. Wash hands.	☐	☐	_____	_____
2. Get disposable face mask, isolation gown, and gloves.	☐	☐	_____	_____
3. Pick up mask by the elastic straps or top strings.	☐	☐	_____	_____
4. Place the mask over your nose and mouth.	☐	☐	_____	_____
a. Pull elastic straps around the ears or				
b. Place top strings over your ears,	☐	☐	_____	_____
c. Tie at the back of head with a bow and repeat with lower strings.	☐	☐	_____	_____
5. Unfold isolation gown so the opening is at the back.	☐	☐	_____	_____
6. Put your arms into the sleeves of the isolation gown.	☐	☐	_____	_____
7. Fit the gown at the neck, making sure your uniform is covered. *By covering all of your uniform, you prevent the uniform from becoming contaminated and do not risk contaminating other residents with your uniform.*	☐	☐	_____	_____
8. Reach behind and tie the neck back with a bow.	☐	☐	_____	_____
9. Grasp the edges of the gown and pull to the back.	☐	☐	_____	_____
10. Overlap the edges of the gown to completely cover your uniform.	☐	☐	_____	_____
11. Tie the waist ties in a bow.	☐	☐	_____	_____
12. Put on gloves.	☐	☐	_____	_____

Procedure	Pass	Redo	Date Competency Met	Instructor Initials
13. Perform procedures for resident.	☐	☐	_____	_____
14. Remove gloves.	☐	☐	_____	_____
15. Wash hands.	☐	☐	_____	_____
16. Untie the gown.	☐	☐	_____	_____
17. Grasp each shoulder of gown at neck to remove sleeves.	☐	☐	_____	_____
18. Turn the sleeves inside out as you remove them from your arms.	☐	☐	_____	_____
19. Roll the gown with the contaminated portion inside. *When gown is inside out and rolled, pathogens are contained.*	☐	☐	_____	_____
20. Discard the gown in a designated container in the room.	☐	☐	_____	_____
21. Wash hands.	☐	☐	_____	_____
22. If the mask has elastic straps, remove them from behind your ears. If the mask has strings, untie the lower strings first, then untie the top strings and remove the mask by the top strings.	☐	☐	_____	_____
23. Discard the mask in a designated container.	☐	☐	_____	_____
24. Wash hands.	☐	☐	_____	_____
25. Use a paper towel to open the door when leaving the room and discard paper towel in the wastebasket inside the room as you leave.	☐	☐	_____	_____

PROCEDURE 8-1: RESPOND TO AN ADULT RESIDENT WHO IS CHOKING

Name _____ **Date** _____

Directions: Practice this procedure, following each step. When you are ready to have your performance evaluated, give this sheet to your instructor.

Procedure	Pass	Redo	Date Competency Met	Instructor Initials
1. Call for nurse and stay with resident.	☐	☐	_____	_____
2. Check if resident is breathing and ask resident if he or she can speak or cough.	☐	☐	_____	_____
3. If not, move behind resident and slide arms under resident's arms and across resident's abdomen.	☐	☐	_____	_____
4. Place your fist between the resident's navel and ribs, thumb side against the abdomen.	☐	☐	_____	_____
5. Grasp your fist with your other hand.	☐	☐	_____	_____
6. Press your fist into the abdomen with quick inward and upward thrusts.	☐	☐	_____	_____
7. Repeat abdominal thrusts until object is expelled.	☐	☐	_____	_____
8. If resident becomes place resident on the floor on his or her back.	☐	☐	_____	_____
9. Tilt resident's head back and check mouth for any visible objects.	☐	☐	_____	_____
10. Perform finger sweep:	☐	☐	_____	_____
a. Open resident's mouth and hold lower jaw and tongue to keep mouth open.	☐	☐	_____	_____
b. Put forefinger of your other hand in mouth and sweep finger from cheek to cheek.	☐	☐	_____	_____
c. Bend your finger and attempt to hook object in airway and pull it up into the mouth.	☐	☐	_____	_____
11. Straddle the resident.	☐	☐	_____	_____
12. Place the heel of one hand above the navel and the other hand on top of the first hand.	☐	☐	_____	_____

Procedure	Pass	Redo	Date Competency Met	Instructor Initials
13. Keep your elbows straight and give three to five quick inward and upward thrusts.	☐	☐	_____	_____
14. Repeat the finger sweep followed by three to five thrusts until airway is cleared or nurse arrives.	☐	☐	_____	_____
15. Follow supervising nurse's directions regarding resident care.	☐	☐	_____	_____
16. Assist nurse with documentation according to facility policy.	☐	☐	_____	_____
17. Check resident frequently for any signs of distress.	☐	☐	_____	_____

PROCEDURE 13-1: MAKE AN UNOCCUPIED BED (OPEN OR CLOSED)

Name _____ **Date** _____

Directions: Practice this procedure, following each step. When you are ready to have your perform-ance evaluated, give this sheet to your instructor.

Procedure	Pass	Redo	Date Competency Met	Instructor Initials
1. Collect clean linen in order of use:	☐	☐	_____	_____
a. mattress pad	☐	☐	_____	_____
b. bottom sheet	☐	☐	_____	_____
c. draw sheet (if used)	☐	☐	_____	_____
d. top sheet	☐	☐	_____	_____
e. bedspread	☐	☐	_____	_____
f. pillowcase	☐	☐	_____	_____
2. Carry linen away from uniform. *Your uniform is considered contaminated and will contaminate the clean linen.*	☐	☐	_____	_____
3. Place linen on clean surface (bedside stand, overbed table, or other clean surface) in order of use.	☐	☐	_____	_____
4. Put bed in flattest position.	☐	☐	_____	_____
5. Remove pillowcase.	☐	☐	_____	_____
6. Strip the bed.	☐	☐	_____	_____
7. Put mattress pad on the bed.	☐	☐	_____	_____
8. Place bottom sheet on the bed. *Shaking linen spreads pathogens.*	☐	☐	_____	_____
a. If using a flat sheet:				
• Put the narrow hem at the bottom of the bed.	☐	☐	_____	_____
• Tuck the sheet under the top of the mattress.	☐	☐	_____	_____
• Make a mitered corner.	☐	☐	_____	_____
• Tuck the sheet under the mattress along the side.	☐	☐	_____	_____
b. If using a fitted sheet, pull the fitted corners over the top and bottom of the mattress on one side.	☐	☐	_____	_____

Procedure	Pass	Redo	Date Competency Met	Instructor Initials
9. If draw sheet is used: a. Place it on top of the sheet about 12 inches from the top edge of the mattress.	☐	☐	_____	_____
b. Tuck the draw sheet under the mattress on one side.	☐	☐	_____	_____
10. Place the top sheet on the center of the bed.	☐	☐	_____	_____
11. Unfold the sheet with as little movement as possible.	☐	☐	_____	_____
12. Center the top sheet with the wide hem even with the top of the mattress and the stitched or seamed side up.	☐	☐	_____	_____
13. Place the blanket over the top sheet.	☐	☐	_____	_____
a. Top edge of blanket should be 6–8 inches below the top edge of the top sheet.	☐	☐	_____	_____
b. Fold the top sheet down over the top of the blanket to make a cuff.	☐	☐	_____	_____
14. Tuck the bottom linen and blanket under the foot of the bed. Make a mitered corner and toe pleat. *Toe pleats provide additional room for the resident's feet and prevent pressure on the toes that could cause skin breakdown.*	☐	☐	_____	_____
15. Move to the other side of the bed. *Complete one side of bed before going to other side of bed to save time and energy.*	☐	☐	_____	_____
16. Unfold and secure clean bottom and top linen.	☐	☐	_____	_____
17. Place the pillow on the bed and put on the pillowcase:	☐	☐	_____	_____
a. Grasp the clean pillowcase at the center of the seamed end.	☐	☐	_____	_____
b. Turn the pillowcase back over that hand.	☐	☐	_____	_____
c. Grasp the pillow at the center with the hand that is inside the pillowcase.	☐	☐	_____	_____
d. Pull the pillowcase down over the pillow with your free hand.	☐	☐	_____	_____

Procedure	Pass	Redo	Date Competency Met	Instructor Initials
e. Line up the seams of the pillowcase with the edges of the pillow.	☐	☐	_____	_____
f. Make sure that the corners of the pillow are in the corners of the pillowcase.	☐	☐	_____	_____
g. Fold the extra material of the pillowcase under the pillow.	☐	☐	_____	_____
18. Place the pillow on the bed so that the open edge is facing away from the door.	☐	☐	_____	_____
19. For an open bed: a. Fanfold the top linen toward the foot of the bed.	☐	☐	_____	_____
b. Be certain that the cuff edge is closest to the head of the bed so the resident who returns to the bed can easily get covered.	☐	☐	_____	_____
20. For a closed bed: a. Place the bedspread over the blanket and the pillow.	☐	☐	_____	_____
b. Tuck the bedspread along the lower edge of the pillow and along the top of the pillow.	☐	☐	_____	_____

PROCEDURE 13-2: MAKE AN OCCUPIED BED

Name _____ Date _____

Directions: Practice this procedure, following each step. When you are ready to have your perform-ance evaluated, give this sheet to your instructor.

Procedure	Pass	Redo	Date Competency Met	Instructor Initials
1. Collect clean linen in order of use:	☐	☐	_____	_____
a. mattress pad	☐	☐	_____	_____
b. bottom sheet	☐	☐	_____	_____
c. draw sheet (if used)	☐	☐	_____	_____
d. top sheet	☐	☐	_____	_____
e. bedspread	☐	☐	_____	_____
f. pillowcase	☐	☐	_____	_____
2. Carry linen away from uniform. *Your uniform is considered contaminated and will contaminate the clean linen.*	☐	☐	_____	_____
3. Place linen on clean surface (bedside stand, overbed table, or other clean surface in order of use).	☐	☐	_____	_____
4. Explain the procedure to the resident.	☐	☐	_____	_____
5. Provide for resident's privacy by pulling the curtain around the bed, closing the door, and closing the window drape.	☐	☐	_____	_____
6. Lower head of bed to a comfortable level for the resident.	☐	☐	_____	_____
7. Raise the side rails and raise the bed to a working height.	☐	☐	_____	_____
8. Lower the side rail on the side of the bed nearest you.	☐	☐	_____	_____
9. Loosen the top linen at the foot of the bed.	☐	☐	_____	_____
10. Remove the blanket.	☐	☐	_____	_____
11. Drape the resident with a bath blanket: a. Unfold the bath blanket over the top sheet.	☐	☐	_____	_____

Procedure	Pass	Redo	Date Competency Met	Instructor Initials
b. Ask the resident to hold the top of the bath blanket or tuck the top edge under the resident's shoulders to keep it in place.	☐	☐	_____	_____
c. Roll the sheet under the bath blanket to the foot of the bed and remove it.	☐	☐	_____	_____
12. Loosen the bottom linen.	☐	☐	_____	_____
13. Turn the resident away from you toward the side rail on the far side of the bed.	☐	☐	_____	_____
14. Roll the bottom lines toward the resident, and tuck it under the resident's body.	☐	☐	_____	_____
15. Put the mattress pad on the bed.	☐	☐	_____	_____
16. Place the bottom sheet on the bed. *Place linen on bed because shaking linen spreads pathogens.*	☐	☐	_____	_____
a. If using a flat sheet: • Put the narrow hem at the bottom of the bed.	☐	☐	_____	_____
• Tuck the sheet under the top of the mattress.	☐	☐	_____	_____
• Make a mitered corner.	☐	☐	_____	_____
• Tuck the sheet under the mattress along the side.	☐	☐	_____	_____
b. If using a fitted sheet, pull the fitted corners over the top and bottom of the mattress on one side.	☐	☐	_____	_____
17. If using a draw sheet, place it on top of the sheet about 12 inches from the top edge of the mattress and tuck it under the mattress on one side.	☐	☐	_____	_____
18. Fold the clean linen toward the resident next to the used linen.	☐	☐	_____	_____
19. Raise the side rail on the side near you.	☐	☐	_____	_____
20. Ask resident to turn onto back and adjust pillow.	☐	☐	_____	_____

Procedure	Pass	Redo	Date Competency Met	Instructor Initials
21. Move to other side of bed, lower side rail, and help resident turn toward the side rail on the far side of bed.	☐	☐	_____	_____
22. Loosen used bottom linen.	☐	☐	_____	_____
23. Roll linen from the head to the foot of the bed, remove, and place with other used linen.	☐	☐	_____	_____
24. Unfold clean bottom linen from beneath the resident, tucking under mattress while pulling it snug.	☐	☐	_____	_____
25. Assist the resident to a comfortable position.	☐	☐	_____	_____
26. Put top sheet over bath blanket and unfold with as little movement as possible.	☐	☐	_____	_____
27. Unfold top sheet with the wide hem toward head of bed.	☐	☐	_____	_____
28. Place blanket over the top sheet about 6–8 inches below the top edge of the top sheet and fold top sheet down over it to form a cuff.	☐	☐	_____	_____
29. Ask the resident to hold the top linen. Roll bath blanket from the head to the foot of the bed and remove.	☐	☐	_____	_____
30. Tuck top linen under the bottom of the mattress and make mitered corners.	☐	☐	_____	_____
31. Raise the side rail.	☐	☐	_____	_____
32. Loosen top linen over resident's feet. *Loosening top linen provides additional room for the resident's feet and prevents pressure on the toes that could cause skin breakdown.*	☐	☐	_____	_____
33. Put clean case on pillow:	☐	☐	_____	_____
a. Grasp the clean pillowcase at the center of the seamed end.	☐	☐	_____	_____
b. Turn the pillowcase back over that hand.	☐	☐	_____	_____

Procedure	Pass	Redo	Date Competency Met	Instructor Initials
c. Grasp the pillow at the center with the hand that is inside the pillowcase.	☐	☐	_____	_____
d. Pull the pillowcase down over the pillow with your free hand.	☐	☐	_____	_____
e. Line up the seams of the pillowcase with the edges of the pillow.	☐	☐	_____	_____
f. Make sure that the corners of the pillow are in the corners of the pillowcase.	☐	☐	_____	_____
g. Fold the extra material of the pillowcase under the pillow.	☐	☐	_____	_____
34. Place pillow under the resident's head with the open edge facing away from the door.	☐	☐	_____	_____
35. Return height of bed to lowest position and lower side rails.	☐	☐	_____	_____
36. Open curtain, window drapes, and door.	☐	☐	_____	_____
37. Dispose of linen in used linen hamper.	☐	☐	_____	_____
38. Be certain that the resident is comfortable, in proper body alignment, and has call signal.	☐	☐	_____	_____

PROCEDURE 16-1: ASSIST RESIDENT TO MOVE TO HEAD OF BED

Name _____ **Date** _____

Directions: Practice this procedure, following each step. When you are ready to have your perform-ance evaluated, give this sheet to your instructor.

Procedure	Pass	Redo	Date Competency Met	Instructor Initials
1. Raise side rails and raise the bed to working height.	☐	☐	_____	_____
2. Lower head of bed.	☐	☐	_____	_____
3. Lean pillow against headboard and lower side rail. *The pillow provides for the resident's safety by preventing resident's head from hitting headboard.*	☐	☐	_____	_____
4. Lower side rail on the side nearest you.	☐	☐	_____	_____
5. Face head of bed, one foot in front of other, 12 inches apart.	☐	☐	_____	_____
6. Keep your knees and back straight.	☐	☐	_____	_____
7. Place one arm under resident's shoulder blades and the other arm under resident's thighs.	☐	☐	_____	_____
8. Ask resident to bend knees, put feet flat on mattress, bend arms, and brace on bed.	☐	☐	_____	_____
9. Tell resident that, on count of three, resident should push with feet and arms as you lift and shift your weight from your back foot to front foot.	☐	☐	_____	_____
10. Place pillow under resident's head and raise side rail.	☐	☐	_____	_____
11. Lower the height of the bed and position side rails as appropriate for the resident.	☐	☐	_____	_____

PROCEDURE 16-2: ASSIST RESIDENT TO MOVE TO HEAD OF BED USING LIFT SHEET AND ASSISTANT

Name _____ **Date** _____

Directions: Practice this procedure, following each step. When you are ready to have your performance evaluated, give this sheet to your instructor.

Procedure	Pass	Redo	Date Competency Met	Instructor Initials
1. Raise side rails and raise the bed to working height.	☐	☐	_____	_____
2. Lower head of bed.	☐	☐	_____	_____
3. Lean pillow against headboard. *The pillow provides for the resident's safety by preventing resident's head from hitting headboard.*	☐	☐	_____	_____
4. You and assistant lower side rails on both sides of bed.	☐	☐	_____	_____
5. Face head of bed, one foot in front of other, 12 inches apart.	☐	☐	_____	_____
6. Keep your knees and back straight.	☐	☐	_____	_____
7. Be sure lift sheet is under resident's shoulders and hips.	☐	☐	_____	_____
8. Roll lift sheet as close as possible to resident's body.	☐	☐	_____	_____
9. Grasp lift sheet with one hand at resident's shoulder and the other at resident's hip.	☐	☐	_____	_____
10. On the count of three, both you and assistant move the resident to the head of the bed by shifting your weight from the back foot to the front foot.	☐	☐	_____	_____
11. Put pillow under resident's head.	☐	☐	_____	_____
12. Unroll, straighten, and tuck the lift sheet under the mattress.	☐	☐	_____	_____
13. Lower the height of the bed and position side rails as appropriate for the resident.	☐	☐	_____	_____

PROCEDURE 16-3: MOVE RESIDENT TO ONE SIDE OF BED

Name _____ **Date** _____

Directions: Practice this procedure, following each step. When you are ready to have your perform-
ance evaluated, give this sheet to your instructor.

Procedure	Pass	Redo	Date Competency Met	Instructor Initials
1. Raise side rails and raise bed to working height.	☐	☐	_____	_____
2. Lower head of bed.	☐	☐	_____	_____
3. Lower side rail. Place your feet apart, one in front of the other, knees bent, back straight.	☐	☐	_____	_____
4. Place resident's arms over chest.	☐	☐	_____	_____
5. Place your arms under resident's shoulders and upper back and move upper section of the body toward you.	☐	☐	_____	_____
6. Place your arms under resident's waist and thighs and move middle of the body toward you.	☐	☐	_____	_____
7. Place your arms under resident's thighs and lower legs and move lower part of the body toward you.	☐	☐	_____	_____
8. Turn resident away from you or raise side rail, lower height of the bed, lower side rails, and begin transfer.	☐	☐	_____	_____

PROCEDURE 16-4: TURN RESIDENT AWAY FROM YOU

Name _____ **Date** _____

Directions: Practice this procedure, following each step. When you are ready to have your performance evaluated, give this sheet to your instructor.

Procedure	Pass	Redo	Date Competency Met	Instructor Initials
1. Place resident in supine position.	☐	☐	_____	_____
2. Raise side rails and raise bed to working height.	☐	☐	_____	_____
3. Lower head of bed.	☐	☐	_____	_____
4. Move resident to the side of the bed nearest you.	☐	☐	_____	_____
5. Bend resident's farthest arm next to head and place other arm across chest.	☐	☐	_____	_____
6. Cross the resident's near leg over the far leg or bend knee slightly. *If resident has a problem with the hip, crossing the leg may be painful. By slightly bending the knee, the leg will turn in the appropriate direction when the resident is turned and will not put stress on the hip joint.*	☐	☐	_____	_____
7. Place one hand under the resident's shoulder blade, and the other hand under the buttocks. *Do not move a resident by grasping a joint because you may pull the joint out of alignment, causing pain and possible injury.*	☐	☐	_____	_____
8. On count of three, roll resident away from you onto side.	☐	☐	_____	_____
9. Lower height of bed and position side rails as appropriate for resident.	☐	☐	_____	_____

PROCEDURE 16-5: TURN RESIDENT TOWARD YOU

Name _____ Date _____

Directions: Practice this procedure, following each step. When you are ready to have your perform-
ance evaluated, give this sheet to your instructor.

Procedure	Pass	Redo	Date Competency Met	Instructor Initials
SAFETY AND INFECTION CONTROL CAUTION: Turn resident away from you whenever possible. If you must turn resident toward you, do not lean against resident during turn because resident may be injured and will be contaminated by your uniform.				
1. Place resident in supine position.	☐	☐	_____	_____
2. Raise side rails and raise bed to working height.	☐	☐	_____	_____
3. Lower head of bed.	☐	☐	_____	_____
4. Lower side rail, move resident to the side of the bed nearest you, and raise side rail.	☐	☐	_____	_____
5. Go to other side of bed.	☐	☐	_____	_____
SAFETY CAUTION: For the resident's safety, leave side rail up when turning resident toward you, if possible, to prevent resident from accidentally rolling off bed.				
6. Bend resident's near arm next to head and place other arm across chest.	☐	☐	_____	_____
7. Cross the resident's far leg over the near leg or bend knee slightly. *If resident has a problem with the hip, crossing the leg may be painful. By slightly bending the knee, the leg will turn in the appropriate direction when the resident is turned and will not put stress on the hip joint.*	☐	☐	_____	_____
8. Reach across without leaning on resident and place one hand under the resident's shoulder blade and the other hand under the buttocks. *Do not move a resident by grasping a joint because you may pull the joint out of alignment, causing pain and possible injury.*	☐	☐	_____	_____
9. On count of three, roll resident toward you onto side.	☐	☐	_____	_____
10. Lower height of bed and leave side rail up. *Never leave the resident rolled to the side of the bed if the side rail is down.*	☐	☐	_____	_____

PROCEDURE 16-6: ASSIST RESIDENT TO SIT ON EDGE OF BED

Name _____ **Date** _____

Directions: Practice this procedure, following each step. When you are ready to have your performance evaluated, give this sheet to your instructor.

Procedure	Pass	Redo	Date Competency Met	Instructor Initials
1. Place bed in lowest height and lock wheels.	☐	☐	_____	_____
2. Move resident to side of bed closest to you.	☐	☐	_____	_____
3. Raise the head of the bed and allow resident to sit up for several minutes. *Allowing resident to sit up for a few minutes before moving to the edge of bed may prevent dizziness from sudden change of posture.*	☐	☐	_____	_____
4. Place one arm under resident's shoulders and the other arm under resident's knees. *Holding the resident under the shoulders and knees allows you to move the body in good alignment. Never pull the resident's legs off the bed or pull resident up by arms, which can cause severe injury.*	☐	☐	_____	_____
5. On count of three, turn resident toward you so legs dangle over side of bed.	☐	☐	_____	_____
6. Tell resident to provide support by pushing fists into the mattress.	☐	☐	_____	_____
7. Stand, blocking the resident's knees, and check resident for dizziness.	☐	☐	_____	_____
8. Be certain resident's feet are flat on the floor.	☐	☐	_____	_____

PROCEDURE 16-7: PIVOT TRANSFER RESIDENT TO WHEELCHAIR

Name _____ **Date** _____

Directions: Practice this procedure, following each step. When you are ready to have your perform-ance evaluated, give this sheet to your instructor.

Procedure	Pass	Redo	Date Competency Met	Instructor Initials
NOTE: Pivot transfer is used for residents who can bear weight and assist with the move.				
1. Put bed at lowest height and lock the wheels.	☐	☐	_____	_____
2. Place wheelchair on resident's strong side, braced firmly against side of bed.	☐	☐	_____	_____
3. Lock wheels and move footrests out of the way.	☐	☐	_____	_____
4. Assist resident to sit on edge of bed.	☐	☐	_____	_____
5. Stand in front of resident and block resident's feet with your feet.	☐	☐	_____	_____
6. Bend your knees and put your knees against resident's knees.	☐	☐	_____	_____
7. Place your hands under resident's arms and under resident's shoulder blades.	☐	☐	_____	_____
8. Ask resident to push on mattress with hands or place hands on your upper arms.	☐	☐	_____	_____
9. On the count of three, help resident into standing position by straightening your knees.	☐	☐	_____	_____
10. Allow resident to gain balance and ask if resident feels dizzy.	☐	☐	_____	_____
11. Taking small steps, pivot resident toward chair.	☐	☐	_____	_____
12. Help resident back up until back of legs touch the seat of the wheelchair.	☐	☐	_____	_____
13. Have resident hold arms of chair if able.	☐	☐	_____	_____
14. Lower resident into wheelchair by bending your knees and leaning forward.	☐	☐	_____	_____
15. Align resident's body and position footrests.	☐	☐	_____	_____

PROCEDURE 16-8: PERFORM RANGE-OF-MOTION EXERCISES

Name _____ Date _____

Directions: Practice this procedure, following each step. When you are ready to have your performance evaluated, give this sheet to your instructor.

Procedure	Pass	Redo	Date Competency Met	Instructor Initials
1. Before beginning procedure, check if joints are swollen, red, or warm or if resident complains of pain.	☐	☐	_____	_____
2. If problem exists, notify the nurse immediately and do not perform procedure unless instructed to do so by the nurse.	☐	☐	_____	_____
3. Support limb above and below joint.	☐	☐	_____	_____
4. Begin exercises at neck then shoulders, elbows, wrists, thumbs, fingers, hips, knees, ankles, and toes.	☐	☐	_____	_____
5. Slowly move joint in all directions it normally moves.	☐	☐	_____	_____
6. Repeat movement as directed by supervising nurse. *The number of times a movement can be repeated depends on the resident's condition and tolerance.*	☐	☐	_____	_____
7. Stop procedure at any sign of pain and report to supervising nurse immediately.	☐	☐	_____	_____

PROCEDURE 17-1: DRAPE AND UNDRAPE RESIDENT

Name _____ **Date** _____

Directions: Practice this procedure, following each step. When you are ready to have your performance evaluated, give this sheet to your instructor.

Procedure	Pass	Redo	Date Competency Met	Instructor Initials
1. Raise side rail, raise bed to working height, and lower side rail on side you are working.	☐	☐	_____	_____
2. Place drape over top linen and unfold.	☐	☐	_____	_____
3. Ask resident to hold drape or tuck drape under resident's shoulders.	☐	☐	_____	_____
4. Roll top linen from head to foot of bed.	☐	☐	_____	_____
5. Perform procedure.	☐	☐	_____	_____
6. Cover resident with top linen.	☐	☐	_____	_____
7. Ask resident to hold top linen or tuck under resident's shoulders.	☐	☐	_____	_____
8. Roll drape from under top linen to foot of bed and remove.	☐	☐	_____	_____
9. Raise side rail.	☐	☐	_____	_____
10. Lower the height of the bed and position side rails as appropriate for resident.	☐	☐	_____	_____

PROCEDURE 17-2: ADMINISTER A BED BATH

Name _____ **Date** _____

Directions: Practice this procedure, following each step. When you are ready to have your perform-
ance evaluated, give this sheet to your instructor.

Procedure	Pass	Redo	Date Competency Met	Instructor Initials
1. Gather supplies including:	☐	☐	_____	_____
a. bed linen	☐	☐	_____	_____
b. drape	☐	☐	_____	_____
c. towels	☐	☐	_____	_____
d. washcloths	☐	☐	_____	_____
e. clean gown	☐	☐	_____	_____
f. waterproof pad	☐	☐	_____	_____
g. bath basin	☐	☐	_____	_____
h. soap	☐	☐	_____	_____
2. Offer resident urinal or bedpan. *Water stimulates the urge to urinate.*	☐	☐	_____	_____
3. Raise side rails before raising bed to working height and lower side rail on side of bed care is being given.	☐	☐	_____	_____
4. Drape resident and remove gown from beneath drape.	☐	☐	_____	_____
5. Fill bath basin with warm water and ask resident to check water temperature.	☐	☐	_____	_____
6. If resident has open lesions or wounds, put on gloves. *Check resident's skin (pressure areas and friction areas) during bed bath.*	☐	☐	_____	_____
7. Fold and wet washcloth.	☐	☐	_____	_____
8. Gently wash eye from inner corner out. Wash other eye using a different part of cloth. *Using soap will irritate eye. Washing eye from inner corner out reduces pressure and pulling on eyelid. Using a different part of the cloth for the other eye reduces the chance of spreading infection.*	☐	☐	_____	_____
9. Wet washcloth and apply soap, if requested.	☐	☐	_____	_____

Procedure	Pass	Redo	Date Competency Met	Instructor Initials
10. Wash, rinse, and pat dry face, neck, ears, and behind ears.	☐	☐	_____	_____
11. Place towel under far arm.	☐	☐	_____	_____
12. Wash, rinse, and pat dry hand, arm, shoulder, and underarm.	☐	☐	_____	_____
13. Repeat steps 11 and 12 with other arm.	☐	☐	_____	_____
14. Place towel over chest and abdomen and lower bath blanket to waist.	☐	☐	_____	_____
15. Lift towel and wash, rinse, and pat dry chest and abdomen.	☐	☐	_____	_____
16. Pull drape up over towel and remove towel.	☐	☐	_____	_____
17. Place towel under far leg.	☐	☐	_____	_____
18. Wash, rinse, and pat dry leg from hip to foot.	☐	☐	_____	_____
19. Repeat steps 17 and 18 with other leg.	☐	☐	_____	_____
20. Change water in basin.	☐	☐	_____	_____
21. Turn resident away from you on to side.	☐	☐	_____	_____
22. Wash, rinse, and pat dry from neck to buttocks and turn resident onto back.	☐	☐	_____	_____
23. Change bath water, put on clean gloves, and use clean washcloth and towel.	☐	☐	_____	_____
24. Provide perineal care.	☐	☐	_____	_____
25. Remove gloves.	☐	☐	_____	_____
26. Wash hands.	☐	☐	_____	_____
27. Help resident put on clean gown.	☐	☐	_____	_____
28. Offer back rub.	☐	☐	_____	_____
29. Change bed linen.	☐	☐	_____	_____
30. Raise side rail, lower the height of the bed, and position side rails as appropriate for resident.	☐	☐	_____	_____

PROCEDURE 17-3: PERFORM PERINEAL CARE

Name _____ **Date** _____

Directions: Practice this procedure, following each step. When you are ready to have your performance evaluated, give this sheet to your instructor.

Procedure	Pass	Redo	Date Competency Met	Instructor Initials
1. Offer resident urinal or bedpan.	☐	☐	_____	_____
2. Assist resident to supine position.	☐	☐	_____	_____
3. Gather supplies:	☐	☐	_____	_____
a. waterproof pad	☐	☐	_____	_____
b. bath basin	☐	☐	_____	_____
c. towels	☐	☐	_____	_____
d. washcloths	☐	☐	_____	_____
e. drape	☐	☐	_____	_____
f. soap	☐	☐	_____	_____
4. Drape resident.	☐	☐	_____	_____
5. Place waterproof pad under resident's hips.	☐	☐	_____	_____
6. Fill bath basin with warm water and ask resident to check water temperature.	☐	☐	_____	_____
7. Put on gloves.	☐	☐	_____	_____
8. Assist resident to spread legs and lift knees if possible.	☐	☐	_____	_____
9. Wet and soap folded washcloth.	☐	☐	_____	_____
10. If resident has catheter:				
a. Check for leakage, secretions, and irritation.	☐	☐	_____	_____
b. Gently wipe catheter from meatus out for 4 inches.	☐	☐	_____	_____
11. For females:				
a. Separate labia.	☐	☐	_____	_____
b. Wash from front to back with one stroke down center of urethral area, then one stroke down each side, using different part of washcloth for each stroke.	☐	☐	_____	_____

Procedure	Pass	Redo	Date Competency Met	Instructor Initials
c. With clean washcloth, rinse in same direction as when washing and thoroughly pat dry.	☐	☐	_____	_____
12. For males: a. Pull back foreskin if male is uncircumcised.	☐	☐	_____	_____
b. Wash and rinse head of penis, beginning at urethra and washing outward.	☐	☐	_____	_____
c. Using a clean washcloth, rinse and dry thoroughly.	☐	☐	_____	_____
d. Put foreskin of uncircumcised male back to normal position.	☐	☐	_____	_____
13. Continue washing down the penis to the scrotum and inner thighs.	☐	☐	_____	_____
14. Use clean washcloth, rinse area, and thoroughly pat dry.	☐	☐	_____	_____
15. Assist resident to turn onto side away from you.	☐	☐	_____	_____
16. Remove any feces with toilet tissue.	☐	☐	_____	_____
17. Wet and soap washcloth.	☐	☐	_____	_____
18. Wash anal area from vagina or scrotum to anal area using different area of cloth for each stroke.	☐	☐	_____	_____
19. Rinse and thoroughly pat dry.	☐	☐	_____	_____
20. Remove waterproof pad and undrape resident.	☐	☐	_____	_____
21. Raise side rail, lower the height of the bed and position side rails as appropriate for resident	☐	☐	_____	_____
22. Remove gloves and wash hands.	☐	☐	_____	_____

PROCEDURE 17-4: ASSIST RESIDENT WITH SHOWER/TUB BATH

Name _____ **Date** _____

Directions: Practice this procedure, following each step. When you are ready to have your perform-ance evaluated, give this sheet to your instructor.

Procedure	Pass	Redo	Date Competency Met	Instructor Initials
1. Gather supplies:	☐	☐	_____	_____
a. towels	☐	☐	_____	_____
b. washcloths	☐	☐	_____	_____
c. soap	☐	☐	_____	_____
d. shampoo	☐	☐	_____	_____
e. shower chair if needed	☐	☐	_____	_____
f. shower cap if needed	☐	☐	_____	_____
g. tub mat	☐	☐	_____	_____
h. personal toilet articles	☐	☐	_____	_____
i. clean clothing	☐	☐	_____	_____
2. Assist resident to bathing area.	☐	☐	_____	_____
3. Clean shower area and shower chair or tub.	☐	☐	_____	_____
4. Stay with resident during entire procedure. *Resident may become weak when bathing.*	☐	☐	_____	_____
5. Help resident to remove clothing and drape resident with bath blanket.	☐	☐	_____	_____
6. Turn on water and ask resident to check water temperature.	☐	☐	_____	_____
7. For shower:				
a. Assist resident into shower chair.	☐	☐	_____	_____
b. Remove drape.	☐	☐	_____	_____
c. Push chair into shower and lock wheels.	☐	☐	_____	_____
8. For tub bath:	☐	☐	_____	_____
a. Place bath mat on floor beside tub.	☐	☐	_____	_____
b. Assist resident into tub.	☐	☐	_____	_____
9. Let resident wash as much as possible, starting with face, and assist as necessary.	☐	☐	_____	_____

Procedure	Pass	Redo	Date Competency Met	Instructor Initials
10. Help resident shampoo and rinse hair, if necessary. *If resident has hair done by beautician, do not wash hair unless directed by nurse.*	☐	☐	_____	_____
11. For shower:				
a. Turn off water.	☐	☐	_____	_____
b. Give resident towel and assist to pat dry.	☐	☐	_____	_____
12. For tub bath:				
a. Drain tub.	☐	☐	_____	_____
b. Help resident out of tub into chair.	☐	☐	_____	_____
c. Give resident towel and assist to pat dry.	☐	☐	_____	_____
13. Help resident dress, comb hair, and return to room.	☐	☐	_____	_____

PROCEDURE 17-5: RUB RESIDENT'S BACK

Name _____ Date _____

Directions: Practice this procedure, following each step. When you are ready to have your perform-ance evaluated, give this sheet to your instructor.

Procedure	Pass	Redo	Date Competency Met	Instructor Initials
1. Gather supplies:	☐	☐	_____	_____
a. towel	☐	☐	_____	_____
b. lotion	☐	☐	_____	_____
c. gloves, if resident has open areas or rash on skin	☐	☐	_____	_____
2. Raise side rails before raising bed to working height, and lower side rail on side of bed care is being given.	☐	☐	_____	_____
3. Turn resident away from you onto side and expose only back and shoulders.	☐	☐	_____	_____
4. Rub lotion between your hands to warm it.	☐	☐	_____	_____
5. Apply lotion to entire back with palms of your hands.	☐	☐	_____	_____
6. Make long, firm strokes along spine from buttocks to shoulders to relax muscles.	☐	☐	_____	_____
7. Make circular strokes on shoulders, upper arms, and down sides of back to buttocks to increase circulation.	☐	☐	_____	_____
8. Observe skin, report abnormalities to nurse, and do not rub reddened areas. *Reddened areas are a sign of decreased circulation and rubbing them may damage skin and underlying structures.*	☐	☐	_____	_____
9. Repeat for 3–5 minutes.	☐	☐	_____	_____
10. Gently pat off excess lotion with towel.	☐	☐	_____	_____
11. Cover resident.	☐	☐	_____	_____
12. Lower height of bed and position side rails as appropriate for resident.	☐	☐	_____	_____

PROCEDURE 17-6: ASSIST RESIDENT WITH ORAL CARE

Name _____ Date _____

Directions: Practice this procedure, following each step. When you are ready to have your performance evaluated, give this sheet to your instructor.

Procedure	Pass	Redo	Date Competency Met	Instructor Initials
1. Gather supplies including:	☐	☐	_____	_____
a. emesis basin	☐	☐	_____	_____
b. towel	☐	☐	_____	_____
c. toothbrush	☐	☐	_____	_____
d. toothpaste	☐	☐	_____	_____
e. mouthwash	☐	☐	_____	_____
f. glass of water with straw if needed	☐	☐	_____	_____
g. gloves	☐	☐	_____	_____
2. Place supplies on overbed table or other clean surface.	☐	☐	_____	_____
3. Raise head of bed so resident is sitting up. *If resident is lying flat or slightly elevated, fluids may drain down back of throat and cause gagging and breathing problems.*	☐	☐	_____	_____
4. Wash hands and put on gloves.	☐	☐	_____	_____
5. Drape towel below resident's chin.	☐	☐	_____	_____
6. Ask resident to rinse mouth with water and spit into emesis basin. *Moistening the mouth before beginning the procedure prevents cracking and other damage to inside of mouth.*	☐	☐	_____	_____
7. Wet brush and put on small amount of toothpaste.	☐	☐	_____	_____
8. Brush all surfaces of upper teeth and then lower teeth. *Brush upper teeth before lower teeth because salivary glands near lower teeth may be stimulated by brushing, will produce too much saliva, and will be uncomfortable for the resident.*	☐	☐	_____	_____
9. Hold emesis basin under resident's chin.	☐	☐	_____	_____

Procedure	Pass	Redo	Date Competency Met	Instructor Initials
10. Have resident rinse mouth with water and spit into emesis basin.	☐	☐	_____	_____
11. If requested, give resident mouthwash half diluted with water.	☐	☐	_____	_____
12. Check teeth, mouth, tongue, and lips for:				
a. odor	☐	☐	_____	_____
b. cracking	☐	☐	_____	_____
c. sores	☐	☐	_____	_____
d. bleeding	☐	☐	_____	_____
e. discoloration	☐	☐	_____	_____
f. loose teeth	☐	☐	_____	_____
13. Remove towel and wipe resident's mouth.	☐	☐	_____	_____
14. Remove supplies and clean equipment according to facility policy.	☐	☐	_____	_____
15. Remove gloves.	☐	☐	_____	_____
16. Wash your hands.	☐	☐	_____	_____
17. Do ending steps:				
a. Be certain resident is comfortable and in good body alignment.	☐	☐	_____	_____
b. Lower height of bed.	☐	☐	_____	_____
c. Position side rails as appropriate for individual resident.	☐	☐	_____	_____
d. Place call light and water on resident's strong side within reach.	☐	☐	_____	_____
e. Open curtains, drapes, and door according to resident's wishes.	☐	☐	_____	_____
f. Check room for safety.	☐	☐	_____	_____
g. Thank resident and ask if anything else is needed.	☐	☐	_____	_____
h. Wash your hands.	☐	☐	_____	_____
i. Report unexpected findings to supervising nurse immediately.	☐	☐	_____	_____
j. Document procedure according to facility policy.	☐	☐	_____	_____

PROCEDURE 17-7: PERFORM ORAL CARE FOR UNCONSCIOUS RESIDENT

Name _____ **Date** _____

Directions: Practice this procedure, following each step. When you are ready to have your perform-
ance evaluated, give this sheet to your instructor.

Procedure	Pass	Redo	Date Competency Met	Instructor Initials
1. Gather equipment:	☐	☐	_____	_____
a. towel	☐	☐	_____	_____
b. emesis basin	☐	☐	_____	_____
c. swabs	☐	☐	_____	_____
d. cleaning solution	☐	☐	_____	_____
e. glass of water	☐	☐	_____	_____
f. padded tongue blade	☐	☐	_____	_____
g. lubricating jelly	☐	☐	_____	_____
h. gloves	☐	☐	_____	_____
2. Place supplies on overbed table or other clean surface.	☐	☐	_____	_____
3. Drape towel over pillow and explain what you are doing to resident. *Even if unconscious, the resident may be able to hear and understand what you say.*	☐	☐	_____	_____
4. Raise side rails before raising bed to working height.	☐	☐	_____	_____
5. Put bed in flattest position and turn resident onto side. *Allows any fluid to drain from mouth, preventing resident from choking or aspirating.*	☐	☐	_____	_____
6. Put on gloves.	☐	☐	_____	_____
7. Place emesis basin under resident's chin.	☐	☐	_____	_____
8. Hold mouth open with padded tongue blade.	☐	☐	_____	_____
9. Dip swab in cleaning solution and wipe:	☐	☐	_____	_____
a. teeth	☐	☐	_____	_____
b. gums	☐	☐	_____	_____
c. tongue	☐	☐	_____	_____
d. all inside surfaces of mouth	☐	☐	_____	_____

Procedure	Pass	Redo	Date Competency Met	Instructor Initials
10. Change swab and repeat as needed.	☐	☐	_____	_____
11. Rinse with clean swab dipped in water.	☐	☐	_____	_____
12. Check teeth, mouth, tongue, and lips for:				
a. odor	☐	☐	_____	_____
b. cracking	☐	☐	_____	_____
c. sores	☐	☐	_____	_____
d. bleeding	☐	☐	_____	_____
e. discoloration	☐	☐	_____	_____
f. loose teeth	☐	☐	_____	_____
13. Cover lips with thin layer of lubricating jelly.	☐	☐	_____	_____
14. Remove towel.	☐	☐	_____	_____
15. Place resident in comfortable position and in good body alignment.	☐	☐	_____	_____
16. Remove gloves.	☐	☐	_____	_____
17. Lower height of bed and position side rails as appropriate for individual resident.	☐	☐	_____	_____

PROCEDURE 17-8: ASSIST RESIDENT WITH DENTURE CARE

Name _____ **Date** _____

Directions: Practice this procedure, following each step. When you are ready to have your performance evaluated, give this sheet to your instructor.

Procedure	Pass	Redo	Date Competency Met	Instructor Initials
1. Gather equipment:	☐	☐	_____	_____
a. towels	☐	☐	_____	_____
b. denture cup	☐	☐	_____	_____
c. emesis basin	☐	☐	_____	_____
d. denture brush or toothbrush	☐	☐	_____	_____
e. denture cleaner	☐	☐	_____	_____
f. mouthwash	☐	☐	_____	_____
g. swabs	☐	☐	_____	_____
2. Raise head of bed so resident is sitting up.	☐	☐	_____	_____
3. Put on gloves.	☐	☐	_____	_____
4. Drape towel under resident's chin.	☐	☐	_____	_____
5. Remove upper denture by gently moving it up and down to release suction. Turn lower dentures slightly to lift out of mouth.	☐	☐	_____	_____
6. Put dentures in emesis basin and take to sink.	☐	☐	_____	_____
7. Line sink with towel and fill halfway with water. *Padding and water will lessen the chance of breaking if denture is dropped.*	☐	☐	_____	_____
8. Never put denture in sink to soak. *The sink is considered dirty and contains pathogens not normally found in the mouth. If the denture is put into the water in the sink, it is grossly contaminated.*	☐	☐	_____	_____
9. Apply denture cleaner to brush, hold denture over sink, and brush all surfaces.	☐	☐	_____	_____
10. Rinse denture in cool water and place in denture cup filled with cool water.	☐	☐	_____	_____
11. Clean resident's mouth with swab, if necessary.	☐	☐	_____	_____

Procedure	Pass	Redo	Date Competency Met	Instructor Initials
12. Help resident rinse mouth with water or mouthwash half diluted with water if requested.	☐	☐	_____	_____
13. Check teeth, mouth, tongue, and lips for:	☐	☐	_____	_____
a. odor	☐	☐	_____	_____
b. cracking	☐	☐	_____	_____
c. sores	☐	☐	_____	_____
d. bleeding	☐	☐	_____	_____
e. discoloration	☐	☐	_____	_____
f. loose teeth	☐	☐	_____	_____
14. Help resident place dentures in mouth if requested.	☐	☐	_____	_____
15. Remove gloves.	☐	☐	_____	_____

PROCEDURE 17-9: SHAVE RESIDENT WITH SAFETY RAZOR

Name _____ Date _____

Directions: Practice this procedure, following each step. When you are ready to have your perform-ance evaluated, give this sheet to your instructor.

Procedure	Pass	Redo	Date Competency Met	Instructor Initials
1. Gather supplies:	☐	☐	_____	_____
a. towel	☐	☐	_____	_____
b. washcloth	☐	☐	_____	_____
c. bath basin	☐	☐	_____	_____
d. shaving cream	☐	☐	_____	_____
e. razor	☐	☐	_____	_____
f. aftershave lotion	☐	☐	_____	_____
2. Raise head of bed so resident is sitting up.	☐	☐	_____	_____
3. Fill bath basin halfway with warm water and ask resident to check water temperature.	☐	☐	_____	_____
4. Drape towel under resident's chin.	☐	☐	_____	_____
5. Put on gloves.	☐	☐	_____	_____
6. Help resident put dentures in mouth, if necessary. *Having the dentures in resident's mouth maintains normal contour of face and makes shaving easier.*	☐	☐	_____	_____
7. Moisten beard with washcloth and put shaving cream over area.	☐	☐	_____	_____
8. Hold skin taut and shave beard in direction of hair growth (downward strokes on face and upward strokes on neck).	☐	☐	_____	_____
9. Always shave away from your fingers. *Shave away from your fingers for safety. Shaving toward your fingers with a razor can cause cuts with the blade that is contaminated with body fluids.*	☐	☐	_____	_____
10. Rinse razor after each stroke.	☐	☐	_____	_____
11. Rinse resident's face and neck and thoroughly pat dry.	☐	☐	_____	_____
12. Apply aftershave lotion if requested and remove towel.	☐	☐	_____	_____
13. Remove gloves.	☐	☐	_____	_____

PROCEDURE 18-1: FEED THE RESIDENT

Name _____ **Date** _____

Directions: Practice this procedure, following each step. When you are ready to have your performance evaluated, give this sheet to your instructor.

Procedure	Pass	Redo	Date Competency Met	Instructor Initials
1. Assist resident with elimination if necessary.	☐	☐	_____	_____
2. Assist resident to wash hands.	☐	☐	_____	_____
3. Place resident in comfortable sitting position.	☐	☐	_____	_____
4. Get meal tray from kitchen cart and check meal card for:	☐	☐	_____	_____
a. name	☐	☐	_____	_____
b. diet	☐	☐	_____	_____
c. likes and dislikes	☐	☐	_____	_____
5. Check tray for:	☐	☐	_____	_____
a. correct food and beverages	☐	☐	_____	_____
b. condiments	☐	☐	_____	_____
c. utensils	☐	☐	_____	_____
6. Sit at resident's eye level.	☐	☐	_____	_____
7. Serve tray with main course closest to resident. *If you stand over resident, he or she may have to tilt head back and bring chin up to eat, the airway is open, and the resident may inhale and choke on food.*	☐	☐	_____	_____
8. Place napkin or clothing protector under resident's chin and across chest, if resident wishes.	☐	☐	_____	_____
9. Describe food for resident.	☐	☐	_____	_____
10. Ask resident what food is wanted.	☐	☐	_____	_____
11. Fill tip of spoon half full with food. *Always use spoon to feed because, if using a fork, you may accidentally poke resident, causing pain and injury.*	☐	☐	_____	_____
12. Gently place food into unaffected side of mouth.	☐	☐	_____	_____

Procedure	Pass	Redo	Date Competency Met	Instructor Initials
13. Allow resident time to chew and swallow.	☐	☐	_____	_____
14. Tell resident what food is being offered and whether it is hot or cold.	☐	☐	_____	_____
15. Offer fluids frequently. Fluids moisten the mouth and throat and help with swallowing.	☐	☐	_____	_____
16. Use different straw for each liquid.	☐	☐	_____	_____
17. Wipe resident's mouth as needed.	☐	☐	_____	_____
18. Encourage resident to do as much as possible.	☐	☐	_____	_____
19. Remove napkin or clothing protector and tray.	☐	☐	_____	_____
20. Measure and record intake if directed by nurse.	☐	☐	_____	_____

PROCEDURE 19-1: ASSIST RESIDENT TO USE A BEDPAN/FRACTURE PAN

Name _____ **Date** _____

Directions: Practice this procedure, following each step. When you are ready to have your performance evaluated, give this sheet to your instructor.

Procedure	Pass	Redo	Date Competency Met	Instructor Initials
1. Lower head of bed.	☐	☐	_____	_____
2. Put on gloves.	☐	☐	_____	_____
3. Turn resident away from you.	☐	☐	_____	_____
4. Place bedpan or fracture pan correctly.	☐	☐	_____	_____
5. Gently roll resident back onto pan and check for correct placement.	☐	☐	_____	_____
6. Raise head of bed to sitting position.	☐	☐	_____	_____
7. Give resident call light and toilet paper.	☐	☐	_____	_____
8. Leave resident and return when called.	☐	☐	_____	_____
9. Lower head of bed.	☐	☐	_____	_____
10. Press bedpan flat on bed and turn resident. *Press the bedpan flat on the bed before turning resident to stabilize the bedpan so it does not spill as the resident rolls off it.*	☐	☐	_____	_____
11. Wipe resident from front to back.	☐	☐	_____	_____
12. Check urine and/or feces for:				
a. color	☐	☐	_____	_____
b. odor	☐	☐	_____	_____
c. amount	☐	☐	_____	_____
d. character (feces) or clarity (urine)	☐	☐	_____	_____
13. Cover bedpan and take into bathroom.	☐	☐	_____	_____
14. If urine and/or feces is abnormal, save and report to supervising nurse immediately.	☐	☐	_____	_____
15. Dispose of urine and/or feces, sanitize pan, and return pan according to facility policy.	☐	☐	_____	_____
16. Remove gloves and wash your hands.	☐	☐	_____	_____
17. Help resident to wash hands.	☐	☐	_____	_____

PROCEDURE 19-2: EMPTY A URINARY DRAINAGE BAG

Name _____ **Date** _____

Directions: Practice this procedure, following each step. When you are ready to have your performance evaluated, give this sheet to your instructor.

Procedure	Pass	Redo	Date Competency Met	Instructor Initials
1. Collect equipment:	☐	☐	_____	_____
a. graduate	☐	☐	_____	_____
b. paper towel	☐	☐	_____	_____
c. gloves	☐	☐	_____	_____
2. Put on gloves.	☐	☐	_____	_____
3. Place paper towel on floor below bag and place graduate on paper towel. *Measurements on the side of the urinary drainage bag may not be accurate.*	☐	☐	_____	_____
4. Detach spout and point it into center of graduate without letting tube touch sides. *The catheter tube will be contaminated if it touches the inside of the graduate and may cause a urinary tract infection.*	☐	☐	_____	_____
5. Unclamp spout and drain urine into graduate.	☐	☐	_____	_____
6. Clamp spout and replace spout in holder.	☐	☐	_____	_____
7. Take graduate to bathroom and check urine for:				
a. color	☐	☐	_____	_____
b. odor	☐	☐	_____	_____
c. clarity	☐	☐	_____	_____
d. amount, by placing graduate on flat surface at eye level and noting amount of urine. *Having graduate at eye level allows for a more accurate reading.*	☐	☐	_____	_____
8. If urine is abnormal, save and report to supervising nurse immediately.	☐	☐	_____	_____
9. Dispose of urine, sanitize graduate, and return graduate according to facility policy.	☐	☐	_____	_____
10. Remove gloves.	☐	☐	_____	_____

PROCEDURE 19-3: COLLECT A ROUTINE URINE SPECIMEN

Name _____ Date _____

Directions: Practice this procedure, following each step. When you are ready to have your performance evaluated, give this sheet to your instructor.

Procedure	Pass	Redo	Date Competency Met	Instructor Initials
1. Gather equipment	☐	☐	_____	_____
a. urine specimen container and lid	☐	☐	_____	_____
b. label	☐	☐	_____	_____
c. plastic bag for specimen	☐	☐	_____	_____
d. laboratory requisition slip	☐	☐	_____	_____
e. gloves	☐	☐	_____	_____
f. clean bedpan or urinal	☐	☐	_____	_____
g. plastic bag or wastebasket for disposal of toilet paper	☐	☐	_____	_____
h. graduate	☐	☐	_____	_____
i. intake and output sheet, if resident has order for intake and output	☐	☐	_____	_____
2. Print resident's name on label and put label on the specimen container.	☐	☐	_____	_____
3. Put on gloves.	☐	☐	_____	_____
4. Ask resident to urinate into a clean bedpan or urinal.	☐	☐	_____	_____
5. Ask resident to put toilet paper in plastic bag or wastebasket.	☐	☐	_____	_____
6. Cover bedpan or urinal and take it to the bathroom.	☐	☐	_____	_____
7. If resident is on intake and output, measure and record the amount of urine.	☐	☐	_____	_____
8. Pour urine into specimen container, filling the container about three-quarters full.	☐	☐	_____	_____
9. Put lid on the specimen container and check label for accuracy.	☐	☐	_____	_____
10. Place the container in a plastic bag for transporting.	☐	☐	_____	_____

Procedure	Pass	Redo	Date Competency Met	Instructor Initials
11. Dispose of urine, sanitize equipment, and return equipment according to facility policy.	☐	☐	_____	_____
12. Remove gloves.	☐	☐	_____	_____
13. Wash your hands.	☐	☐	_____	_____
14. Assist resident to wash hands.	☐	☐	_____	_____
15. Take the labeled specimen container with the requisition slip to the designated area.	☐	☐	_____	_____

PROCEDURE 19-4: ADMINISTER AN ENEMA

Name _____ **Date** _____

Directions: Practice this procedure, following each step. When you are ready to have your perform-ance evaluated, give this sheet to your instructor.

Procedure	Pass	Redo	Date Competency Met	Instructor Initials
CAUTION: DO NOT perform this procedure unless properly trained and authorized. Some states do not permit certified nursing assistants to perform invasive procedures.				
1. Gather equipment:	☐	☐	_____	_____
a. commercially prepared enema or enema bag/bucket with tubing, clamp, and solution ordered by doctor	☐	☐	_____	_____
b. gloves	☐	☐	_____	_____
c. lubricating jelly	☐	☐	_____	_____
d. bed protector	☐	☐	_____	_____
e. toilet tissue	☐	☐	_____	_____
f. bedpan	☐	☐	_____	_____
2. If administering a cleansing or oil retention enema:	☐	☐	_____	_____
a. Prepare solution according to facility policy.	☐	☐	_____	_____
b. Close clamp on tubing and fill bag/bucket with accurate amount of solution.	☐	☐	_____	_____
c. Test temperature of solution to ensure that it is neither too hot nor too cold.	☐	☐	_____	_____
d. Open clamp, allow solution to fill the tubing to remove air, and then close clamp.	☐	☐	_____	_____
3. Position the resident in Sims' position.	☐	☐	_____	_____
4. Protect the bed with disposable pads.	☐	☐	_____	_____
5. Have bedpan within reach.	☐	☐	_____	_____
6. Keep resident covered and expose only the buttocks.	☐	☐	_____	_____
7. Put on gloves.	☐	☐	_____	_____
8. Lubricate the tip (2 to 4 inches) of the enema tubing or tip of prepared enema with lubricating jelly.	☐	☐	_____	_____

Procedure	Pass	Redo	Date Competency Met	Instructor Initials
9. Lift the upper buttock to expose the anal area.	☐	☐	_____	_____
10. Slowly insert tip of tubing 2 to 4 inches using a gentle rotating movement. *Never push against resistance because you may injure resident. Stop procedure and call supervising nurse.*	☐	☐	_____	_____
11. If administering a cleansing or oil retention enema.	☐	☐	_____	_____
a. Open the clamp and raise the enema bucket about 12 to 15 inches above the anus.	☐	☐	_____	_____
b. Allow the solution to flow slowly into anus.	☐	☐	_____	_____
c. If resident complains of discomfort, clamp tubing and wait a minute or so before continuing the flow of solution.	☐	☐	_____	_____
d. When solution is almost gone, clamp the tube and slowly withdraw the tubing.	☐	☐	_____	_____
e. Place the tubing into the enema bucket and do not allow the tip to come into contact with bed or floor.	☐	☐	_____	_____
12. If administering a commercially prepared enema:				
a. Squeeze and roll bottle from the bottom until all solution is used.	☐	☐	_____	_____
b. Place the squeeze bottle, tip first, into original container and discard.	☐	☐	_____	_____
13. Assist the resident onto the bedpan.	☐	☐	_____	_____
14. Encourage the resident to retain the solution as long as possible.	☐	☐	_____	_____
15. Monitor the resident every few minutes.	☐	☐	_____	_____
16. When resident is through:	☐	☐	_____	_____
a. Wearing gloves, remove bedpan.	☐	☐	_____	_____
b. Assist resident to clean perineal area.	☐	☐	_____	_____
c. Remove bed protector.	☐	☐	_____	_____

Procedure	Pass	Redo	Date Competency Met	Instructor Initials
17. Empty bedpan and observe feces for:	☐	☐	_____	_____
a. color	☐	☐	_____	_____
b. odor	☐	☐	_____	_____
c. amount	☐	☐	_____	_____
d. consistency	☐	☐	_____	_____
18. Remove supplies and clean equipment according to facility policy.	☐	☐	_____	_____
19. Remove gloves.	☐	☐	_____	_____
20. Wash your hands.	☐	☐	_____	_____
21. Assist resident to wash hands.	☐	☐	_____	_____

PROCEDURE 19-5: COLLECT A STOOL SPECIMEN

Name _____ Date _____

Directions: Practice this procedure, following each step. When you are ready to have your perform-ance evaluated, give this sheet to your instructor

Procedure	Pass	Redo	Date Competency Met	Instructor Initials
1. Gather equipment:	☐	☐	_____	_____
a. stool specimen container and lid	☐	☐	_____	_____
b. label	☐	☐	_____	_____
c. plastic bag for specimen	☐	☐	_____	_____
d. laboratory requisition slip	☐	☐	_____	_____
e. gloves	☐	☐	_____	_____
f. clean bedpan	☐	☐	_____	_____
g. plastic bag or wastebasket for disposal of toilet paper	☐	☐	_____	_____
h. tongue blades	☐	☐	_____	_____
2. Print resident's name on label and put label on specimen container.	☐	☐	_____	_____
3. Raise side rails before raising bed to working height and lower side rail on side of bed care is being given.	☐	☐	_____	_____
4. Put on gloves.	☐	☐	_____	_____
5. Have resident defecate into a clean bedpan.	☐	☐	_____	_____
6. Provide plastic bag or wastebasket for disposal of toilet paper.	☐	☐	_____	_____
7. Cover bedpan and take it to the bathroom.	☐	☐	_____	_____
8. With a wooden tongue blade, take about 1 to 2 tablespoons of feces from the bedpan from different areas of the stool. To avoid contamination, do not touch the inside of the specimen container or lid.	☐	☐	_____	_____
9. Put lid on the specimen container and check label for accuracy.	☐	☐	_____	_____
10. Place the container in a plastic bag for transporting.	☐	☐	_____	_____

Procedure	Pass	Redo	Date Competency Met	Instructor Initials
11. Dispose of urine, sanitize equipment, and return equipment according to facility policy.	☐	☐	_____	_____
12. Remove gloves.	☐	☐	_____	_____
13. Wash your hands.	☐	☐	_____	_____
14. Assist resident to wash hands.	☐	☐	_____	_____
15. Take the labeled specimen container with the requisition slip to the designated area.	☐	☐	_____	_____

PROCEDURE 20-1: TAKE A TEMPERATURE WITH A GLASS THERMOMETER

Name _____ Date _____

Directions: Practice this procedure, following each step. When you are ready to have your performance evaluated, give this sheet to your instructor.

Procedure	Pass	Redo	Date Competency Met	Instructor Initials
1. Gather equipment:	☐	☐	_____	_____
a. mercury-free or glass thermometer	☐	☐	_____	_____
b. tissue	☐	☐	_____	_____
c. thermometer sheath	☐	☐	_____	_____
d. watch	☐	☐	_____	_____
e. gloves	☐	☐	_____	_____
2. If resident has had hot or cold drinks or has been smoking, wait 20 minutes before taking oral temperature.	☐	☐	_____	_____
3. Position resident comfortably.	☐	☐	_____	_____
4. Rinse thermometer in cool water and dry with clean tissue, if necessary.	☐	☐	_____	_____
5. Hold thermometer at stem end and shake down to below the lowest number. *Holding thermometer by bulb end can result in temperature being inaccurate due to your body heat.*	☐	☐	_____	_____
6. Put on disposable sheath, if available.	☐	☐	_____	_____
a. For oral temperature:				
• Place bulb end of thermometer under resident's tongue and ask resident to close lips.	☐	☐	_____	_____
• Leave in place for at least 3–5 minutes or longer.	☐	☐	_____	_____
b. For rectal temperature:	☐	☐	_____	_____
• Place resident in Sims' position.	☐	☐	_____	_____
• Use gloves.	☐	☐	_____	_____
• Lubricate thermometer.	☐	☐	_____	_____
• Lift the upper buttock and gently insert bulb end of thermometer 1 to $1\frac{1}{2}$ inches into the rectum.	☐	☐	_____	_____
• Hold thermometer in place for at least 3 minutes.	☐	☐	_____	_____

Procedure	Pass	Redo	Date Competency Met	Instructor Initials
c. For axillary temperature:	☐	☐	_____	_____
• Remove resident's arm from sleeve of gown and wipe axillary area with towel.	☐	☐	_____	_____
• Place bulb end of thermometer in center of armpit and fold resident's arm over chest.	☐	☐	_____	_____
• Hold in place for at least 10 minutes.	☐	☐	_____	_____
7. Remove thermometer, wipe with tissue from stem to bulb end, or remove sheath and dispose of tissue and sheath.	☐	☐	_____	_____
8. Hold thermometer by stem end at eye level and slowly rotate until line appears. Accurately read and note temperature.	☐	☐	_____	_____
9. Shake down thermometer, clean it, and store thermometer according to facility policy.	☐	☐	_____	_____
10. Remove gloves.	☐	☐	_____	_____
11. Report unusual reading to supervising nurse immediately.	☐	☐	_____	_____
12. Document procedure according to facility policy, labeling R for rectal temperature and A or Ax for axillary temperature.	☐	☐	_____	_____

PROCEDURE 20-2: TAKE A TEMPERATURE WITH AN ELECTRONIC THERMOMETER

Name _____ **Date** _____

Directions: Practice this procedure, following each step. When you are ready to have your performance evaluated, give this sheet to your instructor.

Procedure	Pass	Redo	Date Competency Met	Instructor Initials
1. Assemble equipment:	☐	☐	_____	_____
a. battery-operated electronic thermometer	☐	☐	_____	_____
b. attachment (blue for oral, red for rectal)	☐	☐	_____	_____
c. disposable probe covers	☐	☐	_____	_____
d. gloves, if necessary	☐	☐	_____	_____
2. If resident has had hot or cold drinks or has been smoking, wait 20 minutes before taking oral temperature.	☐	☐	_____	_____
3. Position resident comfortably.	☐	☐	_____	_____
4. Remove the appropriate probe from its stored position and insert it into the thermometer.	☐	☐	_____	_____
5. Place the probe cover on the probe.	☐	☐	_____	_____
a. For oral temperature:				
• Place probe under resident's tongue and ask resident to close lips.	☐	☐	_____	_____
• Leave in place until electronic thermometer beeps or flashes.	☐	☐	_____	_____
b. For rectal temperature:				
• Place resident in Sims' position.	☐	☐	_____	_____
• Use gloves.	☐	☐	_____	_____
• Lubricate thermometer.	☐	☐	_____	_____
• Lift the upper buttock and gently insert probe $1/2$ inch into rectum.	☐	☐	_____	_____
• Lower upper buttock and hold thermometer in place until electronic thermometer beeps or flashes.	☐	☐	_____	_____
c. For axillary temperature:				
• Remove resident's arm from sleeve of gown and wipe axillary area with towel.	☐	☐	_____	_____

Procedure	Pass	Redo	Date Competency Met	Instructor Initials
• Place probe of thermometer in center of armpit and fold resident's arm over chest.	☐	☐	_____	_____
• Leave in place until electronic thermometer beeps or flashes.	☐	☐	_____	_____
6. Read temperature on the digital display.	☐	☐	_____	_____
7. Eject probe cover into wastebasket without touching it and replace probe in holder.	☐	☐	_____	_____
8. Remove gloves.	☐	☐	_____	_____
9. Return the probe to its stored position. Return the thermometer unit to its storage location.	☐	☐	_____	_____
10. Report unusual reading to supervising nurse immediately.	☐	☐	_____	_____
11. Document procedure according to facility policy, labeling R for rectal temperature and A or Ax for axillary temperature.	☐	☐	_____	_____

PROCEDURE 20-3: TAKE A TEMPERATURE WITH A TYMPANIC THERMOMETER

Name _____ **Date** _____

Directions: Practice this procedure, following each step. When you are ready to have your performance evaluated, give this sheet to your instructor.

Procedure	Pass	Redo	Date Competency Met	Instructor Initials
1. Gather equipment:	☐	☐	_____	_____
a. battery-operated tympanic thermometer	☐	☐	_____	_____
b. disposable probe cover	☐	☐	_____	_____
2. Check that probe is connected to the unit.	☐	☐	_____	_____
3. Insert the cone-shaped end of the thermometer into a probe cover.	☐	☐	_____	_____
4. Position yourself so the resident's ear is directly in front of you.	☐	☐	_____	_____
5. Gently pull ear up and back and insert the probe into the ear canal as far as possible to seal ear canal.	☐	☐	_____	_____
6. Leave in place until electronic thermometer beeps or flashes.	☐	☐	_____	_____
7. Remove the probe from the resident's ear.	☐	☐	_____	_____
8. Accurately note temperature on the digital display.	☐	☐	_____	_____
9. Eject probe cover into wastebasket without touching it and replace probe in holder.	☐	☐	_____	_____
10. Return the tympanic thermometer to the battery charger or base unit.	☐	☐	_____	_____
11. Report unusual reading to supervising nurse immediately.	☐	☐	_____	_____
12. Document procedure according to facility policy.	☐	☐	_____	_____

PROCEDURE 20-4: TAKE RESIDENT'S RADIAL PULSE AND RESPIRATION RATE

Name _____ **Date** _____

Directions: Practice this procedure, following each step. When you are ready to have your perform-ance evaluated, give this sheet to your instructor.

Procedure	Pass	Redo	Date Competency Met	Instructor Initials
1. Use watch with second hand.	☐	☐	_____	_____
2. Place resident's hand on comfortable surface.	☐	☐	_____	_____
3. Feel for pulse on thumb side of wrist with tips of first three fingers. *Do not use your thumb to take a pulse. It has its own pulse that might be confused with the resident's and result in an inaccurate reading.*	☐	☐	_____	_____
4. Count beats for 60 seconds and note:	☐	☐	_____	_____
a. rate—number of beats	☐	☐	_____	_____
b. rhythm—regularity of beats	☐	☐	_____	_____
c. force—strength of beats	☐	☐	_____	_____
5. Continue holding wrist as if feeling for pulse.	☐	☐	_____	_____
6. Count each rise and fall of chest as one respiration.	☐	☐	_____	_____
7. Count respiration for 60 seconds noting:	☐	☐	_____	_____
a. rate—number of breaths	☐	☐	_____	_____
b. regularity—pattern of breathing	☐	☐	_____	_____
c. sound—shallowness or depth of breathing	☐	☐	_____	_____
8. Accurately note pulse and respiration rates.	☐	☐	_____	_____
9. Report unusual reading to supervising nurse immediately.	☐	☐	_____	_____
10. Document procedure according to facility policy.	☐	☐	_____	_____

PROCEDURE 20-5: TAKE RESIDENT'S BLOOD PRESSURE

Name _____ **Date** _____

Directions: Practice this procedure, following each step. When you are ready to have your performance evaluated, give this sheet to your instructor.

Procedure	Pass	Redo	Date Competency Met	Instructor Initials
1. Gather equipment:	☐	☐	_____	_____
a. antiseptic wipe	☐	☐	_____	_____
b. stethoscope	☐	☐	_____	_____
c. sphygmomanometer	☐	☐	_____	_____
2. Have resident rest for approximately 15 minutes before taking blood pressure.	☐	☐	_____	_____
3. Clean earpieces and diaphragm of stethoscope with antiseptic wipe.	☐	☐	_____	_____
4. Uncover resident's arm to shoulder. *Place the cuff on skin, not over clothing, for the most accurate reading.*	☐	☐	_____	_____
5. Rest resident's arm, level with heart, palm upward on comfortable surface.	☐	☐	_____	_____
6. Wrap cuff around upper unaffected arm approximately 1–2 inches above elbow. *Avoid taking blood pressure on affected arm with a wound, cast, IV, an arm that is paralyzed or has skin problems.*	☐	☐	_____	_____
7. Put earpieces of stethoscope snugly into ears.	☐	☐	_____	_____
8. Locate the brachial pulse with your fingertips at the bend of the elbow.	☐	☐	_____	_____
9. Place diaphragm of stethoscope over brachial artery and hold firmly in place, being sure that stethoscope does not touch the cuff. The pressure of the stethoscope on the inflating cuff can alter the reading.	☐	☐	_____	_____

Procedure	Pass	Redo	Date Competency Met	Instructor Initials
10. Close valve on bulb:	☐	☐	_____	_____
a. If blood pressure is known, inflate cuff to 30 mm/hg above the usual systolic reading.	☐	☐	_____	_____
b. If blood pressure is unknown, inflate cuff to 160 mm/hg.	☐	☐	_____	_____
11. Slowly open valve on bulb.	☐	☐	_____	_____
12. Watch gauge and listen for sound of pulse.	☐	☐	_____	_____
13. Note gauge reading at first pulse sound.	☐	☐	_____	_____
14. Note gauge reading when pulse sound disappears. *If you are unable to hear sounds, completely deflate cuff, wait 1 minute, and begin again. DO NOT inflate cuff that has been partially deflated because reading will not be accurate and the skin and underlying structures may be damaged, causing bruising.*	☐	☐	_____	_____
15. Completely deflate and remove cuff.	☐	☐	_____	_____
16. Accurately record systolic and diastolic readings according to current nursing practice.	☐	☐	_____	_____
17. Clean earpieces and diaphragm of stethoscope with antiseptic wipe.	☐	☐	_____	_____
18. Report unusual reading to supervising nurse immediately.	☐	☐	_____	_____
19. Document procedure according to facility policy.	☐	☐	_____	_____

Supplemental Resources

For additional information regarding questions refer to these texts:

Being a Long-Term Care Nursing Assistant, 5th ed. by C. Will-Black & J. Eighmy, 2002, Upper Saddle River, NJ: Prentice Hall

Being a Nursing Assistant, 9th ed. by F. Wolgin, 2005, Upper Saddle River, NJ: Prentice Hall

The Nursing Assistant, 4th ed, by J. Pulliam, 2006, Upper Saddle River, NJ: Prentice Hall

The Long-Term Care Nursing Assistant, 3rd ed. by Grubbs & Blasband, 2005, Upper Saddle River, NJ: Prentice Hall

CHAPTER 1: THE HEALTH CARE SYSTEM AND LONG-TERM CARE

Question	Content	Text
1	The Payment Sources for Long-Term Care	Will-Black, p. 5
2	A Description of Long-Term Care	Grubbs, p. 2
	Introduction to Rehabilitation and Restorative Care	Grubbs, p. 31
3	Restorative Measures to Meet the Resident's Psychosocial Needs	Grubbs, p. 306
4	Responsibilities of the Nursing Assistant	Grubbs, p. 10
5	Introduction to Rehabilitation and Restorative Care	Grubbs, p. 31
6	The Rehabilitation Team	Grubbs, p. 31
7	Physical Therapy Department	Grubbs, p. 31
8	The Care Plan	Grubbs, p. 287
9	The Care Plan	Grubbs, p. 287
10	The Purpose of a Long-Term Care Facility	Grubbs, p. 2

CHAPTER 2: THE ROLE AND RESPONSIBILITIES OF A CERTIFIED NURSING ASSISTANT

Question	Content	Text
1	Guidelines: Personal Hygiene and Appearance	Grubbs, p. 12
2	The Job of the Nursing Assistant	Pulliam, p. 13
	The Health Care Team	Grubbs, p. 4
3	Personal Qualities and Characteristics of the Nursing Assistant	Grubbs, p. 11
4	Residents' Bill of Rights	Grubbs, p. 23
5	Residents' Bill of Rights	Grubbs, p. 23
6	Confidentiality of Resident Information	Will-Black, p. 12
7	The Job of the Nursing Assistant	Pulliam, p. 13
8	Teamwork	Grubbs, p. 14
9	Residents' Bill of Rights	Grubbs, p. 23
10	Planning Work Assignments	Pulliam, p. 20

CHAPTER 3: COMMUNICATION AND INTERPERSONAL SKILLS

Question	Content	Text
1	Communication as a Restorative Measure	Grubbs, p. 271
2	The Right to Personal Privacy and Confidentiality	Grubbs, p. 25
3	Aids to Effective Communication and Relating to People	Wolgin, p. 35
4	Dealing with Families and Visitors	Will-Black, p. 20
5	Communication	Will-Black, p. 14
6	Answering the Call Light	Will-Black, p. 18
7	Guidelines: Communicating with the Vision-Impaired Resident	Grubbs, p. 276

Question	Content	Text
8	Residents' Rights	Will-Black, p. 17
9	Organization of the Department of Nursing	Will-Black, p. 8
10	Guidelines: Age Specific Communication with the Elderly	Grubbs, p. 271

CHAPTER 4: OBSERVING, REPORTING, AND RECORDING

Question	Content	Text
1	Methods of Observation	Pulliam, p. 29
2	Methods of Observation	Pulliam, p. 29
3	Subjective and Objective Reporting	Wolgin, p. 51
4	Commonly Used Abbreviations	Will-Black, p. 108
5	The Patient Chart	Pulliam, p. 30
6	Recording	Grubbs, p. 286
7	Recording	Grubbs, p. 286
8	Recording	Grubbs, p. 286
9	Guidelines: Charting	Pulliam, p. 30
	Reporting Incidents	Pulliam, p. 17
10	Organization of the Department of Nursing	Will-Black, p. 8

CHAPTER 5: INFECTION CONTROL

Question	Content	Text
1	Standard Precautions and New Isolation Procedures	Pulliam, p. 66
2	Transmission-Based Precautions	Grubbs, p. 47
3	Transmission-Based Precautions (Isolation)	Pulliam, p. 68
4	Routes of Transmission	Pulliam, p. 53
5	Aseptic Technique	Pulliam, p. 57
6	Aseptic Technique	Pulliam, p. 57
7	Procedure Handwashing	Wolgin, p. 95
8	Gloves	Wolgin, p. 96
9	Gloves	Wolgin, p. 96
10	Changes in Isolation Strategies	Pulliam, p. 66

CHAPTER 6: BODY MECHANICS AND ALIGNMENT

Question	Content	Text
1	Introduction to Body Mechanics	Pulliam, p. 78
2	Body Mechanics	Grubbs, p. 65

Question	Content	Text
3	Body Mechanics	Will-Black, p. 36
4	Guidelines: Lifting	Will-Black, p. 36
5	Guidelines: Using Correct Body Mechanics	Grubbs, p. 65
6	Guidelines: Body Alignment	Pulliam, p. 172
7	Positioning a Patient in a Chair	Pulliam, p. 178
8	Introduction to Body Mechanics	Pulliam, p. 77
9	Guidelines: Using Correct Body Mechanics	Grubbs, p. 65
10	Body Mechanics	Will-Black, p. 36

CHAPTER 7: SAFETY

Question	Content	Text
1	Understanding the Behavior of Cognitively Impaired Residents	Pulliam, p. 362
2	Preventing Burns	Will-Black, p. 31
3	Major Causes of Fire	Wolgin, p. 120
4	Assisting Patients with Eating	Pulliam, p. 249
5	Using a Wheelchair	Grubbs, p. 136
6	Restraints	Pulliam, p. 79
7	Preventing Burns	Will-Black, p. 31
8	Preventing Burns	Will-Black, p. 31
9	Poisoning	Pulliam, p. 76
10	Fire Safety	Grubbs, p. 68

CHAPTER 8: EMERGENCIES

Question	Content	Text
1	Choking	Pulliam, p. 95
2	Procedure Correcting Airway Obstructions	Will-Black, p. 449
3	Falls	Pulliam, p. 98
4	Hemorrhage	Wolgin, p. 299
5	Seizures	Pulliam, p. 97
6	Seizures	Pulliam, p. 97
7	Nursing Care During a Seizure	Will-Black, p. 320
8	What to Do in an Emergency	Wolgin, p. 286
9	Responding to an Emergency	Pulliam, p. 90
10	Postmortem Care	Wolgin, p. 683

CHAPTER 9: RESIDENTS' RIGHTS

Question	Content	Text
1	Residents' Bill of Rights	Grubbs, p. 25
2	The Patient Unit	Pulliam, p. 203
3	Ethical Code of Conduct	Will-Black, p. 12
4	Abuse of the Resident	Grubbs, p. 26
5	Abuse of the Resident	Grubbs, p. 26
6	Residents' Bill of Rights	Grubbs, p. 23
7	DNR Orders	Pulliam, p. 373
8	Residents' Bill of Rights	Grubbs, p. 25
9	Confidentiality of Resident Information	Will-Black, p. 12
10	Confidentiality of Resident Information	Will-Black, p. 12

CHAPTER 10: FOSTERING INDEPENDENCE

Question	Content	Text
1	Restorative Care and Rehabilitation	Pulliam, p. 291
2	Prostheses and Orthotics	Pulliam, p. 294
3	Prostheses and Orthotics	Pulliam, p. 294
4	Prostheses and Orthotics	Pulliam, p. 294
5	A Restorative Environment	Grubbs, p. 86
6	Prostheses and Orthotics	Pulliam, p. 294
7	Rehabilitation	Will-Black, p. 74
8	Assistive Equipment	Grubbs, p. 33
9	Activities of Daily Living	Pulliam, p. 292
10	Activities of Daily Living	Pulliam, p. 292

CHAPTER 11: THE RESIDENT'S FAMILY

Question	Content	Text
1	Admission	Pulliam, p. 195
2	Admission	Pulliam, p. 195
3	Care of the Elderly	Pulliam, p. 350
4	Care of the Elderly	Pulliam, p. 350
5	Care of the Elderly	Pulliam, p. 350
6	Care of the Elderly	Pulliam, p. 350
7	The Role of the Nursing Assistant in Long-Term Care	Pulliam, p. 352
8	Cultural Awareness	Will-Black, p. 84

Question	Content	Text
9	Developing Interpersonal Skills	Will-Black, p. 85
10	Cultural Awareness	Will-Black, p. 85

CHAPTER 12: PSYCHOSOCIAL NEEDS

Question	Content	Text
1	Psychological Aspects of Aging	Will-Black, p. 77
2	Psychological Aspects of Aging	Will-Black, p. 77
3	Meeting Emotional, Spiritual, and Social Needs	Pulliam, p. 357
4	Basic Needs	Will-Black, p. 79
5	Basic Needs	Grubbs, p. 303
6	Restorative Measures to Meet the Resident's Psychosocial Needs	Grubbs, p. 168
7	Basic Needs	Grubbs, p. 303
8	Basic Needs	Grubbs, p. 303
9	Activities of Daily Living	Pulliam, p. 292
10	Activities of Daily Living	Pulliam, p. 292

CHAPTER 13: THE ENVIRONMENT

Question	Content	Text
1	Admission to a Long-Term Care Facility	Pulliam, p. 196
2	The Resident's Unit	Will-Black, p. 60
3	Care of Personal Belongings	Will-Black, p. 66
4	Care of Personal Belongings	Will-Black, p. 66
5	Care of Personal Belongings	Will-Black, p. 66
6	The Patient's Unit	Wolgin, p. 202
7	Bedmaking	Pulliam, p. 205
8	Procedure 12-2 Opening a Closed Bed	Pulliam, p. 209
9	The Occupied Bed	Will-Black, p. 63
10	A Restorative Environment	Grubbs, p. 86

CHAPTER 14: THE HUMAN BODY

Question	Content	Text
1	Anatomy and Physiology	Will-Black, p. 135
2	Anatomy and Physiology	Will-Black, p. 136

Question	Content	Text
3	Anatomy and Physiology	Will-Black, p. 136
4	Anatomy and Physiology	Will-Black, p. 136
5	Anatomy and Physiology	Will-Black, p. 136
6	Homeostasis	Will-Black, p. 136
7	Observations, Reporting, and Recording	Pulliam, p. 29
8	Observations, Reporting, and Recording	Pulliam, p. 29
9	Development	Wolgin, p. 321
10	Development	Wolgin, p. 321

CHAPTER 15: BODY SYSTEMS

Question	Content	Text
1	The Patient with Breathing Problems	Pulliam, p. 109
2	The Gastrointestinal System	Pulliam, p. 112
3	The Musculoskeletal System	Pulliam, p. 119
4	The Stroke Patient	Pulliam, p. 125
5	The Gastrointestinal System	Pulliam, p. 112
6	The Integumentary System	Pulliam, p. 118
7	Differences Between Right and Left Brain Injuries	Pulliam, p. 125
8	Differences Between Right and Left Brain Injuries	Pulliam, p. 125
9	The Stroke Patient	Pulliam, p. 125
10	The Stroke Patient	Pulliam, p. 125

CHAPTER 16: MOVEMENT AND MOBILITY

Question	Content	Text
1	The Cerebrovascular Accident (Stroke) Patient	Wolgin, p. 542
2	Assisting the Resident in Positioning and Turning	Grubbs, p. 122
3	Procedure Pivot Transfer of the Hemiplegic Resident	Will-Black, p. 211
4	Procedure Pivot Transfer of the Hemiplegic Resident	Will-Black, p. 211
5	Procedure 10-11 Care of Falling Patient	Pulliam, p. 190
6	Guidelines: Caring for a Cerebrovascular Accident Patient	Wolgin, p. 543
7	The Musculoskeletal System	Pulliam, p. 119
8	Encouraging Active Range of Motion	Will-Black, p. 227
9	Encouraging Active Range of Motion	Will-Black, p. 227
10	Guidelines: Applying Restraints	Grubbs, p. 66

CHAPTER 17: PERSONAL CARE

Question	Content	Text
1	Procedure Perineal Care for the Male Patient	Wolgin, p. 267
2	Procedure Perineal Care for the Male Patient	Wolgin, p. 267
3	Dressing the Resident	Will-Black, p. 183
4	Dressing the Resident	Will-Black, p. 183
5	Procedure Dressing and Undressing the Totally Dependent Resident	Will-Black, p. 184
6	Restorative Personal Care and Dressing	Grubbs, p. 177
7	Procedure Care of Dentures	Grubbs, p. 165
8	Oral Hygiene	Pulliam, p. 221
9	Dressing the Resident	Will-Black, p. 184
10	Caring for Eyeglasses and Hearing Aids	Pulliam, p. 232

CHAPTER 18: NUTRITION AND HYDRATION

Question	Content	Text
1	Preparing for Mealtime	Will-Black, p. 256
2	Feeding the Resident Who Cannot Eat Independently	Grubbs, p. 209
3	Assisting the Dependent Resident in Eating	Will-Black, p. 259
4	Feeding the Resident Who Cannot Eat Independently	Grubbs, p. 209
5	Nutrition and the Elderly Resident	Grubbs, p. 204
6	Assisting the Dependent Resident in Eating	Will-Black, p. 259
7	The Dependent Resident	Will-Black, p. 258
8	Assisting Residents with Swallowing Problems	Grubbs, p. 209
9	The Dependent Resident	Will-Black, p. 258
10	Assisting Residents with Swallowing Problems	Grubbs, p. 209

CHAPTER 19: ELIMINATION

Question	Content	Text
1	Providing Privacy	Will-Black, p. 287
2	Urinary Elimination	Grubbs, p. 230
3	Collecting a Routine Urine Specimen	Will-Black, p. 293
4	Providing Privacy	Will-Black, p. 287
5	Procedure Giving Daily Indwelling Catheter Care	Wolgin, p. 476
6	Procedure Giving Daily Indwelling Catheter Care	Wolgin, p. 476
7	Providing Privacy	Will-Black, p. 292
8	General Guidelines	Pulliam, p. 317

Question	Content	Text
9	Enemas	Will-Black, p. 263
10	Procedure 20-5 Giving a Commercial Oil-Retention Enema	Pulliam, p. 319

CHAPTER 20: VITAL SIGNS AND MEASUREMENTS

Question	Content	Text
1	Taking a Patient's Vital Signs	Pulliam, p. 152
2	Measuring Oral Temperature	Pulliam, p. 155
3	Procedure Taking an Oral Temperature Using and Electronic Thermometer	Grubbs, p. 186
4	Measuring the Radial Pulse	Pulliam, p. 161
5	Characteristics of the Pulse	Will-Black, p. 123
6	Respiration	Pulliam, p. 163
7	Respiration	Pulliam, p. 163
8	Guidelines: Measuring a Blood Pressure	Grubbs, p. 195
9	Measuring Weight and Height	Pulliam, p. 166
10	Measuring the Resident's Height	Grubbs, p. 255

CHAPTER 21: RESTORATIVE CARE

Question	Content	Text
1	Introduction	Pulliam, p. 291
2	Prostheses and Orthotics	Pulliam, p. 294
3	Giving Whirlpool or Medicinal Baths	Will-Black, p. 421
4	Giving Whirlpool or Medicinal Baths	Will-Black, p. 421
5	Giving Whirlpool or Medicinal Baths	Will-Black, p. 421
6	Range-of-Motion Exercises	Pulliam, p. 296
7	Range-of-Motion Exercises	Pulliam, p. 296
8	Guidelines for Range-of-Motion Exercises	Pulliam, p. 297
9	Restorative Dining or Self-Feeding Programs	Will-Black, p. 423
10	Caring for the Resident with an Amputation	Will-Black, p. 364

CHAPTER 22: COGNITIVELY IMPAIRED

Question	Content	Text
1	The Geriatric Resident	Grubbs, p. 299
2	Communication as a Restorative Measure	Grubbs, p. 271

Question	Content	Text
3	Communicating with Cognitively Impaired Residents	Pulliam, p. 362
4	Communicating with Cognitively Impaired Residents	Pulliam, p. 362
5	Caring for Residents with Dementia	Pulliam, p. 361
6	Understanding the Behavior of Cognitively Impaired Residents	Pulliam, p. 364
7	Understanding the Behavior of Cognitively Impaired Residents	Pulliam, p. 364
8	Understanding the Behavior of Cognitively Impaired Residents	Pulliam, p. 364
9	Understanding the Behavior of Cognitively Impaired Residents	Pulliam, p. 363
10	Alzheimer's Disease	Will-Black, p. 321

CHAPTER 23: VISUALLY IMPAIRED

Question	Content	Text
1	Diabetes Mellitus	Will-Black, p. 378
2	Communication Impairments	Grubbs, p. 276
3	Answering the Call Light	Will-Black, p. 19
4	Guidelines: Communicating with the Vision-Impaired Resident	Grubbs, p. 276
5	Guidelines: Communicating with the Vision-Impaired Resident	Grubbs, p. 276
6	Guidelines: Communicating with the Vision-Impaired Resident	Grubbs, p. 276
7	Guidelines: Communicating with the Vision-Impaired Resident	Grubbs, p. 276
8	Visual Impairment	Will-Black, p. 153
9	Visual Impairment	Will-Black, p. 153
10	Visual Impairment	Will-Black, p. 154

CHAPTER 24: HEARING IMPAIRED

Question	Content	Text
1	Hearing Loss	Will-Black, p. 154
2	Guidelines: Communicating with the Hearing-Impaired Resident	Grubbs, p. 277
3	Hearing Loss	Will-Black, p. 154
4	Guidelines: Communicating with the Hearing-Impaired Resident	Grubbs, p. 277
5	Hearing Loss	Will-Black, p. 155
6	Hearing Loss	Will-Black, p. 155
7	Guidelines: Assisting the Resident with a Hearing Aid	Grubbs, p. 277
8	Hearing Loss	Will-Black, p. 155
9	Communication Impairments	Grubbs, p. 276
10	Communication Impairments	Grubbs, p. 276

CHAPTER 25: THE DEVELOPMENTALLY DISABLED

Question	Content	Text
1	Nursing Care During a Seizure	Will-Black, p. 320
2	Nursing Care During a Seizure	Will-Black, p. 320
3	Nursing Care During a Seizure	Will-Black, p. 320
4	Nursing Care During a Seizure	Will-Black, p. 320
5	Normalization	Will-Black, p. 402
6	Normalization	Will-Black, p. 402
7	Normalization	Will-Black, p. 402
8	Least Restrictive Alternative	Will-Black, p. 403
9	Data Collection	Will-Black, p. 410
10	Normalization	Will-Black, p. 402

CHAPTER 26: THE ABUSIVE RESIDENT

Question	Content	Text
1	Coping with Difficult Behavior	Pulliam, p. 43
2	Coping with Aggressive Behavior	Will-Black, p. 86
3	Aggressive Behavior	Pulliam, p. 44
4	Dealing with Difficult Behavior	Wolgin, p. 71
5	Aggressive Behavior	Pulliam, p. 44
6	Coping with Aggressive Behavior	Will-Black, p. 86
7	Dealing with Difficult Behavior	Wolgin, p. 71
8	Coping with Difficult Behavior	Pulliam, p. 43
9	Withdrawal and Depression	Pulliam, p. 44
10	Coping with Difficult Behavior	Pulliam, p. 43

CHAPTER 27: THE YOUNG RESIDENT

Question	Content	Text
1	Care Considerations Based on Age Group	Pulliam, p. 40
2	Care Considerations Based on Age Group	Pulliam, p. 41
3	Developmental Tasks and Chronological Age	Wolgin, p. 323
4	Care Considerations Based on Age Group	Pulliam, p. 40
5	Care Considerations Based on Age Group	Pulliam, p. 40
6	Developmental Tasks and Chronological Age	Wolgin, p. 323
7	Developmental Tasks and Chronological Age	Wolgin, p. 323
8	Residents' Bill of Rights	Grubbs, p. 23

Question	Content	Text
9	Developmental Tasks and Chronological Age	Wolgin, p. 323
10	Communicating with Pediatric Patients	Wolgin, p. 626

CHAPTER 28: THE DYING RESIDENT

Question	Content	Text
1	Psychological/Psychosocial Aspects of Caring for a Terminally Ill Patient	Grubbs, p. 676
2	The Dying Resident's Family	Grubbs, p. 375
3	Spiritual Preparation	Pulliam, p. 370
4	Hospice Care	Pulliam, p. 374
5	Hospice Care	Pulliam, p. 374
6	DNR Orders	Pulliam, p. 373
7	Residents' Bill of Rights	Grubbs, p. 23
8	Coping with Staff Stress	Grubbs, p. 376
9	Physical Signs and Symptoms	Will-Black, p. 485
10	The Other Residents	Grubbs, p. 376

Index